ENERGIES
OF
TRANSFORMATION:

A GUIDE
TO
THE KUNDALINI
PROCESS

by

Bonnie Greenwell Ph.D

Cover Art: "Fire Mystery" © 1988 by Judith Cornell
Cover Design: Barbara Gildersleeve

First Edition
Published in March, 1990
By Shakti River Press
a division of
Transpersonal Learning Services
10311 S. DeAnza Blvd. Ste. 2
Cupertino, CA. 95014

Printed by Delta Lithograph
Valencia, CA.

ENERGIES OF TRANSFORMATION:
A GUIDE TO THE KUNDALINI PROCESS

Contents

DEDICATION

THIS BOOK IS DEDICATED TO THE MEMORY OF
MY PARENTS
PERRY ROSWELL YATES AND GERTRUDE RYAN YATES
AND TO MY CHILDREN
TONY, JEFF AND KRISTIN
AND WITH SPECIAL GRATITUDE
TO THE SUBJECTS
WHO GENEROUSLY AND COURAGEOUSLY SHARED THEIR STORIES
IN ORDER THAT OTHERS WHO ENGAGE THIS EXPERIENCE CAN
DISCOVER MORE READILY HOW TO USE IT
FOR TRANSFORMATION

Preface

Perhaps you have wondered about unusual experiences you may have had while meditating, or you have encountered an inexplicable energy that has disrupted and changed your life in dramatic ways. Or you may be a physician, psychotherapist or healer looking for an explanation for symptoms you are unable to categorize adequately using the norms of Western medicine. If so, this book is written to help you recognize and support a unique, universal and ageless process related to spiritual experience and psychological wholeness and identified in ancient times as Kundalini awakening. This experience is impacting the lives of at least hundreds, and possibly thousands, of people annually in this "new" age.

I discovered while working on my Ph.D. in Transpersonal Psychology the profound interface between physical and spiritual energies, and their impact on psychological structures. Plummeted into ecstatic energy, chaotic movements and major shifts in awareness through my own personal process, a combination of neo-Reichian body therapy and intense meditation, I began a search for others who could understand what was happening to me. A friend introduced me to yoga, and as I explored translations of ancient scriptures and the teachings of the yogis whose books I could acquire, I discovered descriptions of the experiences I was having. Seeking deeper understanding of the phenomenon I enrolled in advanced training to become a teacher of Ashtanga Yoga and was graciously allowed to study the unpublished manuscripts of the jnana yoga teacher Baba Hari Dass, an expert on the Yoga Sutras and tantric practices and scriptures.

As I began to discuss this subject among friends and at seminars I discovered that many people today are facing the chaos and change of Kundalini awakening due to spiritual practices, modern therapies which deal with the body and altered states of consciousness, following drug use or near-death experiences, or even spontaneously for no recognizable reason, and that psychologists, physicians and even spiritual teachers often misinterpret their symptoms with grave consequences to them. . It seemed a calling for me to address my dissertation toward this subject, and to gather together as much information from as many sources as possible about how to support and nurture this process to its ideal fruition, which according to Eastern scriptures is a changed perspective of the nature of existence, expanded consciousness and bliss.

I've explored over 200 manuscripts to gather the bits and pieces that each had to offer about this ancient and esoteric experience, which must be imbedded very deeply in the psyche to have been recorded since the very beginning of records. I've interviewed dozens of Westerners who have described this process and how it impacted their lives, and ten of these cases are described in depth in this manuscript.

I am extremely grateful to the Institute of Transpersonal Psychology for supporting my decision to use this material to write a dissertation on viii

such a non-traditional topic, and to committee members, Dr. Jill Mellick, Dr. Robert Frager and Dr. Ron Jones, who understand implicitly the connections between spirituality and psychology, and model it in their lives. Portions of this volume were first published in that dissertation <u>Kundalini: A Study of Eastern and Western Perspectives and Experiences and their Implications for Transpersonal Psychotherapists</u> (Jan. 1988). I wish also to acknowledge the contributions of mentors and friends including my husband Bill, Dr. Gay Hendricks, Dr. Jim Spencer, Dr. Jonathan Hart, Baba Hari Dass and the yogis at Mt. Madonna Center in Watsonville, CA., all of whom made it possible for me to do this work.

The title for this book emerged during a committee meeting for the planning of a conference about Kundalini, called Energies of Transformation, held by the Spiritual Emergence Network in March of 1990. I am grateful to whomever came up with it but none of us remember who said it first! Energies of transformation have been described under various names in the esoteric practices of every culture and the phrase reflects the universality of this process and the multiplicity of its impact.

Many Sanscrit terms are used in this manuscript but for the ease of western readers phonetic marks and italics are omitted as much as possible, and definitions are usually provided when Sanscrit words are used. English clearly offers a poor translation for Sanscrit however, as this beautiful ancient language has a much more expansive vocabulary related to spiritual philosophy and phenomena, with many fine nuances that are lacking in English.

The term "Kundalini" has been capitalized throughout because this energy/consciousness has been personified as a Goddess in the scriptures, and I have found it sustains my spiritual and creative process to interact with her as such. I have also used numerous references, a practice not too comfortable for the reader, but essential to the work, for this book is standing on the shoulders of hundreds who have written before about this subject, ranging from small treasures of obscure scriptural translations to encyclopedic volumes such as those of Sri Aurobindo. Hopefully it will entice you to read more Eastern literature, especially if you are in a Kundalini process, as it is nurturing for the soul. Also, I hope to demonstrate by including such a vast number of scholars and teachers that this is not an abnormal or deranged process simply because it is unknown to the average practitioner of western medicine, but has been described by some of the most remarkably talented and intelligent people of every age. There is ample cross-cultural validation for it, and a wide range of scriptures that define and support the positive transformative impact it can have on someone's life.

If you have fallen into the maelstrom of this process either with intention or inadvertently, I hope the context and guidelines offered here will serve you well.

CHAPTER ONE

KUNDALINI: AWAKENING TO RADICAL SPIRITUALITY

> Suddenly energy moved up from the bottom of
> my spine to my heart and exploded like a
> neutron bomb going off in my chest. I ex-
> panded spherically in tiny pieces, which were all
> that remained of me, like bits of energy
> traveling fast through warp speed to the ends of
> the universe...I became waves of energy passing
> on and on past the edges of the universe.
> Nothing was left. . . . Rob.

This book is about the subtle energy of the life force, the
pure consciousness beyond mind and the ecstatic experience of
spiritual awakening. It also tells of physical collapse, psychic chaos,
and personality upheaval, elements of human transformation that
uproot us to the core, and cause us to "know" we have been touched
by powers greater than ourselves. It tells the stories of individuals
across the ages who have discovered and integrated an experience that
pushes the edges of their sanity and their divinity. And it is a guide
for survival and transformation.

It appears that when people pray, meditate or turn inward
with great intensity to find "God" what they may ultimately experience is the *sat-chit-ananda* of the ancient Indian scriptures. *Sat* is
existence or beingness, the substance or essence that is all things; in
Eastern scriptures prior to creation there was only *sat*, one, without a
second,undivided. It exists always and everywhere. *Chit* is cosmic
intelligence or knowledge that fills everything, a consciousness
without personal identity. *Ananda* is ecstatic bliss. Indian pandits

identify these three qualities as the essential nature of existence. Direct intuition of them becomes possible following the eruption of Kundalini energy, which is latent in each of us. When this primal, intense energy awakens it seems to move with intentionality through body and psyche and is believed by eastern mystics to have the power to transform a person at the cellular level. When one feels the first intense waves of this energy/consciousness, and is tossed into the physical, psychological and spiritual chaos that follow, it is called Kundalini awakening.

If you have awakened this energy, whether through discipline and spiritual practice, as a consequence of breathwork or other intense therapies, following a near-death experience or other traumatic event, or inexplicably, for no reason at all that you can understand, you are connecting with evolutionary energetic and psychic forces. These energies carry consciousness with them just as waves in the air can carry radio signals, and in some people cause the equivalent of a psychic Armageddon, where the boundaries that have contained self-identity are pushed open and new possibilities emerge. People who have experienced the sudden awakening of Kundalini energy describe it in many ways:

> While meditating I felt suddenly as if I had broken through a layer of ice and could feel myself dancing above an ocean of bliss, feeling my toes touching it, feeling intense thrills, warm, flowing from my toes up Through my body, flowing everywhere. Then I was plunged into this ocean and lost awareness of what was happening. It was indescribable. . . .Jay

> I woke up one night unable to breathe. I felt as if I was being electrocuted. My body was paralyzed.I could not even move a finger or cry out for help.I was wide awake and terrified. Two giant hands were squeezing my chest, preventing me from breathing. I felt certain I was the victim of a freak accident involving lightning or wiring. . . .Beth.

> I reached for a book of Yogananda's, to look up a quote. I felt as if someone put a heavy hand on my shoulder and pressed me down to the floor and stretched me out. Waves of ecstatic

energy flooded through me and my mind was
lost in energy and light. I stayed like this for
about four hours. . . . Chris.

While these experiences are remarkable as singular events in
someone's life, they are identifiable as Kundalini experiences because
they are the beginnings of processes lasting months and years in
which a broad range of additional events occurred. There are many
phenomena that accompany this awakening of spiritual energy/
consciousness. They fall into roughly seven categories of experience:
kriyas (involuntary movements); body sensations and symptoms;
spontaneous yogic postures and breathing; emotional upheavals;
extrasensory input -- visual, auditory and olfactory; psychic and
occult phenomena; and samadhi or satori experiences. Major changes
in perspective and lifestyle frequently accompany such an awakening.

Often the first flush of Kundalini is felt as energy moving
up from the base of the spine where, according to esoteric literature,
it has been coiled into a latent form since birth.   It may flood the
body like a geyser, crawl slowly upward in a spiral motion like a
snake, or flow in a steady stream up the spine and through the crown
of the head. The body vibrates or feels charged by energetic and (if
fortunate) ecstatic sensations. The nervous system may be overwhelmed by intense heat, sounds, or light. The energy may then
seem to fade away. Or it may linger and remake the man or woman,
from the ground up as it were, into a new person. This new person
may struggle for years with physical and psychological upheavals, as
if every latent or incomplete physical and emotional condition in the
body/mind system must be addressed and resolved. This "radical"
spiritual experience seems to arise from the deepest roots of the Self,
and sweeps one into revolutionary personality and physiological
changes. The intensity of this movement has been described in some
yogic scriptures as the rush of a divine goddess, Shakti, who is
released and charging upward through the system to be reunited with
her lover, Siva, the universal consciousness that awaits her. This demanding goddess, the creatrix and sustainer of the human being,
initiates a struggle to free human consciousness from worldly preoccupations, and she produces a wide range of psychic and
physiological phenomena, promotes ecstatic experience and agonizing
self-confrontation, and demands the reorientation of one's life.

After centuries of hiding in nearly every culture on the globe
as a secret esoteric truth, the Kundalini experience is reported more
and more frequently among modern spiritual seekers and appears to be
occurring even among people who do not follow spiritual practices.

When this happens to those who have neither a context for nor understanding of the correlations between physical and mystical experiences it can leave them bewildered and frightened, even psychologically fragmented. And when they turn to traditional physicians, psychotherapists or church advisors their anxiety is compounded because of the general lack of understanding in western culture regarding spirituality and its relationship to energy.

Although there is clearly significant impact on the physical and psychological being of one who is experiencing it, spiritual awakening need not be a fragmenting nor painful event. There is ample evidence that its' nature is primarily of expanded consciousness and bliss, which is felt consistently once the process has stabilized. This book is written to support those who have had or want to have this experience, and for those who wish to help them integrate and stabilize it. It is helpful to view this as a process: a series of actions, changes and functions intended to strengthen the body and character in order to build a vehicle strong enough to contain spiritual energy and insight. Most yogis believe a great deal of structure must be created in the body/mind complex through yoga practices, self-discipline and moderate living before it is safe to awaken this process. Many Westerners find themselves with the challenge of navigating this transformation with no structure prepared to contain it.

Kundalini Awakening in the West

In recent years the awakening of Kundalini energy is occurring more commonly or is reported more often by individuals in western society who experience it either spontaneously or as a result of certain spiritual practices or therapeutic processes. Many factors may be influencing this eruption of spiritual consciousness, including the fact that wide-spread meditation and energy-raising practices have been available in the West since their introduction in the 1930's by eastern yogis such as Paramahansa Yogananda (Kriya Yoga), Swami Muktananda (Siddha Yoga), Shri Brahmananda Sarasvati (Dr. Ramamurti Mishra), Maharishi Mahesh Yogi, who founded the Transcendental Meditation movement (TM), Yogi Amrit Desai, Swami Sivananda, Swami Prabhavananda, Bhagvan Rajneesh, Yogi Bhajan (Kundalini Yoga) and many others.

Since the 1960's Zen styles of meditation have also spread rapidly in the West, inspired by teachers such as Alan Watts, Philip Kapleau, and Kennett Roshi and organizations such as the Insight Meditation Society. Many Sufi orders in the west teach forms of energization and meditation practices. Most recently Tibetan yoga and tantric practices have also merged into western culture, often under the tutelage of lamas and monks forced to bring secret disciplines into profane societies in order to prevent the extinction of their ancient knowledge.

Classical scriptures indicate that these kinds of practices prepare the mind and body to experience and integrate an altered state of consciousness that will transform the spiritual, physical and emotional life. All sincere meditation processes promote such transpersonal states of consciousness, even those associated with schools that do not describe nor encourage experiences with Kundalini energy. Although some people who meditate have a conscious intention of awakening Kundalini, many others find this energy phenomena inexplicable because Kundalini is not recognized within the spiritual traditions they follow.

In addition to the thousands of people practicing meditation or yogic breathing exercises (called pranayama) with little understanding of the depths to which the practices may lead them, many people are exploring new forms of therapy and bodywork that utilize the breath in ways similar to ancient yogic techniques for awakening Kundalini. Others have experienced altered states while under the influence of drugs such as LSD and ADMA, which sometimes open consciousness to the possibility of radical spiritual emergence. Drug experiences are generally not considered by spiritual teachers to be valid as mystical experiences but they have opened many minds to the range of potential lying dormant in the psyche, and a number of western writers have credited such insights with leading them into a search for a spiritual perspective, seeking safer ways to expand and stabilize these kinds of experiences.

Not only spiritual teachers but psychotherapists, psychics, body therapists and other kinds of educators have promoted meditation practices, varieties of tantric practices, training for out-of-body experiences, breathing processes such as Rebirthing, Holotropic Therapy and Radiance Breathwork, and Reichian and neo-Reichian bodywork. Hatha yoga exercises, Tai Chi and Aikido classes are available in most communities. All of these practices tend to activate and amplify certain kinds of energies previously latent or less active in the physical system. Deep relaxation processes, biofeedback, imagery and gentler styles of bodywork can also deeply affect the subtle body energy system, in which Kundalini is a major factor. Some therapists and sociologists have researched near-death experiences and reported radical shifts in energy and consciousness that often accompany them. Other researchers report people who seem to become spiritually awakened through dreams. A 1988 Harris poll indicated that close to 4.5 million Americans meditate. It is probable that most of these people have been exposed to at least a nominal number of processes that can awaken the spiritual Self, the energy of Kundalini.

Perhaps the awakening of Kundalini in the West is also a psychic response occurring in greater numbers at this juncture in history because of the growing disillusion and fear regarding traditional models of power and success in western society. . . fear of death, of nuclear or natural disasters, of alienation, of deprivation. Spiritual consciousness and hope is a natural balancing element for such dark musings. Awareness of pain and suffering in the world motivated the Buddha's search, and such awareness is more and more difficult to repress and avoid.

All of these factors -- exposure to many practices, especially meditation, and deep concern about the meaning of life -- can be found in the histories of people who report Kundalini symptoms. Yet one can never predict who will awaken this energy. Openness of mind, heart and/or body seems to promote it. This means it is helpful if psychological and emotional conflicts are minimal and the body is free of blocks and tensions. It is well to have few attachments regarding worldly concerns.

Love -- passionate love for a divine Being or spiritual guide one has never even seen -- can lead one into this experience. This is well-documented by the Bhakti and Sufi poets who wrote enraptured songs and poems in celebration of the Divine, and love of Jesus is clearly the path of many of the Christian mystics as well. Many people have had at least some exposure to a spiritual teacher such as Swami Muktananda, Da Free John and others, who sometimes awaken one's Kundalini through a transmission of energy (called shaktipat in the yogic tradition).   In some traditions, most notably that of Siddha Yoga (the Yoga of the Masters), Kundalini is activated by the guru. Once transmitted, the seed can lie dormant in the follower until the right moment, when he or she is awakened, perhaps lifetimes later. Other schools of yoga teach that one can prepare for this process for lifetimes, but that the awakening is ultimately an act of grace.

In the ancient traditions those who awakened Kundalini were always advised and supervised by a teacher or guru, who by his/her nature could see into and recognize the unique needs of each devotee. Because of this the classical literature was not inclined to address the problems of Kundalini, nor search out general recommendations for their solutions. This does not mean difficulties did not exist, especially for those following yoga practices without supervision. Many traumatic symptoms were described in Gopi Krishna's autobiography, published in 1974. He was surprised to have thousands of people identifying with his problems and writing him for advice regarding their own experiences. The following of practices that lead to a direct experience of "God" is not a new or radical idea, but is in fact one of the oldest ideas recorded in spiritual literature, being a primary focus of ancient Vedantic and yogic philosophies. It is also a cornerstone of shamanic rituals in many cultures. But it is a radical spiritual movement for anyone raised under the influence of western psychology and religion, which holds the ego as central to the self, and prefers a God-archetype that is a myth of the all-knowing and impeccably-judging father. Thus to traditional western psychology, being religious implies a regression to a child-like state (submission to the father or merging with the mother); and to fundamentalist Christians, introspection and altered-states of awareness are full of risk and therefore evil, because people may have experiences antithetical to the doctrine. These kinds of convictions cannot be supported by those who delve deeply into their own psyches, and find there a tremendous urge toward spiritual liberation, or a desire to know "God" directly, which pulls them paradoxically more deeply into themselves, until they penetrate beyond awareness of form and thought.

In addition to exploring traditional eastern paths, many people are discovering new methods of finding spiritual meaning and integration. Many Westerners have a facility for experimentation and plunge actively into the mysteries of science or religion with little concern for consequences. Some are practicing with great intensity one or another process to encourage Kundalini awakening, believing it will bring them peace, bliss, transformation, wisdom, power or a wide variety of outcomes.

Because of my research and my work as a transpersonal psychotherapist I frequently discover new friends and clients who come to me to talk of their radical experiences of spiritual emergence. They are generally sane and rational individuals, talking of energy, out-of-body experiences, overwhelming physical and emotional upheavals, transcendent or spontaneous sexual experiences, psychic awareness, consciousness, light and bliss. They are struggling with all the inevitable conditions that occur when the transpersonal or collective Self confronts the ego-self. They are trying to develop a spiritual lifestyle and support a unitive perspective in a culture that is too preoccupied with economics and conflict to acknowledge the existence of mysticism, and relegates it to the ramblings of inconsequential and possibly "dysfunctional" saints in ecclesiastic history books.

Those who have these experiences are forming a quiet counter-culture of individuals who know that ego-consciousness is only part of the capacity of the human condition, and the lesser part at that. Within this counter-culture are such unlikely companions as physicists, therapists, gurus, movie stars, housewives, business consultants, teachers, artists, psychics, writers, students and more. They have come to this point through spiritual practices, meditation programs, near-death experiences, or because of breathwork or Reichian-based body therapies, acupressure, and biofeedback. A few simply wake at night as if caught on a electrical wire, and are challenged to discover the meaning of it. If the heart is very open they may feel uncontrollably in love, yet with no love-object, unless there is a vision of Jesus, Lord Krishna, or another guide or saint to contain the projection. Some feel wired and charged with massive energy, followed later by depletion and exhaustion. Others feel they are being make love to by the divine, or experiencing "cosmic orgasms"

This charge reorients the spiritual life and practices of the individual, and a life so altered   is another aspect of radical spirituality. It is a spirituality of the entire body-mind-soul, and once fully engaged one's view of oneself and the world is radically and irrevocably altered. It also holds the potential, according to Gopi Krishna, to turn one into a genius, having access to universal wisdom and inspiration. He believed this is the consequence of the deep biological changes in the brain which can be developed over years of living with this process, and he saw it as the hope for the future of the planet.

Tranformational Energy Across Cultures

There is ample evidence that the concept of spiritual awakening is not simply a phenomenon of the yogic experience, but is a process known cross-culturally by those who engage in mystical or occult practices. Such practices enable people to connect with energy, light and higher consciousness, in order to bring forth what can broadly be defined as the energies of transformation. Allusions to such experiences can be found in the mystical esoteric teachings and practices of many cultures -- Assyrian, Egyptian, Celtic, Greek, Taoist, Tibetan, Judaic, American Indian, Alaskan, Australian, and

African shamanism, Gnosticism, Sufism, and Christian mysticism. Theosophists, Freemasons, Rosicrucians and the alchemists also reportedly have had secret practices for awakening energy.

In Taoism *chi* is stimulated to great heights with practices that circulate light and energy through the body in specific patterns. In the ancient T'ai I Chin Hua Tsung Chih, translated in The Secret of the Golden Flower (Wilhelm, 1931), connection with the primal spirit of the inner Self allows one to "overcome the polar opposites of light and darkness and tarry no longer in the three worlds (earth, heaven and hell)."[1] In Taoist practices, in order to experience "primal spirit" one must subjugate ordinary consciousness or ego through the circulation of light.

> If one practises the circulation of the light, one must forget both body and heart.The heart must die, the spirit live. When the spirit lives, the breath will begin to circulate in a wonderful way. This is what the Master called the very best. Then the spirit must be allowed to dive down into the abdomen (solar plexus). The energy then has intercourse with spirit, and spirit unites with the energy and crystallizes itself. This is the method of starting the work. In time the primal spirit transforms itself in the swelling of life into the true energy. At that time,the method of the turning of the millwheel must be applied, in order to distill it so that it becomes the Elixir of Life. That is the method of concentrated work.[2]

This work also describes a "backward-flowing method" of turning sexual desire downward, and in the moment of release, using the mind to lead the energy back upwards so that it penetrates the "crucible of the creative" (the third eye, between the eyebrows). This is similar to those practices of tantric and Tibetan yoga that focus on awakening energy at the base of the spine, then move it upwards into the third eye or through the crown of the head.

Other Taoist breathing and energy practices utilize the breath to circulate streams of energy during prescribed time intervals, indicating that inhalation is to be accompanied by the sinking of the abdomen and exhalation by the lifting of it, with the emphasis on creating a "backward-flowing movement". Thus while inhaling the "lower energy-gate" is opened and energy rises upward along the spinal cord; and while exhaling, the "upper energy-gate" is closed and the stream of energy flows downward along the front line of the body. These practices are said to create in time an embryo which is "in reality the spiritual breath-energy of the ego". The spirit must penetrate the "breath-energy" (the soul), then the "breath-energy" envelops the spirit. "When the energy is strong enough and the embryo is round and complete it comes out of the top of the head." [3]

Shamans were also known to use initiatory experiences involving healing trances and light. According to Metzner (1986) "The explorer Rasmussen quotes an Eskimo shaman as saying, 'Every real shaman has to feel *qaumaneq,* a light within the body, inside his head or brain, something that gleams like fire, that enables him to see in the dark, and with closed eyes see into things which are hidden, and also into the future".[4]

Waters (Book of the Hopi, 1963) indicates that the Hopi Indians of North America have always known about Kundalini, and the subtle body, a complex invisible energy system which explains the Kundalini process in East Indian terms. The Hopi taught:

> The living body of man and the living body of
> the earth were constructed in the same way.
> Through each ran an axis. Man's axis being the
> backbone, the vertebral column, which
> controlled the equilibrium of his movements
> and his functions. Along this axis were several
> vibratory centers which echoed the primordial
> sound of life throughout the universe or sounded
> a warning if anything went wrong.[5]

Hopis described the soft spot at the top of the head as the "'open door' through which (one) received his life and communicated with his Creator" and which hardened during the last phase of creation, then reopened at death to allow the soul to exit. They identified a thinking center, which lay below the soft spot; the throat center, as the source of vibration and sound; the heart center, as the source of goodness and purpose; and the solar plexus center, which was "the throne in man of the Creator himself. From it He directed all the functions of man".[6]

Some African cultures also have teachings and rituals associated with the raising of energy. Kripananda cited evidence of African cultures who performed rituals that suggest awareness of

Kundalini energy or an experience akin to it, describing the practices of the !Kung Bushmen of Africa as studied and filmed by John Marshall on an expedition under the auspices of Harvard University. The majority of tribe members learned to perform intense dances which heat up energy (*n/um*), in order to attain a transcendent state (*kia*) that they believed allowed them to participate in eternity. *N/um*, which is initiated and controlled by a *n/um* master, rises from the base of the spine to the skull where *kia* then occurs. The report stated that this energy was seen not as a physical substance but as "energy or power, a kind of supernatural potency whose activation paves the way for curing." Kripananda said the experience is described by some participants as feeling as though they have a hole in their heads about two inches wide, which extends like an empty column down the spine.[7]

This dance is echoed in another ancient rite of "royal consecration" or "Baptism of Water" described by Eliade in <u>Yoga: Immortality and Freedom</u> (1969). A mandala is draw by means of two cords or by laying down colored rice powder: a white circle traces its outer limits, and the inner circle is composed of five different colors. In the center stand images of gods, vases of incense, flowers, and branches laid out in the form of triangles (which encourage the descent of the gods). The disciple draws a small mandala around the feet of the guru, and offers himself and a girl as a gift. The guru then puts five drops of sacred substances on his tongue, gives him appropriate mantras, and consecrates the incense, after which he brings on "possession by the furious god". The initiate recites the mantras and

> ...inhales vigorously, whereupon Vajrapani, the angry god, takes possession of him and he begins to sing and dance, imitating the traditional gestures of wrathful divinities. This rite allows the forces of the unconscious to invade the disciple, who, by confronting them burns all fear and timidity. Then, chiefly by mudras, he invokes the five peaceful divinities, the Saktis of the five Tathagatas, and becomes calm again. [8]

At this point the initiate is blindfolded, throws a flower into the mandala, and the section into which it falls indicates the deity most especially favorable to him. He then begins a "march toward the center" of the mandala, which corresponds to approaching "the center of the world." Here he is in a sacred space, outside of time, and performs a series of meditations which "help him to find the gods in his own heart", and to realize in a vision "the eternal process of periodic creation and destruction of worlds, and this allows him to enter the rhythms of the cosmic great time and to understand its emptiness."[9]

Many of the aspects of these rituals are reenacted by Westerners doing breathwork, when they hyperventilate, move their hands in mudras, and plunge mentally into altered states of consciousness where they may encounter sensations and visions as diverse as fighting off monsters, performing ritual dances and seeing inner guides or deities. The experiences of becoming aware of "the gods in one's own heart", of the destruction the worlds, of "entering the rhythm of cosmic great time" and of understanding emptiness are also frequently described as part of the experience of spiritual awakening, and will be evident in many of the personal accounts recorded in later chapters of this book.

More scientifically-oriented, the Alchemists pursued a search for the secret of life and a transformative substance which could turn base metals into gold. Undoubtedly they sought Kundalini, the life force which could transform the ordinary conditions of human embodiment. Swiss psychiatrist C. G. Jung believed they were "projecting upon matter and chemical transformation the whole gamut of the deep unconscious."[10] European alchemist Paracelsus spoke of "the light of nature" and claimed that psychic perception and clairvoyant dreams were caused by this light. It enables one to "search out supernatural things". These lights were described as "fiery sparks" coming from the world soul and as "seeds of a world to come", sprinkled throughout the great cosmos.[11]

Yet it appears that Kundalini is not a physical property that can be identified through scientific methods. It is not housed in the physical body in the way one ordinarily thinks of it, which is why Western medicine has failed to recognize it. Instead, it is part of the subtle body, a less visible energy system.

Kripananda says the Cabala, the system of exoteric Hebrew theosophy, indicates 22 graphs that are used as letters in the Hebrew alphabet and are 22 proper names originally used to designate different states or structures of the one cosmic energy, which is the essence of all there is. He quotes Suares who wrote that the decoding of Genesis is actually a process of penetrating an unknown world of cosmic energies, and stated that the names in the Book of Genesis, when read according to the Cabalistic code, are actually abstract formulas of cosmic energy focused in the human psyche. Suares said that in certain traditions the serpent in the Garden of Eden was actually called Kundalini, and is the resurrection of Aleph, the principle of all that is and all that is not, from its earthly entombment.[12]

According to Elaine Pagels, (1979) the Gnostic Gospels, 52 (extant) texts from the early centuries of Christianity, included secret mystic gospels, poems, descriptions of the origin of the universe, myths, magic and instruction for mystical practices. They advocated seeking God by taking oneself as the starting point, described the Self and the Divine as identical, spoke of enlightenment and included techniques of spiritual discipline and meditation. One text suggests a chant of sacred words and vowels which bring one into an ecstatic state.   Pagels describes visions, ecstatic experiences and out-of-body experiences recorded by a writer called Allogenes, who saw "holy powers" that offered him specific instruction, which suggests involvement with the energies of Kundalini:

> O Allo(g)enes, behold your blessedness. . . in
> silence, wherein you know yourself as you are,
> and seeking yourself, ascend to the Vitality that
> you will see moving. And if it is impossible
> for you to stand, fear nothing; but if you wish
> to stand, ascend to the Existence, and you will
> find it standing and stilling itself. . . And when
> you receive a revelation. . . and you become
> afraid in that place, withdraw back because of
> the energies. And when you have become
> perfect in that place, still yourself. [13]

Later Christian mystics often described experiences which correlate with yogic definitions of experiences related to Kundalini, although generally body sensations were not described. Hildegard of Bingen (1098--1179) left a remarkable record of spiritual illuminations in her writing and art which corresponds in some ways to visions and experiences of the yogis. She drew a vision of "a most quiet light and in it burning with flashing fire the form of a man in sapphire blue" which is similar to Swami Muktananda's vision of a blue pearl, in the heart of which is a blue God. (Indian gods Krishna and Rama are both blue beings.) Hildegard frequently related fire and flashing lights to the mystic experience. In one place she described the Trinity as "The Father is brightness and this brightness has a flashing forth and in this flashing forth is fire and these three are one". She calls the Creator a "living light", the Son "flash of light", the Spirit," fire which binds all things together, tieing together eternity and equality so that they are one -- this is like tying a bundle together, everything would fall apart otherwise."[14] This is very similar to the yogic concept of Kundalini, which is seen as the source and substance of all consciousness and creation, containing everything, and as residual energy holding the physical being in stasis until its eruption.

Also in a way similar to many Indian mystics, writing became an essential response of the spiritual process for Hildegard. "Beaten down by many kinds of illnesses, I put my hand to writing. Once I did this, a deep and profound exposition of books came over me. I received the strength to rise up from my sick bed, and under that power I continued to carry out the work to the end, using all of ten years to do it". She also wrote about breath: "If we human beings whose natural disposition may correspond to that breath of the world inhale this altered air and exhale it once again so that the soul can receive this breath and carry it even further into the body's interior, then the humors of our organism are altered ."[15]

Other Christians whose work and descriptions of personal experiences echo portions of yogic scriptures are Meister Eckhart, St. Catherine of Genoa, St. Catherine of Siena, St. John of the Cross, St. Paul, St. Teresa, Teilhard de Chardin, Jacob Boheme and Emanuel Swedenborg, to mention only a few.

Theosophy, a metaphysical system that attracted thousands of people at the turn of the century, incorporated and elaborated on Tibetan and yogic practices, and detailed an extensive philosophy related to the subtle body, and seven rays of energy and healing. The Theosophists contributed greatly to the publishing and popularizing of Eastern books and teachings in the West, and although their descriptions of the subtle body vary slightly from yogic theory, and are frequently maligned by Eastern scholars because of this, many of their teachings are still widely read and practiced. Krishnamurti, a prominent Indian teacher of the 20th century, whose Kundalini experiences were described in two biographies, spent most of his childhood being trained and initiated in Theosophical practices, although he later severed his philosophical alignment with them.

Some spiritual groups encourage the activation and flow of energy or the cultivation of psychic openness in the body during specific forms of their devotional practices -- among these are the Quakers, Shakers, Subud, and some charismatic groups. The shaking phenomenon that may occur during these practices appears similar to a Kundalini experience, but it is more likely a sign of heightened pranic activity. (Pranic energy, more clearly defined in chapter three, operates all the directional movement and activities of the physical system, can be expanded through a variety of practices, and is much more easily contacted than the latent Kundalini energy.) I have talked with a number of people who experience this phenomenon of shaking involuntarily, especially during bodywork or meditation. Many have experienced it once, following a stressful event. Others have felt it during Subud practices (a trance-like spiritual practice which encourages the movement of energy and body motions, and appears to open psychic and healing potentials), while receiving or performing healing, and at other times. It may be important to distinguish these experiences from Kundalini awakening as it is described in the yogic and mystical literature.

Whether trance states that arouse energy during environmentally controlled rituals (such as described by Kripananda and Eliade) are a true arousal of Kundalini is also questionable, since the experiences seem to be contained within specific boundaries and do not necessarily promote a life-long series of changes in consciousness. I would assume that for shamans and medicine people, as opposed to those who simply participated in tribal ritual, a more permanent energy shift was activated, and in fact there are close correlations between descriptions of shamanic initiations and Kundalini awakenings. Communal rituals appear to heighten access to the psychic and healing phenomena associated with Kundalini, and may represent a way in which primitive cultures could temporarily raise pranic energy and perhaps increase alpha levels of their brain-waves in order to gain insights for cultures which had not yet developed intellectual function.

All of the observable movements in these practices, as well as in those who have awakened Kundalini, are pranic releases, but a genuine Kundalini experience continuously promotes major changes in both mind and body. It is possible that pranic energy may increase gradually before an awakening, or Kundalini may release small amounts of energy, like steam from a pressure cooker, during states of intense altered consciousness, and return back to her resting place afterwards. But once there is a full awakening the subject will experience her activity constantly, until transformation is complete.

After studying many cases of Kundalini awakening in the literature and conducting dozens of personal interviews I have concluded that this experience often occurs in stages. Most people report a preliminary experience of strong energy and spiritual awareness, bliss or samadhi experiences, years before a more intense and difficult encounter with Kundalini. These preliminary experiences or occasional movements and releases of energy may spontaneously prepare one for the later awakening.   Although many practices may provide preparation for an awakening there is little evidence to indicate a consistency in what practices will awaken Kundalini, and there seems to be a significant factor of either "grace" or psychic preparedness over which the aspirant has little control.

There are hundreds of kinds of experiences that appear to be associated with pranic energy and Kundalini, and many cultural and spiritual practices worth examining in order to authenticate the universal application of this process.   But it is the eastern yogis who have most thoroughly and conscientiously documented these events and developed teachings regarding them.   Their scriptures contain clearly articulated paths relevant to spiritual attainment, and report the most expansive range of experiences.

Kundalini as the Great Goddess

As noted earlier, some of the classical literature of Kundalini describes her as the great goddess. In The Laksmi Tantra , an ancient Pancaratra text (the oldest surviving Visnuite sect in India) there is a dialogue between Laksmi, another name for the goddess Kundalini, and Sakra, a devotee. It is told that Sakra did divine penance by standing motionless on a piece of wood on one foot, observing silence and subsisting on air alone for 2000 years, with hands, gaze and face turned upward to the sky.

The goddess then appeared and he asked to know the nature of truth.   She identified herself as Kundalini and all other goddesses as well, advocated her worship as the Great-Mother Goddess, and explained Sakti (another term for Kundalini) as a supra-metaphysical principle. She presented a detailed guide on how to live a spiritual life which included rituals, meditation, constantly engaging in the repetition of mantra, practicing loyalty, self-restraint, sobriety, intelligence, non-violence, self-control and generosity. She advocated meditating in the first part of the night, sleeping the remaining two parts, and waking in the latter half to repeat the same cycle. She recommended reading scriptures in the afternoon in order to realize the Self, without being distracted by greed, attachment or hatred. She suggested one accept only that much of such scriptures as depicts something about oneself. [16]

This beautiful scripture describes in detail the essential role of Kundalini (or Shakti) in human existence, inseparable from Siva, and the creator of all form. It describes the levels of experience of the

jiva, or individual embodied soul, and indicates that Kundalini decides
when her grace will descend to awaken one to higher consciousness.
It presents the design of the material universe, and the process of
God-realization in the soul. The nature of letters, sound and mantra
(repetitive Sanscrit prayers and tones) are explained. The purpose of
mudras (yogic hand movements that affect concentration, energy and
consciousness) and their function in the scheme of creation is
presented. Kundalini is characterized as motivated by the urge to
create. "With a billionth fraction of myself I voluntarily embark on
creation by differentiating myself in two separate (particles) of which
one is conscious and the other is the objects of its knowledge." [17]

The joy and love of the goddess for her creation resonates
throughout this text, and it would be reassuring to anyone on a spiritual path. It conveys a sense of the Great Mother Goddess within
each being who knows the deeper truths of the soul purpose. In the
following passages Laksmi describes herself to Sakta.

> The way to obtain liberation from the bondage
> of the material world is to worship Laksmi, the
> Visnu-Sakti. One should abandon all other
> activity and concentrate solely on propitiating
> the Goddess either directly, or indirectly through
> Visnu, in order to obtain spiritual release. [18]

> Every manifestation of God is through Sakti's
> manifestation. She is God's supreme will and
> acts under his direction. The universe is the
> manifestation of Sakti. . .

> I, the eternal Goddess, am the object of all the
> Vedas; I am the life-principle of the universe
> and the potent force behind all creation. . .

> I am recognized by the wise as the bliss and
> tranquility inherent in each state of being. . .
> (After) discovering me and propitiating me the
> jiva (individual soul) washes away all klesas
> (evil tendencies) and blows away the dust of
> impressions; whereas the jiva, that has (thus)
> already severed its fetters through meditations
> (yoga) fuses with true knowledge and attains

me, who am Laksmi and whose nature is
supreme bliss. [19]

I am Goddess Narajani, ever co-operating in
performing the functions of Narayana, who
consists of jnana (knowledge), ananda (bliss)
and kriya (activity); and I, too, consist of
knowledge, bliss and activity. There is not a
single place nor moment when it is possible for
me to exist without Him, or for Him to exist
without me. [20]

Laksmi also describes the state of the jiva or soul who attains union with her, giving encouragement to those struggling
through the awakening and integrating stages of the process. She
cites some of the gains of this experience as freedom from all re-
striction and limitations, awareness that no single material or immaterial object exists that is not infused with I-hood, and perfect
tranquility. The conscious Sakti is described as flawless and pure,
consisting of consciousness and bliss.

Laksmi describes the jiva as doing five things when contained in the human body: it makes contact with objects, gets attached, ceases attachment of one for another, has an impression left
behind, and eradicates the impression. This destruction, like fire, has
the propensity to destroy everything within reach. This describes to
some extent what one is primarily experiencing once the Kundalini is
fully awakened. It is the change of consciousness from the being
who is attached, to the one who has destroyed everything within
reach. The fire which demolishes the ordinary psychic orientation
does not have to be felt physically, it is a psychic fire as well,
burning away the former parameters of identification. She says
"When in consequence of the advent of pure knowledge the jiva dis-
cards its limitations, then freed from every shackle it becomes illu-
minated." [21]

Although the boon of illumination is appealing to
Westerners, they have many defenses against burning away ego
attachments, and it is a major upheaval of consciousness to discover
that many of the former interests and involvements of life have
become irrelevant. There is a tendency not to consider seriously the
demands for change instigated by a spiritual life and to hope that
"enlightenment" is all accomplished in some nice, neat, and all-
inclusive meditation experience. The truth is that   mystical

experiences force people to find radically new meanings in human experiences, and encourage them to live in a style that is completely indifferent to ego satisfactions. This experience is akin to falling in love with a goddess who is utterly fascinating and obsessively demanding of all of one's attention, forgoing any other temptation or attachment.

Sakti or Kundalini is said to help one become liberated in two ways -- creating the means to experience liberation, and instilling the inclination to seek her favor to obtain emancipation. In other words the Self creates the means of its own liberation, and instills in one the desire to become free. Laksmi proposes a method of self-surrender in this tantra, with advice that might be useful to spiritual aspirants or those who wish a gentler relationship with Kundalini. (For it is often fear, resistance and misinterpretation of what is happening that makes this process painful.) She advises one to resolve to conform to God's desire, to abandon all acts that displease God, to have a firm conviction God will protect those who choose God as sole protector, and to practice self-surrender and humility. Thereby one becomes free of misfortunes such as fear, sorrow, exhaustion, selfish activity and desire, self-interest and pride, and is sheltered in God alone. One becomes benevolent toward all beings, based on the conviction "I exist in all beings"; and will drop all hostility and arrogance. She recommends prayer and the deeprooted conviction God will protect you. [22]

This tantra is unique in the literature of Kundalini because it is feminine and because it is specific in terms of recommendations for those who seek a relationship with Her. It presents a god and a goddess archetype that are supportive and nurturing of the process, being part of all living things and the sole protectors during this time of transition. It is useful to remember that in the Eastern cosmology the image of "God" bears little resemblance to the Christian archetype, although similar kinds of advice is found in all spiritual traditions. One might think of this "God" as a quality of all-encompassing consciousness of which we are all a part and which we can trust implicitly as being the sole source and sustenance of our lives. To surrender to this God is to surrender to the Tao, to trust that everything is already perfect, even that which ego does not accept nor understand. Humility is the non-assertion of ego against this flow.

Yet even should one follow the scriptures precisely, and surrender to the Tao perfectly, it seems likely that every experience with Kundalini would still be individualized, just as there are numerous facets to her creation. A significant factor of my findings was that there are many ways one can be opened to this process, with responses that are varied and unpredictable. Each story is unique, and yet there is a resonance of common features that make Kundalini experiences recognizable. Individual encounters with her are as unique as individual faces. We always recognize it is a face we are looking at, but the differences between faces are more striking than the similarities. It is not so easy to recognize Kundalini, until one knows her well, but it is important we don't misjudge her, because the wrong approach to treatment can strangle the potential of the emergent Self.

The Goddess & the Self

Now I have identified Kundalini both as the Self and as a goddess, and in fact both positions are clearly supported in eastern scriptures. She is a goddess, also identified as Shakti in her more cosmic condition, because she is that which creates form, which molds through an intricate energy arrangement the form of each living being. It is said that when Kundalini awakens she rushes upward, through the spine, in order to reunite with her beloved in all his splendor. But in fact, she can never be separate from him, only expanded into more and more awareness and expression of him. Both are intrinsically interwoven into every atom of the universe. How can this goddess then also be the Self?

The goddess is a personification, an archetype, representing our personal innate connection with the Source of All, with eternal-existence, with wisdom beyond that of which the mind can conceive. She is the creative or form-producing agent of the Divine, residing in each living being. This energy of Kundalini has created a template and activated each of us as unique individuals who bring into the world varied conditions --thought-forms, energies, mental and emotional characteristics, physical strengths and vulnerabilities, potentials. In eastern theory this form of "us" is activated through our nadis, a complex network of invisible energy flows, and our five kosas (sheaths) contained in three subtle bodies. All of the energy we normally have access to, be it to move, dance, swallow, belch, eliminate, speak, is part of the activity of this energy, distributed through a network of 720,000 nadis (or up to 72 million, depending on which esoteric source one uses) in energy forms called pranas in eastern scripture.

Prana is known as *Chi* or *Ki* in Chinese and Japanese medicine, respectively, and methods of managing it, balancing it, and enhancing it have been well known in eastern cultures for thousands of years. Yet it remains enigmatic in the West. According to the Indian subtle body system the residual energy, after our systems are complete, coils 3 1/2 times at the base of the spine, and goes into a dormant state. Our minds become engaged in the process of living, and we identify with our bodies, our genetic heritage and our mental, sensate and emotional processes, separating from any awareness of the Self, or the Soul, or the source of our existence, however one wishes to identify it.

The word "self" is used in several forms in psychology. The most common is to place the "self" as a central unifying aspect of the psyche around which one forms identity and creates experience, commonly correlated with the ego. The awareness of and stability of this self is based on early childhood experiences, according to many western theorists. This is indeed a useful model, and practices that strengthen the sense of this self are very important for enhancing one's psychological health and sense of wholeness. Some therapists would view the Self as a more highly evolved center in the psyche, superior to the ego, not entangled in the emotional traumas and conditioned responses of the psyche, but nonetheless a "personal" entity.

C. G. Jung identified the "Self" as a center of consciousness separate from ego, which possesses an absolute authority in the psyche, and around which all other factors, both conscious and unconscious, circumambulate. According to Jungian analyst Esther Harding, when the Self functions strongly in a human being it produces a preoccupation with the inner, subjective life, and exerts a non-personal compelling power over the individual. She says it is expressed in such terms as "finding the God within." [23]

Harding believed this Self can never entirely replace the ego, as continuation demands some egoic sense. However as egoic consciousness is pre-empted by the nonpersonal Self biological desire is relegated to a subservient possession, with the instincts becoming relative, their energy transferred in part from the biological to the psychic sphere.

Jung's perspective is very similar to eastern views of Self, but we might say that in the East the Self is viewed more intensely, or more profoundly. It is the center of all one's experience, the very reason for the existence. This Self is the core of one's being, of which the personal self is only a reflection, and the Kundalini energy/consciousness is it's essence. The Self is the consciousness, wisdom and intention of our creation and predetermines what is brought into our experiences, emotions and minds, while we remain unaware.

This Self is more primal (that is, pre-existing, although unlikely to be conscious in it's pre-existent state), essential and eternal, than the personality self. It is more difficult to connect with consciously, although it may spontaneously reveal itself at times, providing awe-filled moments like many described in mystical literature. It may appear in visions or numinous dreams, through experiences of light or bliss during meditation and at other rare moments, or flood one with sudden knowing and recognition of profound truths or ecstasy.

It seems that experiences of the Self are sometimes accompanied by archetypal encounters with gods and goddesses, saints relevant (or even non-relevant) to the tradition of the subject, or transforming symbols such as those often encountered in a the deep Jungian analytical process. In such cases the Self is leading consciousness into archetypal realms, providing bridges through which we can come to understand the core of our experience as humans, along with the potential of the numinous. These archetypal forces determine the patterns that we live out in our lives. At higher stages of spiritual evolution this higher Self loses its "personal-ity", and becomes the Self of all, and one experiences the interrelatedness of all creation as one Self.   The experience of individuation moves consciousness from a false and adapted self into the knowing of the personal Self and ultimately into glimpses of the collective Self, while the Kundalini experience tends to move consciousness from the personal Self into the collective Self.

Kundalini & Western Therapies

Another Jungian analyst, Erich Neumann (1961), writing of numinous experiences and their impact on the psyche, could well have been describing Kundalini when he said:

> The numinous content possesses a fascination,
> a richness beyond the power of consciousness to
> apprehend and organize, a charge of energy sur-
> passing consciousness. Hence the encounter
> with it always leads to an upheaval of the total
> personality and not only of consciousness. In
> every confrontation of the ego with the
> numinous, a situation arises in which the ego

> gets 'beside itself', it falls or is wrenched out of
> its shell of consciousness and comes back to
> itself only in changed form. [24]

Neumann clearly knew the spiritual processes of the psyche, and his words suggest the reasons why the Kundalini process is sometimes put in the hands of a therapist, for those experiencing it sense they are changing radically. They may feel disengaged from their former sense of self, engage in erratic or irrational behaviors, see visions, or make involuntary movements that they formerly identified only with the mentally ill. Besieged as well with physical changes, pains and random symptoms, they often wonder if they are dying, or are guilty of psychosomatic excesses.

The issue of Kundalini awakening should be an area of special concern to therapists who see clients with spiritual concerns or practices because persons experiencing it are frequently mistakenly diagnosed and inadequately treated. The average therapist or physician has not heard of it and has no spiritual context with which to integrate it. Gopi Krishna wrote of a friend who experienced the symptoms and went to a psychologist who told him the phenomenon was "quite unknown in the domain of psychology and must be a delusion of some sort or an unconscious impulse finding its way into surface consciousness". He claimed there are countless cases of spontaneous awakening of Kundalini that go unnoticed, or that trail off into insanity because the experience is not understood and proper advice is not available. "Apart from psychosis" says Krishna," there are also many people in whom the awakening of Kundalini leads to neurosis and other psychic disorders. They lead an unbalanced life without crossing the border into the territory of the incurably insane. There are also others who, while having the experiences, manage to continue in the normal tenor of their lives."[25]

In addition to the possibility of seeing clients who have inadvertently awakened Kundalini, some therapists, particularly those trained in the transpersonal model, use methods with the breath and concentration that are similar to ancient yogic methods for opening this energy. One of the most common of these is breathwork. Breathing exercises are also used in behavior therapy (as in the process of progressive relaxation), as a preparation for most biofeedback training, to correct irregular breathing patterns, and to treat hypertension. Thomas Wolfe, reported using biofeedback equipment to reach altered states in which he believes his Kundalini energy awakened.[26]

I have personally seen pranic energy movements similar to those occurring with Kundalini awakening occur during and subsequent to transpersonal therapy sessions involving Holotropic Therapy (a form of breathwork), as taught by Dr. Stanislav and Christina Grof, and Radiance Breathwork, as taught by Drs. Gay and Kathlyn Hendricks. During these neo-Reichian bodywork processes clients following Grof's methods will lie down and deeply relax, with eyes closed, focus on breathing and breathe more quickly than usual, accompanied by intense music for periods of up to two hours. Usually this process is done in a group, with a partner sitting beside the breather as a quiet support system.

According to Grof, as tensions in the body collect bands of intense constriction tend to develop in regions associated with the chakras, and also along the arms, hands, legs and feet, causing pressure or even pain. Grof discounts the typical medical response to this "hyperventilation syndrome", which has been treated with tranquilizers, injections of calcium, and a paper bag placed over the face when it occurs in neurotic patients. He says the use of hyperventilation for self-exploration and therapy proves this response incorrect. "With continued breathing, the bands of tight constriction, as well as the carpopedal spasm (contractions of hands and feet), tend to relax instead of increasing, and the individual eventually reaches an extremely peaceful and serene condition associated with visions of light and feelings of love and connectedness". [27]   He reports that this exercise stimulates deep shifts in consciousness so that a client may go into altered states which release archetypal images; memories of early life, birth, pre-natal, or past-lives; free-flowing emotions; yogic postures and mudras; ancient and exotic dance movements and rituals; and major energy releases.

> In a group of randomly selected individuals. . . at least one out of three can reach transpersonal states of consciousness within an hour of the first session. It is quite common for participants to report authentic experiences of the embryonal state or even conception, elements of the collective or racial unconscious, identification with human or animal ancestors, or reliving of past incarnation memory. Equally frequent are encounters with archetypal images of deities or demons and complex mythological sequences. The spectrum of experiences that are available for an average participant include telepathic

flashes, experiences of leaving the body, and astral projection.[28]

These are also experiences that frequently accompany Kundalini awakening, and it is apparent that some people who do breathwork may open into the Kundalini experience in the same ways that people who practice yoga and pranayama breathing exercises may also awaken it. It is also likely that different kinds of breathing rhythms access different areas of consciousness, as the breath impacts various parts of the body/mind system. Tantric yogis teach that breathing through the left or right nostrils, or through both nostrils simultaneously, the rate of the breath, and the portions of the nostrils the breath touches all have significant affect on health, longevity, moods, the outcome of activities undertaken, and one's state of consciousness. An entire science of diagnosis for both physical and psychological conditions exists which is based on observation of the breathing patterns, and mastery of the breath is believed to lead to mastery in life.

This discussion of breath has several implications for a therapist, in addition to pointing out the possibility that therapy involving breathing techniques inadvertently (or deliberately!) may awaken pranic or Kundalini activity. If a range of breathing rhythms and patterns activate varied states of consciousness it would seem possible for people who have knowledge of the system to activate specific kinds of psychological processes. This information might also explain the wide range of spontaneous emotional and physiological activity that one observes in persons doing Holotropic or Radiance Breathwork, as well as in hypnotherapy, acupressure and other forms of bodywork. Another consideration for a therapist treating a person with unpleasant symptoms is that through proper understanding of pranayama (yogic breathing) techniques the system may be warmed up or cooled down, or brought into a better balance. Because of the use of breathing techniques in many transpersonal therapy practices, and because many Westerners are currently practicing Eastern meditation and breathing techniques, it is becoming imperative for therapists to have a solid understanding of the Kundalini process.

Eastern-Western Synthesis of Radical Spiritual Experiences

This book is an attempt to synthesize the concepts of eastern spirituality and subtle physiology with the new experiences and conditions now appearing in the West. The similarities cross-culturally of spiritual awakening are evident in examining excerpts from classical and modern yogic literature, biographies and autobiographies of persons from eastern and western cultures, and the stories of western subjects who were interviewed regarding their personal experiences with Kundalini. Like a prism these resources reflect from many perspectives the nature of this experience and allow us to observe the spiritual, physical, emotional, and behavioral changes associated with it. We can glean from the stories ways in which individuals may initiate and respond to this process and theorize about the kinds of support most beneficial for the integration of this process.

Indirectly I am exploring the question of how ego consciousness and spiritual awareness may be synthesized in an individual who feels drawn to know the Self, but is entangled in the perplexities of dissolving ego-consciousness in a society that views this as insanity. I am presenting what I observe as a new paradigm, one that uses eastern and western modalities to engage the transpersonal Self, and new models for the experience and integration of spiritual consciousness in both cultures. The teachings of the East are rich in understanding of the supraconscious elements of the human psyche. Western theologians and psychotherapists must release the rigidity of their adherence to western perspectives and open to the possibility that a profound wisdom about spiritual matters existed thousands of years before Christ. It is possible that the ancients cared far more about these pathways and openings to the Self than the majority of modern intellectuals, scientists and even clergy who have pursued mastery of the universe on their own terms since the Crusades. And it is fortunate that some mystics have chosen to safeguard this wisdom until such times as a sufficient number of people were willing to integrate it back into the culture.

Now is clearly the time in the West, not only to honor and value this wisdom, but to experiment and explore the evolution of a new paradigm in order to master spiritual awareness and revitalize an ailing society. I suspect those of us having this experience now will eventually create a new model, bringing forth the wisdom of the East and integrating it with the experimental and creative aspects of the

West, to provide groundwork for the future emergence of wide-spread spiritual experience My sense is that we are forerunners of an evolving spiritual consciousness -- paradoxically, because in fact this is in no way a new experience, is in fact the most ancient of recorded experiences.

In the following chapters we will explore these experiences from many ancient and modern perspectives, identify the range of conditions associated with it, suggest eastern and western metaphysical and biological approaches to the phenomena, reveal personal accounts of the experience over a five hundred year span, and describe supportive approaches that will assist people engaged in this process.

References: Chapter 1

1 Wilhelm, R, (1931). The Secret of the golden flower. New York: Harper, Brace & World, p. 25.

2 Op. cit., p. 30.

3 Op. cit., p. 73.

4 Metzner, R. (1986). Opening to inner light. Los Angeles: J. P. Tarcher, p. 79.

5 Waters, F.(1963) Book of the Hopi. Middlesex, England: Penguin, p.9.

6 Op. cit., p. 10.

7 Grof, S. (Editor) (1984) Ancient wisdom: Modern science. Albany: State of University of New York, pp. 82-83.

8 Eliade, M. (1969) . Yoga, immortality and freedom. New York: Bollingen, p. 224.

9 Op. cit., p. 225.

10 Martin, P. (1955) Experiment in depth. London: Lowe & Brydone, p. 99.

11 Metzner,R, Op. cit., pp. 79-89.

12 Grof, S. Op. cit., pp. 80-81.

13 Pagels, E. (1979) The Gnostic gospels. New York: Vintage, p. 167.

14 Hildegard of Bingen (Ed: Matthew Fox) (1985). Illuminations of Hildegard of Bingen. Sante Fe: Bear & Co., p. 23.

15 Op. cit.

16 Gupta, S. (1971) The Laksmi Tantra -- A Pancaratra text. Leiden, Netherlands: E. J. Brill, p.78.

17 Op. cit., p. 70.

18 Op. cit. p. xix. (Vishnu is the aspect of God as sustainer of the
       universe.)
19 Op. cit., p. 78.
20 Op. cit., p. 49.
21 Op. cit., p. 71.
22 Op. cit., p. 94.
23 Harding, E. (1947/1963) Psychic energy: Its source and its
       transformation, Princeton: Princeton University, p. 24.
24 Neumann, E. (1961) "Mystical Man" Spring. New York:
       Analytical Psychology Club. p. 15.
25 Krishna, G. (1974) Higher consciousness: The evolutionary thrust
       of Kundalini. New York: Julian, p. 149.
26 Wolfe, W. (1978) And the sun is up: Kundalini rises in the West.
       Red Rock, New York: Academy Hill.
27 Grof, S. (1985) Beyond the brain: Birth, death and transcendence
       in psychotherapy . Albany: State University of New York,
       p. 388.
28 Op. cit., p. 389.

CHAPTER TWO

ACROSS THE SPECTRUM: EXPERIENCES WITH KUNDALINI

The experiences that occur during the months and years of a Kundalini process are physiological, emotional, psychic and life-changing in their impact. They touch every sense and absorb people in dramatic episodes that can be alternatively painful, humorous and ecstatic. Every individual seems to follow a unique pattern, unpredictable and varying in intensity and duration. For some people symptoms occur primarily in the middle of the night, when defenses are down and the psyche is in a state of relaxation. Others may feel tormented with painful physical problems that defy diagnosis and symptoms that move inexplicably from one body organ to another. A few report flights of emotions and waves of orgasmic-like sensations. The conditions observed during Kundalini awakening fall into seven categories which will be outlined in depth in this chapter.

1. Pranic activity or kriyas: intense involuntary body movements, shaking, vibrations, jerking, and the sensation of electricity, tingling, and rushes of energy flooding the body. The term kriya is sometimes defined in yoga as "the power of assuming any and every form."[1]

2. Physiological problems: these may include the activation of latent illness or pseudo illness, apparent heart problems, gastro-intestinal disorders, nervous problems, eating disorders, and pains occurring in various parts of the body, especially along the spine

and in the head and other difficulties that usually prove difficult to diagnose and treat.

3. Yogic phenomena: the body may involuntarily perform yogic postures (asanas) or hand movements (mudras) that the subject has never before seen, and the psyche may produce symbolic images or the mind produce chants, Sanscrit words, tones and a variety of specific sounds commonly recorded in the yogic tradition.

4. Psychological and emotional upheavals: there can be an intensification of any unresolved psychological tendencies and issues, fear of death or insanity, mood swings, and overwhelming waves of anxiety, anger, guilt, or depression as well as intense compassion, unconditional love, and heightened sensitivity to the moods of others.

5. Extrasensory experiences: these may include visual input (lights, symbols, images of entities, the reviewing of what appears to be other lives, and visions) or auditory input (hearing a voice, music, or phrase) or olfactory (perhaps smelling sandlewood, perfume or incense).

6. Parapsychological experiences: psychic awareness, unusual synchronicities, healing abilities, and psychokinesis are the most commonly reported occult phenomena.

7. Samadhi or satori experiences: absorption of consciousness into mystical states of unity, peace, light or energy; less intensive trance states; tranquility, joy, and overwhelming waves of bliss occurring during or after meditation or spontaneously at other times.

Physiological Dimensions of the Kundalini Process

My whole body changed -- my pulse raced and my heart pounded and I was hungry all the time. But I felt I could barely eat enough and in one week I lost seven pounds. . . subject, Beth.

I had drenching night sweats, every night for weeks, so heavy I would have to change the bedding several times a night. . . subject, Jay.

> My body, particularly the right side, would
> frequently go into spastic movements I could
> not control. . . subject, Mark.

Generally a Kundalini experience is first identified because of the unusual physiological activity it generates. It is difficult for western medicine to grasp the connection between body symptoms and mysticism, even though a cursory glance at the writing of Christian mystics makes it clear that they commonly endured dramatic physical problems. These have been considered a consequence of a weak physical disposition by those who have no framework for understanding the relationship between energy, the body and religious experience. If we can theorize that spiritual awakening involves an intense movement of energy and a restructuring of the physical system in order to handle it, then we can begin to appreciate the impact on the body and the strain of the system trying to integrate it..

I have grouped the pranic activity and physical phenomena reported in the literature and among western subjects into six categories--pranic activities or kriyas, internal physical sensations, visual problems, changes in eating patterns, temperature changes, and symptoms of physical illness or pseudo-illness.

Pranic Activities (Kriyas)
Involuntary jerks, shaking, vibrating, spasms.
Contractions, especially of the anus, abdomen and throat
(the yogic "locks" or bandhas).
Sudden movements of the arms, legs or head.
Involuntary dancing, hopping, spinning.
Falling down, or becoming frozen in action, stiffness,
rigidity.
Running madly at breakneck speed.
Jerking as a major flood of energy comes up the body
originating from the big toe, the foot or the
base of the spine.

Internal Physical Sensations
Ecstatic, blissful sensations, mild or intense, lasting a few
minutes or a few months.
Feeling intoxicated, detached, slightly out-of-body.
Falling into a trance, staring into space.
Increased pulse rate.
Feeling as if plugged into an electric socket,

tingling, itching.
Nervous energy, tension, throbbing; sometimes alternated
with lethargy.
Nausea, abdominal pain.
Feeling a snake is inside, especially in the abdomen or
crawling up the spine.
Chest pains as if having a heart attack.
Chronic or temporary pains all over the body, for which no
diagnosis can be made.
Backaches and sharp pain along spine.
Headaches, feeling of energy buzzing in head, tingling,
itching, or bugs crawling on scalp.
Electrical sensations in head, feeling scalp is being opened.
Numbness in hands, arms or feet.
Pain or electrical sensations in big toe, darkening
of toenail or losing toenail.
Intense sexual energy; spontaneous orgasms,either
genital or described as "whole body" or
"brain orgasms."
Sucking sensations at the cervix; itching in
perineal area.
Body feeling light as air; out-of-body experiences.
Extremely sensitive hearing -- hearing voices at a great
distance or hearing as if a color is associated
with each tone.
Vibrations and energy coming out of the ears.
Hearing and feeling deep inner sounds.
Hyperactivity followed by exhaustion.
Hair standing on end.
The stomach swelling, as if pregnant.
The lungs spontaneously filling with air.
A sweet nectar taste coming down into the throat
(amrita).

Visual Problems
Eyelids closing temporarily and refusing to open.
Temporary blindness.
Diminished vision.
Extreme sensitivity to light.
Acute vision -- seeing everything as if colors are
very intense.
Seeing auras.
Eyes burning.

Twitching between the brows, or attention riveted
on the "third eye".

Changes in Eating Patterns

Major appetite swings -- may include inability to eat at all
for several days or weeks or having a voracious
appetite. May have little or no impact on weight.
Tendency to eliminate meat, intoxicants and drugs from diet.

Temperature Changes

Hot flashes, sometimes with profuse sweating. Heat may
stream from the body or feel like intense burning.
Night sweats.
Flashes of freezing cold, sometimes alternating with heat
flashes.
Hot and cold sensations in various body parts,
especially the hands or the base of the spine.

Illness or Pseudo-Illness

Apparent heart attacks, usually false alarms; complaints the
heart is not beating.
Stomach disorders and other digestive tract problems.
Migraine headaches.
Symptoms similar to epilepsy or Parkinson's disease.
Sincere conviction one is dying, with a range of vague pains
and complaints.
Eruption of latent illness.
Floating pains, congestions, digestive problems
and other complaints fluctuating in a variety
of body organs, remitting without treatment.
Pain along spleen meridian, probably due to over-
stimulation.
Symptoms of adrenal exhaustion.

These symptoms tend to be erratic, they may occur only in the middle of the night or come and go without provocation and they are generally unresponsive to medical treatment. Their frequency and endurance are impossible to predict. Some people have little physical response during Kundalini awakening and others react primarily with intense physical reactions. Some of the most advanced yogis have reported very intense symptoms although generally these conditions are endured for only a short period, several days or weeks.

It is possible that people with previous physical injuries experience pain at the site of earlier traumas, and that those with unresolved emotional blocks may experience pain in those body areas where tension is stored. Body therapists generally associate pain with resistance or contraction at the site. Relief may occur if one can surrender to this process, and relax into the energy flow. In many cases physical difficulties seem to abate within a year or two, if not sooner, although awareness of sensations and energy flow remains. Some people report that the body maintains a consistent level of internal vibration and never feels quite ordinary again, and that by tuning into it they can deepen their meditative state or produce bliss at will. Many practices such as meditation, hatha yoga, physical exercise, chanting, body therapies, breathing exercises, as well as dietary and social restrictions seems to increase, decrease or redistribute this energy.

Generally kriyas or involuntary jerks and movements do not cause pain, and although they may be uncomfortable or embarrassing if they come at inconvenient times, people usually become accustomed to them and learn to consider their presence a reassurance that the spiritual energy is still with them. They are often accompanied by sensations of bliss either during their movement or after it. They are reportedly more intense during meditation, breathwork, body therapy, sexual activity and in periods of stress. There is often (but not always) some degree of control over them, so that a person may shift the body, or try a yoga posture or breath, or put awareness on another activity and they diminish. It is also possible to use breath and visualizations to change the patterns and intensity of kriyas.

Yogi Baba Hari Dass has said that Kundalini is the rising consciousness of Self and that all of the energy or movement manifestations are only the indirect effects of pranic energy movement in one who has not mastered control of pranic energies through proper pranayama practices, diet and disciplined living.[2] Other yogis also equate unusual pranic activity with insufficient purification. Madhusudandasji once wrote that there are two kinds of kriyas -- one for purification, and one for the manifestation of joy.[3]

Gopi Krishna wrote extensively about the physical problems associated with Kundalini and said "When we admit that a regular biological process is at work in the brain to invest it with an expanded state of consciousness. . . it is easy to see that the emergence of the higher state of consciousness with complete clarity and precision cannot be possible all at once. Like other processes of growth it must be attended by ups and downs, divisions and distortions, to be smoothed out and straightened in the course of time."[4] He called approaches to higher consciousness that ignored the biologic aspects of transcendent experience "puerile and unrealistic" and stated "There is hardly any understanding that for the transpersonal manifestations of consciousness the active participation of brain and body is essential. . . It is reasonable to assume that any deep change in psychological state would be accompanied by change in the human organism and would be attended by subtle or even tangible changes in the brain and nervous system."[5]

There is controversy in the literature regarding the illness associated with Kundalini. Classical references suggest the body will eventually become free from all disease and ill health; however, it is clear that gurus and spiritual teachers are as susceptible to cancer, diabetes, heart disease and other illness as the general population. It is possible that the intensification of pranic energy activates latent illness in some who awaken Kundalini and promotes a healthier physical system in others, depending on predisposing factors which may be related to genetics or karma, depending on your perspective. Although it appears that much of the apparent illness that emerges in the process passes without conclusive diagnosis or treatment it is advisable to consider a medical examination for serious problems.

Involuntary Yogic Activities

> One morning I felt a tug at the end of my right finger as I did the Salute to the sun (a hatha yoga pose) and then as I bent over one leg the muscle contracted under my right knee. I leaned over my left leg to get more leverage. suddenly my right hand grasped the leg and yanked it. It was so painful my mouth flew open to scream,but out of it came a soft sound -- "ta" . . . subject, Mark.

> My body kept bending over backwards, my face
> nearly flat on the ground. . . subject, Karen.

Westerners who have awakened Kundalini may be quite astonished to discover themselves spontaneously moving into a yogic asana, a posture of the hatha yoga tradition, which they may never have seen or learned and could not do in a normal state of consciousness. It feels as if the body takes on a purposeful movement and flow that presses and bends them into form without the cooperation of the conscious mind. I have speculated that this occurs because of an unconscious force that knows exactly what the body needs to release a block, and that yoga postures may have originally sprung from such movements of ancient spiritual masters. It is also possible the genetic, past-life or collective pool of experience is merging from the unconscious at such moments in order to attract attention or gain new awareness for the person so afflicted. It is not usually a painful experience, just puzzling.

In a similar way some people perform hand mudras, symbolic gestures that represent the evolution of the universe and the eventual involution of individual consciousness back to its divine source. These graceful movements are said to center and calm the mind, and to have a significant impact on the energy system. They are part of yogic worship, signs of devotion to the cosmic source. There are many mudras and each has a specific meaning related to the creative process of nature and human life.

Unusual breath sequences also appear unexpectedly during this process. The manipulation of the breath has many purposes in yoga including control of various body organs, movement of prana to the base of the spine to stimulate Kundalini, quieting the mind, heating or cooling the body, healing specific ailments, producing activity and intensity or mental calm and relaxation, developing yogic powers and other tasks. Tibetan yogis may spend days unclothed in sub-zero weather practicing certain breathing practices that produce heat. Such skills constitute a science in the yogic tradition for the breath directs, expands or diminishes prana, the primary energy of the physical system.

People experiencing Kundalini awakening sometimes report breathing in unusual patterns, perhaps very rapidly or very shallowly, or not breathing at all for extended periods. This can be frightening for those who do not understand the usefulness of such patterns, and it is rare for Westerners to have such training. Perhaps these patterns are stimulated by physiological needs, or connections with memories in the collective unconscious, or triggered for specific healing purposes unknown to the conscious mind. They often occur during intense meditation practices.

A relationship with Kundalini is very much a relationship with an "otherness" within oneself that often demonstrates what appears to be intentionality all its own. Those engaged in this process have several choices -- to study yoga and come to understand these events; to accept them without much concern, trusting there is some value in the unconscious impulse, or being willing to play the game if that is all it is; or to resist and become angry about the invasion. In the latter circumstance they are likely to experience the greatest difficulties of Kundalini awakening -- fear, panic, contraction and other disruptive emotions.

Still another mystery of the process is the Sanscrit words or sounds that sometimes emit from the subject who has awakened Kundalini, and the occasional movement of awareness into inner music or sound. It is unnerving to speak when one is not consciously directing it and even more distracting when it is a foreign language that emerges. Since Sanscrit is reportedly the language of the origin of the universe -- the words through which creation was created, (remember "And the Word was God..."?) it must be indeed a deeply embedded primary structure of the collective unconscious. Such sounds may come to open us, to soothe us, to create new forms within us, to reunite us with primary material which lies between us and our origins. By the time someone is experiencing this phenomena he/she may be at very primitive levels of the deep unconscious or very refined levels of the superconscious essence, penetrating genetic or psychic layers in order to let go of the human condition. Perhaps these sounds are the original sources of language.

Yogic and Tantric schools teach the resonance of certain sounds with the awakening of specific chakras, and the sound of Om or Aum as the basic hum of the universe, containing all within it. Aum represents the three states of consciousness -- the waking, the dream-state and the dream-less state. Sanscrit chants and mantras are based on particular tones and forms of sound that are said to have specific results. Certain mantras, usually lengthy and complicated ones, are believed to actually create forms or results in the material world if they are recited the correct number of times (sometimes in the millions) with appropriate devotion and breathing cadences. This is how much of the magic of yogic powers is believed to occur. Like the science of breath, the science of sound and vibration is a major cornerstone of esoteric yoga practices.

Surat Shabd Yoga, as described by Kirpal Singh,[6] specifically teaches how to connect with inner sound or the "radiant sound current". An aspirant is initiated with a specially charged mantra and meditates on it while focusing on the third eye center (the sixth chakra). The idea is that spiritual current descends from above into the third eye and from there spreads throughout the body. Through concentration at this point the yogi connects with this current directly, perceiving transcendent light and sound, and making the practices of yoga which depend on prana and mind unnecessary. When contacting this spiritual energy the sensory currents are automatically drawn upward but the motor currents in the body are left untouched, so that the entry into samadhi and the return from it become more natural and less disruptive to accomplish.

The transcendent sound and light into which the yogi merges are the essence of divine spirit so this is considered to be a more direct method of awakening than those that focus on Kundalini and pranic energies. It bypasses completely the need for the strict physiological practices common to other schools of yoga. If transcendent sound and light is thus the primary essence of divine energy, before it is transmuted into the physiologic and biologic systems, being swept by inner music and sound would be a natural correlate of Kundalini processes as energy penetrates the third eye, and one is moving towards dissolution of identification with the body.

Hazrat Inayat Khan, a great Sufi master, has called the creation the "Music of God". He wrote that all of space is filled with abstract sound, with vibrations too refined to be audible to the human ear or eye. He said:

> This Sound of the Abstract is always going on within, around and about man. Those who are able to hear it and meditate on it are relieved from all worries, anxieties, sorrows, fears and diseases, and the soul is freed from the captivity of the senses and the physical body, and becomes part of the All-pervading Consciousness.
>
> This Sound develops through and into ten different aspects, because of Its manifestation through the different tubes of the body (Nadis), and sounds like thunder, the roaring of the sea, the jingling of bells, the buzzing of bees, the twittering of sparrows, the vina, the flute, the sound of Shankha (conch shell) are

heard, until It finally becomes Hu, the most
sacred of all sounds, be they from man, bird,
beast or thing.[7]

In addition to hearing such sounds, spontaneously repeating
mantras, or making tones that resonate with various chakras, certain
yogic images and symbols may arise during this process. Yogis
have attributed specific lotuses, colors, lights, gods and goddesses,
symbols, and animals to each of the chakras and these images have
been reported by meditators   as well as those engaged in body
therapy, breathwork, trance states, psychedelic drug use and other
altered states of consciousness. I know of no studies to correlate
specific chakra openings with these images in Westerners, but they
are so extensively in agreement in Eastern literature we must suppose
they are seen frequently in spiritual aspirants there. Anandamayi Ma,
who was not formerly trained as a yogi, was said to have produced
spontaneously these images and facts related to all the chakras exactly
as recorded in ancient esoteric texts, even though she had no prior
interest in, nor knowledge of them. Brugh Joy reports much of his
knowledge of chakras coming to him in a similar spontaneous way
long before he knew anything about Eastern philosophy and subtle
body theory. He wrote that he was quite astonished to find a book
one day which outlined what he had been discovering independently.[8]

Not everyone who awakens Kundalini will report these kinds
of yogic experiences, and some will have them and have no idea what
they are, perhaps not even associating them with the process. What
they suggest to me is that the science and wisdom of yoga was not
created from the intellects of the ancient Rishis and teachers, but was
more likely "channeled" through their personal supra-conscious
processes, and that yoga practices therefore are not a product of the
Hindus, but a product of the Kundalini itself, bringing forth a method
for others to use to unravel the egoic structures of the psyche.

Emotional & Psychological
Responses to Kundalini

I saw the world in a new way -- and it was
warped and uncontrollable and I was unable to
be rational. I was manic-depressive, with mood
swings from euphoria to total contraction,
expansion to suicidal, and thinking the energy

> would probably kill me anyhow. . . subject, Rob.

> I started having uncontrollable bouts of weeping all of a sudden. The bout would begin in a state of great pain. I would weep and sob uncontrollably in a most pathetic way. Then I would come to my own automatically. B.S. Goel[9]

> As I walked through New York City, I tried to touch people and bless them. I saw terrible faces in the clouds above the city. When the cab drove to the airport the hood flew up and I freaked out, gave the driver all my money, and walked the rest of the way. At the airport I was intensely confused and collapsed at the ticket counter. . . .subject, Mark.

Some of the more difficult emotional conditions that may accompany a Kundalini awakening have led some clinicians to consider this process a psychosis, a neurological disorder or a manic-depressive illness. Most individuals do not have problems this severe, but do feel beset by unpredictable emotions and anxieties that may bring them into therapy.

Emotional Conditions Most Commonly Reported
>Intense emotional swings
>Depression, anxiety, anger, guilt.
>A belief one is dying.
>Temporary mental confusion and difficulty with work tasks.
>Ritualistic behaviors.
>Inability to sleep.
>Impulsive desires to uproot one's life.
>Intense sexual drives that are uncharacteristic for the client.
>Temporary gender identity issues.
>Belief that people are influencing one's energy field, or subject is influencing others.
>Feeling a connection with entities or guides from other dimensions.
>Psychotic-like symptoms, i.e. seeing visions, or lights or hearing sounds.

Borderline symptoms i.e. scattered thoughts, indecisiveness, boundary issues.
Narcissistic symptoms, especially grandiosity and inflation.
Falling into trance or semi-conscious states of consciousness.

Because of the similarity of some of these symptoms to a psychotic break, and the lack of any other diagnostic category available to therapists to categorize hallucinatory experiences, the relationship of Kundalini to psychosis has been explored by several writers. Gopi Krishna, Lee Sannella, Itzak Bentov, and others suggest that some psychotic breaks are related to this experience having gone awry or having been inappropriately treated. Bentov estimated as many as 25% to 30% of all institutionalized schizophrenics may be victims of this misunderstanding.[10] Psychiatrists John Perry and R. D. Laing have done remarkable work in bringing people with psychotic symptoms through a transformative spiritual healing process, which raises questions and confusions about the relationship of such episodes to Kundalini. An excellent exploration of their perspectives is available in the anthology Spiritual Emergency (Grof and Grof, 1989).

I do not believe that Kundalini causes psychosis, or conversely, that the spiritual components of a psychotic experience are proof that Kundalini has awakened. But it may be possible for the two experiences to occur simultaneously due to weak ego boundaries and the facility in touching non-ordinary states of awareness that is often manifest during a psychotic illness. It is also possible that disturbed and erratic energy fields present in psychosis may activate physiological symptoms similar to those activated by the awakened movement of Kundalini. And I agree with Bentov and others who have observed that Kundalini is frequently misdiagnosed, leading to inappropriate treatment that may increase the potentiality for a psychotic break, or cause a long-term ego fragility that is debilitating for the patient. Lee Sannella, an ophthalmologist and psychiatrist did a pioneering study currently published as The Kundalini Experience (1988) to differentiate between the two experiences.[11]

Frequently people fear they are mentally ill when kriyas and unfamiliar internal sensations manifest, or because they see visions or make strange sounds. If they have no context with which to understand these conditions and if they are misdiagnosed or treated with psychotropic drugs they may develop serious mental problems, identifying themselves as mentally ill and feeling mentally confused because of drug reactions. It is important to understand the powerful psychological impact of spiritual practices and openings, and their potentiality for plunging individuals into the crisis identified by transpersonal therapists as spiritual emergency. The Mother, who worked closely with Aurobindo and headed his organization for many years, wrote of the psychological impact of yoga practices:

> Yoga in its process of purification will lay bare and throw up all hidden impulses and desires in you. And you must learn not to hide things nor leave them aside, you have to face them and conquer them and remould them. The first effect of yoga is to take away the mental control, and the hungers that lie dormant are suddenly set free, they rush up and invade the being. So long as this mental control has not been replaced by divine control there is a period of transition when your sincerity and surrender will be put to the test.[12]

Aurobindo has also written of the psychological effects of the spiritual life.

> In ordinary life people accept the vital movements, anger, desire, greed, sex, etc, as natural, allowable and legitimate things, part of human nature. . . spiritual life demands the mastery of these . . . this is why struggle is felt more -- intense struggle between the spiritual mind and vital movements which rebel and hang onto old ways. . . as for sadhana (spiritual practices) raising up these things, the truth is many things are unconscious because the vital hides them from the mind and gratifies them unconsciously. . .in yoga the secret motive is pulled out, exposed and got rid of. Also some things suppressed in nature may erupt to be expressed in nervous forms or disorders of the mind or vital or body -- psychoanalysis exaggerates this -- in sadhana one must be conscious of these and eliminate them. They

don't need to be acted on, only raised to consciousness.[13]

Aurobindo believed it was not the push toward divine union that led one to madness, but the way people with certain predispositions responded to certain energies. He said that only in three cases had he ever witnessed a case of collapse in yoga. He described the people involved as suffering respectively from sexual aberration, exaggerated ambition and megalomania, and an unbalanced and weak nervous system derived from following unruly impulses without using a strong will to restrain them. He claimed that where emotional problems were present the cause was a predisposition due to heredity, natal or birth circumstances, or insufficient nervous balance. Anxiety or excessive stress in meditation would not bring on nervous problems without these predisposing weaknesses.[14]

Issues related to the prior mental stability of spiritual aspirants are more prevalent in the West than in the East, where proper preparation and mental attitude are considered prerequisites for the practice of yoga. Several western therapists have addressed differences between meditation practitioners in the two cultures. Engler cited a number of studies of western and eastern students of Vipassana meditation that suggest spiritual progress is relatively more slow in Westerners. He attributed this to western students becoming fixated on the psychodynamic level of experience, as well as by an increase in fantasy, daydreaming, reverie, imagery, incessant thinking and emotional lability when practicing meditation. He observed a tendency to become absorbed in the content of awareness rather than simply observing process. In addition he described them as developing more intense transference to teachers, subject to rapid and extreme oscillations between omnipotence and devaluation.

Engler observed that many who become interested in Buddhism and attended meditation retreats had a tendency toward avoidance of essential developmental tasks and to use meditation practice as a short-cut solution for resolving personal problems. "The Buddhist teaching that I neither have nor am an enduring self is often misinterpreted to mean that I do not need to struggle with the tasks of identity formation or with finding out who I am, what my capabilities are, what my needs are, what my responsibilities are, how I am related to other selves, and what I should or could do with my life."[15]

He concluded at their worst these vulnerabilities and disturbances of personal identity are pathological, and that many of these students function at or close to a borderline or narcissistic level of ego organization, in the sense of personality organization and functioning. When this is so, embracing ideals related to egolessness can become a justification for the essential lack of self in the personality, and the person can misconstrue personal emptiness as enlightenment. In addition, one may cathect the ideal of enlightenment as the peak of personal perfection, erasing all mental problems, making one complete and invulnerable. This may reinforce the narcissistic striving for perfection, and the desire to feel oneself superior to everyone else.

When issues such as borderline or narcissistic pathology are brought to the spiritual quest or when Kundalini experiences occur spontaneously in such a person, one may anticipate major difficulties with ego identity and spiritual integration. It is possible that some of the extreme mental fragmentation or apparent psychotic conditions attributed to spiritual awakening may fall into this category. These people are not capable of completing the deeper work of transformation until they have done the preliminary tasks of structuring a personal identity and resolving their personality disorder. A gradual weaning away from the spiritual practices and the projections related to them may need to occur before personal development can happen. But the vast majority of people who are reacting intensely and emotionally to Kundalini do not fall into this category.

Other complications of meditation practices have been noted by clinicians, according to Epstein and Lieff.[16] These include intense depersonalization experiences, sometimes with precipitating anxiety attacks, tension, agitation and restlessness, extreme euphoria, and grandiose fantasies. Walsh and Roche[17] identified psychotic episodes characterized by paranoia, agitation and suicide attempts, brought on in three individuals with a history of schizophrenia following their participation in intensive meditation retreats which included fasting and sleep deprivation. Glueck[18] identified psychotic episodes reported after Transcendental Meditation (TM) training in two young psychiatric patients with previous LSD experiences.

Psychologist David Lukoff has recommended the diagnosis of "mystical experience with psychotic features" for psychiatric patients who demonstrate psychotic conditions with an overlay of mystical experience, urging clinicians to develop alternative strategies to assist them. It appears to him that some people become psychotic in response to awakening experiences associated with spiritual practices, and it may be possible in such cases for the psychosis to become part of a growth process, and a positive outcome to occur if appropriate treatment modalities are used. Lukoff suggests an approach that allows individuals a "wide latitude of freedom for expressing their beliefs, affects, and symbolic imagery" and placing them in a "sanctuary-type environment" such as a private home or non-hospital setting that is part of a religious community, where 24-hour care is provided by friends and relatives.[19]

Erich Neumann has written that "For the ego, the mystical encounter with the non-ego is always a borderline experience, for in it the ego always moves toward something lying outside of consciousness and its rationally communicable world. This area situated outside of consciousness is indeed, from the viewpoint of the total personality which it has transformed, the creative area par excellence, but from the viewpoint of consciousness it is an area of nothingness." [20] This would make the Kundalini process most difficult, if not impossible for people with borderline or psychotic pathology because they would become stuck in the pathology; but it is important to remember that clients may occasionally exhibit borderline or psychotic symptoms when undergoing this encounter with the numinous, even when that is not their ordinary personality style.

Aside from the risk of being labeled mentally ill, people are vulnerable to erratic emotional upheavals, as Aurobindo and The Mother suggested, during the Kundalini process. Some of the more troublesome emotions of this process are fear, doubt, anger, depression, and irrational love projections (falling in love with someone who seems completely inappropriate, or becoming completely enamored with a guru, teacher or therapist).

Not everyone experiences all of these conditions. It is wise to remember the uniqueness of an individual's life and previous inner work, self-discipline, intellect and emotional tendencies and possibly past-lives may all have an influence on the patterns that emerge. It appears to me from the research I have conducted that individuals are likely to experience an intensification of personality issues they have always had at some level, rather than an entire onslaught of new issues.

One of the more common emotional issues is fear of death. Many people have reported extreme attacks of death-anxiety, convinced that some somatic problem is the beginning of the end of their life. Anxiety attacks precipitated by these concerns often occur. The ego is confronting a death-like collapse which most likely accounts for the preoccupation with physical death during this process.

Another commonly reported condition is extreme and unpredictable mood swings, from deep depression to euphoria, sometimes occurring several times a day, at other times lasting for weeks. This is often associated with the bliss and conscious awareness of transcendent realities, followed by the painful awareness that one is little attached to the events and pleasures of ordinary living that were once satisfying. Sometimes the experience is more akin to the classical "dark night of the soul" when contact with the numinous feelings and experiences has vanished, and one no longer knows for certain it was real, or doubts intensely it will ever return. Irina Tweedie was caught in this experience when she wrote in her journal:

> All seems dark and lifeless. There is no purpose anywhere or in anything. No God to pray to. No hope. Nothing at all. A deep-seated rebellion fills the mind. . . only this time it mattered less than usual.[21]

The consequence of such an abandonment by the numinous is enormous emptiness until the task of full awakening has been completed, because chances are the person has changed to the extent that few or no ordinary pleasures hold appeal. Spiritual teachers say this is the time when there is the greatest need to cling to the memory and the vision of the early experiences, and to intensify the spiritual practices, somehow trusting there is a next step to the process. The emotional ups and downs might also be viewed as the swings between ego and Self-consciousness that are inevitable until one has stabilized the energy and the consciousness which is shattering the formerly-known system. Living a life that is resonant with the emerging spiritual consciousness, resolving latent psychological and emotional patterns and issues, and following consistent spiritual practices assist in this stabilizing. Therapeutic measures that address the emotional upheavals of Kundalini will be further expanded in a later chapter of this book.

Visions and Sounds -- Hallucination or Divine Intervention?

> Sometimes I fell into a hypnogogic state, and suddenly entered into a third or fourth dimension, rather like wearing 3-D glasses where dimensionality shifted somewhere such as the Astral Plane. I saw incredibly beautiful nature scenes. . .subject, Margaret.

At times I felt there were monsters walking around, and I heard footsteps. I feel my guide was creating these experiences to desensitize me and help me overcome my fear of being alone and having monsters outside. . . subject, Nan.

Standing in the garden, with an obviously discernible form, made of subtle energy but without any kind of visibility, was the Virgin, Mary, Mother of Christ. . .Da Free John/ Jones[22]

I felt Sai Baba's presence occasionally, and smelled a certain perfume when he was there. . . subject, Jayne

I woke up in a state of ecstasy in the middle of the night and a voice said "this is really Kundalini, we're just taking it very easy on you!". . . subject, Chris

Encountering visions and hearing occasional voices are experiences quite common during the process of Kundalini awakening, along with perceptions of luminosity both in the external and the dream worlds. Such reports are commonly found in all mystical literature and scriptures, including the Bible, and are a significant aspect of shamanic cultures, yet are rarely taken seriously by modern intellectuals. Sometimes they are reported as part of transformative states of consciousness described in psychological literature, and are even encouraged through the vehicles of active imagination, guided imagery, past-life regression, and other altered state processes. Psychedelic drugs produce them. They pop up unexpectedly during meditation, but one is usually advised to allow them to pass, as they are viewed as a temporary and insignificant stage of the process. Since visions and discarnate voices are also common to the psychotic state, the spiritual initiate is vulnerable to misunderstanding and the administration of psychotropic medication when they are reported, so mystics in modern society are well-advised to keep their visions to themselves, unless they can prove there is a good excuse for them -- using a controlled "imagination" process or a drug.

The extensive work that Carl Jung and other analysts have done with dreams and active imagination is pioneering in its' tendency to take seriously the spiritual nature of certain images produced by the unconscious that may lead individuals to wholeness. It is notable that many of the images produced by patients engaged in the individuation process correlate with images produced by those experiencing Kundalini awakening. Images of monsters and disasters, gods and goddesses, great lights, newborn beings, and symbols of crosses, swords, serpents, fire, water, light, a blue pearl, crystals, triangles (sometimes intersected), circles, and spirals are among those often produced in vision, dream and art related to these transformative processes. In addition some people see visions of the inner-workings of their bodies; have visitations by guides, gurus or teachers occurring either visually or through a felt-sense or through hearing; or experience visions or voices bringing precognitive awareness.

Visions are images or scenes that are witnessed as if they were taking place, either externally or internally, but that are clearly out of the context of ordinary reality. They may occur while in waking consciousness, in meditation, or in the state of "tandra", a dream-like yogic state of sleepiness, which is similar to a hypnogogic state. People sometimes awake at night to a vision or voice, but may also experience them spontaneously during waking consciousness. They are reported often in times of stress, or great psychic upheaval, as well as in times of transformation.

Kennett Roshi described a vision as follows:

> It superimposed itself on what was around me. I tried to close my eyes on occasion and I was absolutely forced not to . . . so that I would stay in a context that I knew. I knew that I was in the room and at the same time I was quite genuinely moving and doing things. I was aware of things going on around me, conversed with people, and did not leave my body.[23]

In this case the vision occurred as something outside of herself, while she observed from a conscious state.

Edward Thornton, a Western businessman and mystic, wrote a diary in which he described visions occurring both in meditation and waking states. His first vision appeared while he was in a conscious state, as did several subsequent visions. During an air-raid, having just finished meditation, he gazed into the darkness of a room and saw "a great dark lake surrounded by gloomy mountains. Out of the lake there emerged a naked man. He was fettered from neck, waist and, ankles in chains, and was trying to drag himself out of the water on to the shore. He was dragging himself with, what seemed to me, superhuman strength, and I felt sure that he would reach dry land. The man had obviously been submerged in the water, and was now entering a new element. But the foreboding mountains and the gloom of the dark lake did not give me the impression of a very happy future." [24]

Thornton's visions and dreams progressively carried themes involving symbolic births in elements related to each chakra. Late at night after meditation he had an exterior vision: "It was night, and above me the full moon was shining brightly in a clear sky. Before me was a vast altar on the top of which stood a bowl of fire. The flames were rising upwards to the moon.   All this took place in a wooded glade." [25] Four nights later, he had another exterior vision-- "I saw three gold candlesticks with a gold chalice enveloped in fire above them. This vision had an overwhelming effect on me, and I was held by what I can only describe as holy awe. This does not mean that I was in any way afraid, for the experience was more like that of a rapture." [26]   After this most of his visionary experiences were interior, occurring with his eyes closed, during meditation. In the last meditation vision recorded in his book he "beheld a total eclipse of the sun. From behind the dark image of the moon flames of fire were emerging from the hidden sun." [27]

In daily meditations during the time he experienced visions, he was "aware of a luminous point which seemed to hold my attention. It appeared to come from the very center of my being deep within myself. As time went on this luminous point developed, and I began to see four rays, or tongues of light issuing from it in the four cardinal directions. These interior visions culminated on June 28, 1944 when eight tongues of light emanating from the central luminous point, yet not seeming to touch it, were enclosed in a circle of Chartres blue. The four tongues pointing in the cardinal directions were slightly larger than the other four lying between them." [28]

This image is very similar to one of Kennett Roshi's (1977) who reports "There are five golden columns of light coming out of my body. They move up and are now coming out of the lotus blossom upon my head, arranged towards the back of it." [29] She works over a period of time with movement in and out of these columns, following the advice of the inner Self. Later they came from the Buddha mark on her forehead or from the five points of the lotus, or they formed the column at the base of the spine. She is told the meaning of all five.

> They truly are the aspects of the monk; the first is earth penetrating heaven; the second, the knot of eternity; the third, heaven penetrating earth; the fourth, the putting on of the golden robe which is within the fountain of the Buddha's Wisdom, the bathing within its radiance; the fifth, the ability to die whilst sitting and standing which transcends both peasant and sage' -- the right to go to heaven or hell if the intention is right -- to help all living things.[30]

Yogic literature attempts to define reasons for visionary states of consciousness. Gopi Krishna believed "in the heightened state of consciousness engendered by the awakened Kundalini, visionary experiences become more pronounced. The whole icongraphic system of Hatha Yoga is based on this possibility." [31] He points out that yogis learn to visualize the upgoing current, chakras, the lotuses and letters of the alphabet which accompany each chakra, along with their respective deities, mantra sounds, hues and colors. One can expect proneness to visionary states in one with an awakened Kundalini, because it makes figments of the imagination more vivid. He believes visions and hallucination occur in the intermediate stage of the Kundalini process before the brain is completely attuned to the higher functions, and that higher stages of consciousness are devoid of visions. He says the average adult suddenly experiencing happiness, awe and wonder needs a formative vision conforming to his preexisting ideas and concepts or he might be completely lost, bewildered and confused.

Krishna's views contrast with the reports of many mystics, noted for their visionary ecstasies. Many of these are known to us from history, including St. Paul and Joan of Arc. Carl Jung has reported visions, and Emanual Swedenborg writes about them. Almost all the yogis in the biographical literature reviewed for this book reported some kinds of visions. It is an act of courage to write of such experiences, in a society that might invalidate one's work because of them.

Many yogis claim a certain reality for some visual experiences. These images are no more maya (delusion) than is

ordinary reality, both being reflections of the mind. Swami
Sivananda states:

> The beings and objects with whom you are in
> touch in meditation belong to the astral
> world.They are similar to human beings minus
> a physical overcoat. . . they have desires,
> cravings, love, hatred just as human beings
> have. . . they have powers. . . if lustrous they
> are Devatas (Gods) of mental or higher planes
> who come to give you Darshan and encourage
> you. [32]

One may feel pushed from the physical body into the new
plane and need help in separating from the body and going above
body-consciousness, according to Sivananda. One may see the sky or
physical forms of people. These visions are either one's own mental
reactions or are realities of finer planes of matter. He advises using
discrimination and common sense in responding to them. The case
histories I have studied reveal that many people who experience
Kundalini do seem to be assisted by spiritual guides and teachers from
another dimension.

Aurobindo believed one should never interfere with images
which rise from within because their occurrence is a sign that inner
planes of consciousness are opening and to inhibit them would mean
to inhibit the expansion of consciousness and experience. He said:

> Inner vision is vivid like actual sight, always
> precise and contains a truth in it. The inner
> vision can see objects, but it can see instead the
> vibration of the forces which act through the
> object. The mental visions are meant to bring
> in the mind the influence of the things they
> represent. The cosmic vision is the seeing of
> the universal movements -- it has nothing to do
> with the psychic necessarily.[33]

Aurobindo also said visions are valued by people because
they are a contact with other worlds or inner worlds and all that is
there.

> . . . these are regions of immense riches which
> far surpass the physical plane as it is at present.
> One enters into a larger freer self and a larger
> more plastic world. . . . These things have not
> the effect of a mere imagination. . . but if fully
> followed out bring a constant growth of the
> being and the consciousness and its richness of
> experience and its scope. [34]

He said visions "can give a first contact with the Divine in
his forms and powers; it can be the opening of a communion with
the Divine, of the hearing of the Voice that guides, of the Presence as
well as the Image in the heart, of many other things that bring what
man seeks through religion or yoga."[35]

Yogis often refer to visions when describing meditative
experiences. Vivekananda writes that "Haloes are symbols of inner
light and can be seen by the Yogi. Sometimes we may see a face as
if surrounded by flames and in them read the character and judge
without erring. We may have our Ishta come to us as a vision, and
this symbol will be the one upon which we can rest steadily and fully
concentrate our mind."[36]

Kennett Roshi, the Abbess of a Zen monastery at Mt.
Shasta, in California, in a radical departure from Buddhist tradition,
reported a major series of visions occurring during her third kensho
experience, which took place over several months, and forced her to
look at many opposites slowly and deliberately. Among the images
in her visions were mountains, lotuses, pillars, fountains, darkness
and light. She saw and resolved strands of karma from past lives, and
went through a series of mystical visions and initiation experiences
with other monks and Buddhist saints. She believes this type of
kensho needs much explanation and documentation because almost
nothing is written of it, and that it is in no way exclusive to her.
Almost anyone who trains seriously, and who not only tries to live
by Buddhist precepts but cleans up the negative patterns of both
present and past lives can experience this kensho. Regarding the
relationship of the phenomena that arise in meditation to
kensho she wrote:

> It has been taught in the West that all
> experiences, visual or otherwise, during
> meditation should be regarded as makyo and
> taken no notice of whatsoever. Whether this is

true for all who have not had a first kensho, it
is not necessarily true for those who have the
little flashes of what I here call the On-Going
Fugen kensho and not true at all for those
having the third kensho. The Zen masters of
old did not talk about the valid experiences,
however, for fear that new trainees would mistake makyo for the real thing.[37]

The important thing is to observe, and learn from the visual
experience and avoid attachment either to having an experience or not
having it. Enlightenment, which she defines as an ongoing process,
brings numerous kensho experiences, which may or may not include
visions. Visions make no difference to the depth of the enlightenment experience. She suspects most people who have led
spiritually focused lives will go through the type of visual experience
she describes in her book during their final illness and shortly before
their death. But the Zen master has learned to meditate properly and
overcome fear of death so is able to go intensely into training and
meditation to achieve this experience without having to die.[38]

Indian Guru Swami Muktananda has described both fearful
and blissful visions in his autobiography.

While meditating in the state of tandra (a
conscious but dream-like state), I visited many
different inner worlds. In meditation I traveled
to the world of the moon, the world of departed
spiritism, to heaven and hell, and to the world
of the Siddhas (the yoga masters), which is
inhabited by great saints and sages of all
traditions. After seeing these worlds, I came to
realize that the descriptions of the different
planes of existence which one reads in the
scriptures and in the writings of the ancient
sages and yogis are absolutely true, all these
worlds are extremely subtle; they cannot be
seen with the physical eyes.[39]

The vision of the blue pearl is the most significant vision a
yogi can attain, according to Muktananda. It is the divine light of
consciousness which swells within everyone, or the actual form of

the Self, the form of God which lives within us. He said this vision puts an end to bondage, and makes the yogi realize perfection.

Visions may also occur unexpectedly, and their presence seem out of context to the avowed spiritual beliefs of the recipient. Da Free John describes this event in the garden of Muktananda's ashram in India:

> I had been pulling weeds for perhaps half an hour when, suddenly I felt a familiar Presence, as if a friend was standing behind me I stood up and looked behind my shoulder. Standing in the garden, with an obviously discernible form, made of subtle energy but without any kind of visibility, was the Virgin, Mary, Mother of Christ.[40]

His first impulse was laughter, as he had spent years of total non-sympathy for Christianity, and had no attraction toward Catholic symbols. He had thought "the Virgin" was only a religious symbol, a secondary creation of the church. Yet he felt compelled to honor her presence, and he found himself growing in love and devotion as she continued to meet with him. "Just as her presence was not physical, but subtle, her communication to me was internal, as I had earlier known it with Baba." [41]

Free John spent several days chanting the "Hail Mary" as a mantra and then she appeared and showed him the image of Christ's face. "It appeared visibly in my heart, and she seemed only to uncover it. That image and the feelings it awakened in me seemed to me to have been hidden and suppressed there since my childhood. I was in love with Christ!" [42]

"As these experiences increased I began to resist them mightily. I thought I must be deluded, I tried to meditate in the usual way, but always Mary and Christ would appear to guide and instruct me." [43]

Ultimately he was told to leave the ashram and go on a pilgrimage to the Christian holy places, which he did. He came to feel that this experience was a manifestation of the Kundalini shakti working independently in him, and that this indicated he was no longer dependent on the presence of his teacher, Muktananda, or the ashram in order to have experiences with the shakti.

In addition to images of deities and guides, dreams and visions of destruction are quite common during times of psychic upheaval and change. These may follow themes of personal destruction, such as dismemberment, torture or death; or of world destruction in the form of earthquakes, nuclear war, and other cataclysmic events. Jungian psychiatrist John Weir Perry wrote that "when a transformation of one's inner culture is under way, dissolution of the world image is the harbinger of change."

> The energy that had been bound up in the structures of the old self-image and world image, in the issues of who one is and what sort of world one lives in, is immense. In dreams or visions, nuclear explosion is a frequent expression of this enormous charge of psychic energy that is loose during a renewal process and raises havoc for a period of time, though one's own nature is struggling to break through one may feel that who one is and what one values is up for grabs.[44]

Perry, who is a pioneer in using innovative approaches to psychotic processes, believes these images indicate a crisis which is apt to keep one in a state of fear until resolved. People in this kind of crisis may feel isolated because communication about these experiences is often misunderstood by professionals, who want to suppress the process and make one conform to the ways of the former self and the world. He sees this fear and an accompanying rage as producing the biochemical effects to the brain that many doctors "prefer to see as the primary cause of psychological disorder". He also states:

> This biased and mechanistic diagnosis does not hold up, however, since it is now well known that if a person undergoing this turmoil is given love,understanding,and encouragement, the spiritual crisis soon resolves itself without the need for interruption by suppressive medication. The most fragmented 'thought disorder' can become quite coherent and orderly within a short time if someone is present to respond to it with compassion. Such a relationship is far better than a tranquilizer in most instances. A haven where there is attentiveness to inner experiences and where, removed from the context of daily life, one can

examine one's whole existence, is also advantageous.[45]

Following the production of fragmentation and anxiety-producing destructive images, the psychic energy may reincarnate into fresh new forms, and visions of birth and new worlds, or memories of early childhood experiences may emerge, according to Perry.

Experiences of Light

One night I felt the energy rise to my neck, closed my eyes and looked inward, and I saw golden energy swirling incessantly around my organs. It seemed to move with determination and intelligence around each organ, as if familiar with my anatomy, bathing me in a glistening sheen . . . subject, Beth.

Sometimes I wake up at night with little flashing bolts of lights in my head, which feel expanded beyond my skull. . . or there is a glow slightly beginning above me which penetrates into my head that is a subtle white or slightly goldish color. . . subject, Jay.

I see different colored lights when meditating. When my state of being shifts I may see flashes of color, as if there is a dark sky with pinholes through which luminescent blue and purple come through and grow a bit. At times the world looks luminous. . . subject, Rob.

Experiences of light are commonly reported by meditators, mystics and many other people during altered states of consciousness. A variety of light phenomena are associated with various stages of meditation in yoga, but meditators are usually advised by teachers to pay little attention to them. They are not indicative of "enlightenment" despite the fact they seem to many people to be major experiences, often convincing them for the first time of another level of awareness beyond the customary parameters of their minds.

Red, white, blue, green, or a mixture of colors may appear; these colors are called "tanmatric" lights by the yogis. The tanmatras are subtle elements or energies from which derive the senses (sound, touch, sight, taste, smell) and the five elements (ether, air, fire, water, earth). They are associated with the spectrum of colors perceived at certain depths of awareness, and yogis are advised not to become distracted by them if they wish to move on to deeper spiritual experiences.

Four specific colored lights of red, white, black and blue have been identified by Swami Muktananda, who said that Vedanta scriptures described them as having specific sizes (physical body, thumb, finger-tip and lentil-size respectively) and identified them as representations of four bodies (the gross, subtle, causal and supracausal, further outlined in chapter three) and the four states of consciousness (waking, dream, deep sleep and transcendent). He said that the sequence of visions of these lights indicates different stages of the spiritual journey.[46]

Aurobindo has stated that the appearance of fire, lights (either in masses or in symbolic forms), flowers, sun and moon symbols are commonly seen by most people who follow spiritual practices, and he believed they indicated the movement or action of inner forces. He said that sparks or movements of light indicated the play of forces in or around consciousness, and fire indicated a dynamic action. He said the mind did not necessarily have to be quiet or concentrated in order to see lights, as it depended only on the opening of the subtle vision of the sixth chakra. This is an opening often quickly accessed by meditators or easily developed in others who may have an inborn facility for psychic experience. He associated various colors with a variety of forces, saying that when the light appeared outside of the person it indicated the touch or influence of an external force, and when it occurred internally it meant that power had penetrated, and was frequently active in the individual's nature.

Although he stated it was not always easy to define exactly the symbolism of colors because of the complexity and variability of shades and combinations of colors, he did identify some colors with specific forces. He described golden light as always representing divine truth, and a certain shade of blue as indicating spiritual force. Yellow indicates the mind is growing brighter, reaching toward the golden light of truth. Orange or red-gold is generally the light of the higher forces as they are present in the physical being, but orange is also the color of occult knowledge, and crimson indicates the light of love in the physical body. (Paradoxically, orange-red is also commonly associated with muladhara, the base chakra). Some greens are associated with life and a strong action of the life-force, as well as the emotional life. Green may be connected with work and action, and can also indicate emotional generosity, activity with abundant vital energy behind it, or the force of health. Violet light represents divine compassion, and can also suggest the inflowing of divine grace, while purple is the color of vital powers, and lavender-blue may represent the intuitive mind. White light indicates the divine consciousness in which all others are contained and manifested, and may also indicate a force of purity.[47]

Aurobindo also described images of the sun as symbolic of the concentrated light of truth, perceived directly. A red sun indicates that "true, illumined physical consciousness will replace the obscure and ignorant physical consciousness in which people ordinarily live". The moon indicates spiritual consciousness, or may suggest the flow of bliss. Visions of stars represent the promise of a light or creation in consciousness which is yet to come. Waves of colors represent a dynamic rush of forces into awareness. Visions of the dawn always mean an opening of some kind -- something not yet fully present to consciousness, and the night symbolizes ignorance.[48]

Aurobindo also wrote in The Life Divine more specifically of light as a transformative element of consciousness, indicating that one who has quieted the mind and heart, life and body, can become open to a powerful downward flow of light that stimulates the luminous inner force of transformation. He called this force the illumined Mind, where the clarity of spiritual intelligence is superceded by an intense splendor and illumination of the spirit that brings with it a "fiery ardor of realization and a rapturous ecstasy of knowledge." He said that this experience is usually accompanied by a downpour of inwardly visible light.[49]

There are few expositions in yogic literature on color and symbol as specific and detailed as those of Aurobindo's, although classical yogic and Christian scriptures are ripe with the abundance of light symbols and images when describing ecstatic experiences. Ralph Metzner, writing in Opening to Inner Light (1966), found these descriptions so profuse in the literature that he stated:

> The basic feature of the experience of enlightenment appears to be a sensing, feeling and knowing that one's body, heart and mind are being infused, usually from "above" with inner light of a spiritual nature. Light coming in from above is a literal, direct perception in

many instances of body enlightenment, and in some light-yoga practices, as noted, the light-energy is channeled into the body from above.[50]

Thus it seems that a wide range of light phenomena occur through every stage of spiritual practice, and these can be significant indicators of both inner movement and contact with external sources that encourage and abet the psychic elements of change. It is so easy, however, for the mind to delude itself at each step of spiritual process, bringing with it inflation, and creating excuses to evade the genuinely difficult challenges of spiritual evolution. Therefore the wisest course is to accept the experiences of light without attachment, continue one's spiritual practices without expectations of repeating such experiences, and refuse to settle for light (and the bliss which often accompanies it) as the completion of the journey. Understanding that constitutes a profound inner knowing (as opposed to an idea or thought), and a genuine shift of consciousness, along with a stabilized inner peace, are more propitious indicators of what the ancients called "enlightenment". Illumination, in the final analysis, is that of the entire mind and being. It may be revealed in a body that emits light, be accompanied in some steps by the words of perceived beings of light, or occur along with a profuse merging into light, but the experience of light in itself is not "it" just as the experience of sexual union is not complete knowledge of the truth of every facet of the beloved.

Psychic Phenomena & Yogic Powers

Walking on the beach at night I saw a crow pass over the moon, flying rapidly, about 60 miles per hour. I wanted a photo of it and focused my mental energy on communicating with it. It came back and hovered with wings outstretched before the moon, leaving immediately after the picture was shot . . . subject, Rob.

I see and hear entities when working with clients, and they give me advice about healing them. Once I smelled a Havana cigar while meditating, and looked up to see a big,

> craggy Englishman. He dictated some information for his wife, who was a friend of a houseguest of mine, although I did know at the time she was a widow. It made no sense to me, but she knew exactly what I was talking about .. subject, Sarah.

A final category of information often related to Kundalini is the powers associated with it such as psychic ability, expanded creativity, heightened intelligence, healing, abilities to read and influence the minds of others, the ability of consciousness to leave the body and similar paranormal experiences. Some yogis have been observed to walk on nails, water or fire, or live underground with no air or food for extended periods of time. (This does not indicate spiritual advancement, only mastery of concentration and certain senses; many Westerners have mastered fire-walking in recent years.) Sai Baba, a modern Indian guru, is said by many to have the power to materialize objects. There is evidence that several masters could transfer their bodies from one place to another, or be seen in two distant places simultaneously. (This indicates mastery of subtle body energies.) Although there are tantric yoga sects that emphasize the development of powers in the yogic tradition, most of the literature does not emphasize it, and often one is warned that the desire for power or preoccupation with it divert one from the true purpose of the spiritual path, union with God. Anandamurti wrote:

> When an aspirant wants occult powers he may or may not get occult powers, but it is sure that he will not get (cosmic consciousness and bliss) . . . if you want to get occult powers, go outer and outer: if you want Paramapurusa, go inner and inner and inner and inner.
>
> Occult powers, like all other powers, are transitory, temporary in nature . . . as soon as you die, the occult power will be taken away from you. But Paramapurusa will remain with you even at that time, as that property is of a permanent nature.
>
> Occult power is also an ordinary power. The general public does not possess that ordinary power, that's why they think it is a super-natural power. Gold is also an ordinary metal, but because it is a bit rare, that's why it

is costly. . . It's just like that. . . There is
nothing supernatural in this world -- everything is natural.[51]

**Commonly reported paranormal experiences related to
Kundalini awakening:**
Psychic awareness.
Precognitive visions or a felt-sense knowledge about events
    or people.
Seeing or feeling auras.
Synchronistic events in which one feels something is a
    perfect coincidence, divinely initiated, or providing
    a timely affirmation or warning.
The ability to do some degree of hands-on healing.
The ability to use one's energy to balance disturbed energy
    fields in others (such as someone who is having a
    negative reaction to drugs).
Spontaneous remembrance of past lives.
Increased comprehension of spiritual scriptures.
Feeling the ability to influence someone else's mind.
Channeling poetry, art, books and other information (a pro-
    cess which seems to bring in information indepen-
    dently of the intellect, as if from an outside entity).
Instinctive intuitive awareness of what one needs to do.
Feeling aware of the presence of a light being or teacher
    from another dimension.
Psychokinetic experiences (disturbing electrical or battery-
    operated appliances, or having objects move, crack
    or break near them while in intense inward states of
    consciousness).
Out-of-body experiences.
An expanded vision of reality.

In addition to these unconventional activities many people
report awakened creativity, and begin to write or produce art, at least
as a temporary stage of the process. This seems to serve a healing and
integrative function in their lives. Aurobindo has correlated a great
outburst of creative expression with the "luminous consciousness"
which emerges in spiritual awakening. He said:

        I have seen both in myself and others a sudden
        flowering of capacities in every kind of activity
        come by the opening of consciousness, -- so

> that one who laboured long without the least
> success to express himself in rhythm becomes
> a master of poetic language and cadences in a
> day. It is a question of the right silence of the
> mind and the right openness to the Word that is
> trying to express itself -- for the Word is there
> ready formed in those inner planes where all
> artistic forms take birth, but it is the trans-
> mitting mind that must change and become a
> perfect channel and not an obstacle.[52]

He cites Shakespeare as as an example of one who
abundantly illustrates this principle, and also cites the art of Rem-
brandt, the musical composition of Cesar Franck, and the work of
Wordsworth as representative of the quality of the illumined mind,
which brings in a vibration which goes "straight to the heart".[53]

Some people have occult powers without other indicators of
enlightenment, or spiritual awareness, perhaps as natural gifts
brought in at birth, or developed by teachers who had mastered a
particular speciality, such as healing, or engaging in out-of-body
experiences. These probably indicate particular chakras which are
more highly charged than in people with more ordinary capacities,
generally the sixth chakra. It is also possible some people with such
abilities have more awareness of pranic energy and can control or
direct it more readily than others. Many who develop some of these
conditions or abilities during the course of their spiritual process feel
they are gifts that should be used to create health or well-being for
others.

Most likely the dangers are not so much in using the occult,
as in becoming fascinated by it or attached to it, and particularly in
using it to accomplish egoic goals, which can distract one from
further advancement and awareness. There are numerous stories in
India of persons with occult powers using them for manipulation,
revenge, personal power and other preoccupations of the lower-chakra
energies, which indicates such powers can be developed prematurely
and used to the detriment of one on the spiritual path, creating
lifetimes of negative karma to be resolved. The challenge of the
occult for one who wishes to become enlightened is to keep it in a
perspective similar to that of other innate abilities or talents we
possess as humans: that is, using it without attachment, for purposes
which are not self-serving, and being willing to surrender it along
with other egoic positions in order to attain greater depths of spiritual
awareness.

The Samadhi Experience

> All I wanted was to merge and have no separate
> identity -- having a separate identity was
> painful. I had a desperate feeling for unity
> which wouldn't end... subject Nan.

> During samadhi her face lost all freshness of
> life; the body appeared to be very frail and weak
> and in her general appearance there was no ex-
> pression whatever of either joy or pain. . . . she
> said "It is a state beyond all conscious and
> supra-conscious planes--a state of complete
> immobilization of all thoughts, emotions and
> activities, both physical and mental -- a state
> that transcends all the phases of life here be-
> low" Sri Anandamayi Ma. (Bhaiji)[54]

In the classical yogic literature Kundalini is primarily
correlated with samadhi or enlightenment experiences. The yogi
Keshavadas wrote "Samadhi is the aim of all yogas. This is a
superconscious state where the soul is united with God. By attaining
that universal consciousness, all doubts are dispelled, karma extin-
guished, and bliss and eternal peace are experienced". [55]

This spiritual awakening has also been described as the
perception of the Self. According to the ancient Svetasvataropanisad
(translated by Tyagisananda):

> As oil in sesame seeds, as butter in curds, as
> water in underground springs, as fire in wood,
> even so this Self is perceived in the self. He
> who, by means of truthfulness, self-control and
> concentration, looks again and again for the
> Self, which is all-pervading like butter
> contained in milk, which is rooted in self-
> knowledge and meditation, he becomes that
> Supreme Brahman, the destroyer of
> ignorance.[56]

Another swami, Madhusudandasji , wrote:

> When the Kundalini is aroused (one) progresses
> very rapidly on the path of spiritual evolution.
> He realizes the full potential of body and mind,
> attains inner peace, harmony and integration,
> and ultimately experiences the sublime truth of
> unity in diversity -- the fact that all life is one
> seamless fabric.[57]

There are various levels of the samadhi experience, and there are variations in the scriptures and the writings of yogis regarding the numbers of them and their names. According to the Yoga Sutras, while in the first level, called collectively stages of Sabija Samadhi one investigates and masters knowledge about ordinary objects, sense perceptions, reasoning and awareness regarding gross and subtle bodies. Under this category are four stages of Samprajnata Samadhi, successive levels of realization, that must be practiced before it is possible to experience the two kinds of Nirbija Samadhi, the more advanced levels. Concentrative and meditative practices lead to their experience.

In (1) Savitarka and (2) Nirvitarka Samadhis, one recognizes the true nature of a gross object, directly perceiving the five elements that comprise it, and releases attraction to it. Savitarka is the recognition with deliberation, Nirvitarka, without, (one is merged with the object, and has cast away all knowledge of it). Certain meditation practices that emphasize focusing on an object until one is merged with it support the development of this level of samadhi experience. People experiencing these states may report feeling merged with a candle, tree, or rock, with another person, or with a wide expanse of nature. As these kinds of experiences occur people lose attachment to the thoughts that bind them to body-consciousness and become more able to perceive they are not their physical or gross bodies. These are impressions commonly reported during Kundalini processes, and are believed by some yogis to correspond to the movement of Kundalini from the base to the throat chakra. It is also probable that many people who have these experiences as a result of intense concentration have not yet awakened Kundalini.

In (3) Savichara and (4) Nirvichara Samadhis the mind penetrates deeper as one maintains an unbroken samadhi state and one recognizes the nature of subtle objects. This is a leap in consciousness, and one now perceives a reality beyond ordinary reality, whether with reflection, or without (again, while merging), respectively. These may include experiences of one's own subtle body, or visions of the subtle body or energy fields of other people or objects. They are states we would expect to see occur in one who has awakened Kundalini, particularly as it moves through the sixth and seventh chakras. In this stage one may experience oneself as the subtle body, have access to subtle body memories of other lives, have extra-sensory awareness, and feel various kinds of bliss associated with the dissolution of identification with what yogis call the tanmatras, or subtle elements that control the senses. The nature of space and time is revealed, and life is seen as a play of forces. At the level of Nirvichara all conditions become undifferentiated, attractions to pleasure and pain fall away, and the illusions of life are pierced.

The ability to experience additional stages of (5)Sananda and (6)Sasmita Samadhis follow. The distinguishing characteristics of these samadhis are the experiences of various intensities of bliss. Egoic and intellectual awareness dissolve as one merges into these states. Some yogis say it is the dissolution of those energies which create egoic consciousness that causes the intense blissful stages, and it is easy to become stuck in this stage of Samadhi because it is so intensely pleasurable, and gives an illusion of completion. All existence is experienced as ecstatic bliss. The workings of intellect and its role in creating the material world are perceived in the stage of Sananda. In Samsita, the ego is cast away and one realizes "I am that I am", awareness beyond the ego. The "I" who is receiving the bliss (and all of manifestation) is realized as an illusion, as not-real in and of itself, but as a reflection of the impulses of cosmic reality. Some scriptures indicate that those who try to stay in this state will eventually lose it, unless they move on to more expanded stages of knowledge.

Complete union with God, universal consciousness, and freedom from all karma are associated with the deepest levels, which are called Nirbija states and are experiences beyond the Kundalini experience, usually associated with levels of consciousness beyond the sahasrara, or crown chakra. According to the scriptures of Samkya Yoga the levels of Samadhi at these states are (7) Asamprajnata. a samadhi of superconsciousness without conscious awareness; (8) Dharma Megha described by Taimini in The Science of Yoga as "the final Samadhi in which the yogi shakes himself free from the world of dharmas (properties, characteristics or functions) which obscure reality like a cloud", and the stage in which the cycle of one's individuality is finished, karma is finished, and complete and irreversible Self-realization occurs; and finally, (9) Kaivalya, or perfect liberation, (also known as Sahaj Samadhi or Nirvikalpa Samadhi), a stage of supreme experience and infinite knowledge even the Sutras do not attempt to describe. This is a transcendental state beyond awareness of gross or subtle bodies, beyond duality, time, space or causality, in which all desire for the material world ceases.

Taimini says "It is impossible to imagine this state in which the light of consciousness illuminates itself instead of illuminating other objects outside itself but the student, at least, should not make the mistake of imagining it as a state in which the yogi finds himself immersed in a sea of nebulous bliss and knowledge. Each successive stage of unfoldment of consciousness increases tremendously its vividness and clarity and brings about an added influx of knowledge and power. It is absurd to suppose therefore that in the last stage which marks the climax of this unfoldment, consciousness lapses suddenly into a vague and nebulous state."[58]

Some spiritual teachers, however, do not describe this stage as the complete and final goal of the journey, but only a stage itself of the ever-expanding potential of consciousness. In some traditions the capacity to move spiritual energy from other dimensions into the human plane, and to experience the Divine in every aspect of the human condition are later stages which follow liberation.

The ending of karma is an appealing concept to many who believe in reincarnation, implying complete freedom of choice regarding incarnation thereafter. Karma represents the entanglement of the ego and the personality on the wheel of causality, the patterns of cause and effect, and the personality tendencies and attachments (sanskaras) that govern one's life. The karmic patterns brought into consciousness at birth are believed in some traditions to be specifically predetermined from experiences and choices in past lives, and by other traditions to be obtained from what might be thought of as a collective karmic pool through which the soul either chooses or is burdened with certain traits and tasks on its way into life. Either way all beings are called upon to experience this karma and create positive karma through their thoughts and actions during their lifetimes. How can samadhi free one from this process?

It is not a magical experience, like redemption or a blessing that comes unearned. It is instead the reasonable consequence of seeing clearly who one is, of reuniting with the primary unitive consciousness of the universe and releasing all attachment to the body-mind identity, even forgetting it, and existing completely in the moment. It is not an idea, nor an understanding of who one is, and has nothing to do with the intellect. It must be a direct experience, a complete letting go. Even so, having this experience momentarily, in snatches of blissful contemplation, does not automatically free one from karma. One must live it and die in this state of non-attachment. There must be no trace of identity or desire to hook one's consciousness during the dying process. This is the only way the soul can become free from the cycle of karma. This is what The Tibetan Book of the Dead attempts to lead one through, and the reason Tibetan and Hindu yogic traditions encourage practicing for death. Of course, as Ken Wilber has pointed out in The Atman Project (1980) all major psychic and spiritual evolutions require a similar kind of dying to one's previous attachments and identity, so as we progressively develop spiritually we practice and become more capable of dying in a state of liberation.[59]

In the yogic tradition, Kundalini is the Self which is aware of its divinity, of its primary relationship and union with the creation in its state of formlessness. This state is composed of *sat-chit-ananda* -- being, consciousness and bliss. Kundalini awakening is essential if one is to know higher levels of samadhi. But preliminary experiences, often identified as samadhi or satori (in the Zen tradition) give hints of this later condition, motivate one on the path toward the final goal, and prepare the mind for what is to come. These begin with experiences of loss of self-awareness, absorption with objects, experiences of unity, merging into light or energy phenomena, connections with the archetypal energies through voices or visions that seem to translate messages from other planes of existence into human consciousness, and other altered states. These experiences are stepping-stones toward an ultimate awakening or surrender. They are flashes of Self-experiences, widening consciousness, enabling one to integrate a piece at a time the concept of letting go of personal identity, tempting one to reunite with a primary state of beingness, consciousness and bliss.

The more one has of these "smaller" samadhis, the greater one's sense of acceptance of life and death as they are, and the smaller the attachment to ego goals. It is these flashes of insight into the nature of ego-death and the vastness of universal consciousness that trigger personality changes (and anxiety) in many who have meditated or used drugs. One cannot stay so attached to ego-goals after grasping even small aspects of this truth. The psyche begins to rearrange itself! But in order to complete the spiritual journey it is essential to resist identifying these experiences as attainment or enlightenment, and to surrender each experience for the next, neither clinging to it nor attaching oneself at any step of the journey.

People who have awakened Kundalini universally have this awareness and report occasional glimpses of this perspective of consciousness. Many find themselves drawn more and more toward a desire to know unitive consciousness. It may not feel at all like an intellectual choice or decision. It is as if some part of them compulsively pulls them into meditation, or into processes aimed at releasing egoic identifications and merging into awareness of the Self. It is possible, but not common, to have awakened Kundalini and only experience samadhi; and it is possible to have some kinds of samadhi experiences, such as feeling merged with an object of contemplation, or feeling a powerful surge of union in looking at a beautiful sunset, without having awakened Kundalini. But people who have intensive and repeated high-level samadhi experiences through disciplined spiritual practices have undoubtedly awakened this energy, even if they do not show any of the other physical or emotional conditions reported in the Kundalini experience.

Vedantic and yogic scriptures indicate that in ancient times deeper level samadhi experiences were the more common path to spiritual consciousness, and it was not until the Kali Yuga (the age of Iron or materialism) that physical methods of awakening and experiencing this energy (such as Hatha Yoga, tantric practices, and pranayama) had to be employed. They were developed to help more sensually-oriented races of people awaken their bodies in preparation for spiritual awareness. It is more challenging in this age for individuals to release physical, emotional and intellectual attachments and identifications.

People who are experiencing Kundalini awakening can integrate and focus their process by understanding and seeking samadhi experiences, and opening to Kundalini as a spiritual guide, giving it attention and respect. Without this, they will probably not feel the inherent bliss and ecstasy that the process potentially holds. If they can identify themselves as spiritual seekers, value the energy as the awakening of the Self, and follow spiritual practices consistently it seems inevitable that the process will become more smooth and more integrated over a period of time.Krishnamurti wrote in the later years of his life of an ecstasy that never left him. "I am full of something tremendous. I can't tell you in words what is like a bubbling joy, a living silence, an intense awareness like a living flame." [60] This is an outcome of samadhi.

Commentary on the "Symptoms"

There are clearly a wide range of "symptoms" and experiences related to Kundalini awakening, and fortunately no one seems to have the necessity of experiencing every one of them. But it is sometimes difficult to diagnose Kundalini, because many of these "symptoms" are not exclusive to the Kundalini process. Many people have demonstrated psychic, intellectual or creative abilities without spiritual awakening, and many more have exhibited any or all of the physical and mental symptoms, such as heat flashes, shaking, eating irregularities and seeing lights or visual phenomena. These happenings may occur in anyone because of stress, mental or physical illness, in response to meditation, or due to other circumstances of ordinary life, a fact making it difficult to correlate them specifically with Kundalini awakening.

However, when many of these conditions occur together in someone with no previous indicators of serious mental illness or physical disability, when the conditions were precipitated by a dramatic movement of energy such as described in yogic definitions of Kundalini awakening, and when the experiences fall in several of the categories identified, they indicate a high probability of Kundalini awakening, particularly if there is evidence of samadhi or increased spiritual awareness. Since this energy cannot yet be mechanically measured, and is generally unfamiliar to Western science, it cannot be scientifically defined and determined. But until more studies of probable Kundalini subjects are available there will not be an adequate data base for understanding this phenomenon in the West.

In the meantime, there are more and more published accounts available by spiritual teachers, mystics, and others in the East and West which tell of the depth and power of their personal encounters with Kundalini. By reviewing many of these one can sense both the similarities and the uniqueness of each individual experience. Like refracted rays of light, each story is a reflection from a single source, yet has its own characteristic dimensions and qualities. Because Western theologians and scientists have so dogmatically separated religious experience from scientific inquiry both schools have failed to grasp the implications of discovering correlates between heightened physical energies and human potentialities for spiritual emergence and creative transformation.

The following two chapters contain metaphysical and biological perspectives that may explain some of the symptoms of the Kundalini process, and present frameworks for speculation and research. Chapter five offers a collection of excerpts from stories told by Eastern and Western mystics and teachers about their experiences. Chapter six is comprised of ten case histories that indicate the impact of this radical experience on people who live ordinary lives in the West. Through these stories you will see the similarities of emotional, physical and spiritual processes as Kundalini is awakened, expressing Herself within the framework of unique historical, cultural and personality variables.

References: Chapter 2

1   Singh, J. (1979) _Siva sutras: the yoga of supreme identity_ . Delhi: Motilal Barsidass, p. xxii.

2   Hari Dass, B. Personal communication Mt. Madonna Center, Watsonville, CA., 9/18/87.

3   Mahusudandasji, D. (1979) Shakti: Hidden treasure of power, Vol. 1. Pasadena: Dhyanyoga Center, p. 12.

4   Krishna, G.(1975) The awakening of Kundalini. New York: Kundalini Research Foundation, p. 69.

5   Op. cit., p. 22.

6   Singh, K. (1961) _The Crown of Life_. New Hampshire: Sat Sandesh Books. pp. 155-163.

7   Op. cit., p. 217.

8   Joy, B. (1979) Joy's way. Los Angeles: J. P. Tarcher.

9   Goel B. S. (1985) Third eye and Kundalini. India: Third Eye Foundation, p. 67.

10 Bentov, I, (1977) Stalking the wild pendulum , New York:Bantam, p. 213.

11 Sannella, L. (1976) Kundalini -- Psychosis or transcendence? San Francisco: H. S. Dakin.

12 Anonymous (1912) Words of The Mother. Pondicherry: Sri Aurobindo Ashram, p. 43.

13 Aurobindo, S.(1950) Letters of Sri Aurobindo, first series, Bombay: Sri Aurobindo Ashram, p. 176.

14 Aurobindo,S. (1971) Letters on Yoga, 4 parts Pondicherry, Sri Aurobindo International University Center, p. 1767.

15 Engler, J. (1984) Therapeutic aims in psychotherapy and meditation: Developmental stages in the representation of the self. Journal of Transpersonal Psychology, 16 (1) p. 35.

16 Epstein, M. and Lieff, J. (1981) Psychiatric complications of meditation practice Journal of Transpersonal Psychology, 13, (2). pp. 137-145.

17 Walsh, R. and Roche,L. (1979) Precipitation of acute psychotic episodes by intensive meditation in individuals with a

history of schizophrenia. American Journal of Psychiatry. 136. pp. 1085-1086.

[18] Carpenter, J. (1977) "Meditation, esoteric traditions: Contributions to psychotherapy." American Journal of Psychotherapy, 31, 394-404.

[19] Lukoff, D. (1985) "The diagnosis of mystical experiences with psychotic features. " Journal of Transpersonal Psychology, 17, (2), p. 176-177.

[20] Erich Neumann (1961) "Mystical man." Spring. N.Y. Analytical Psychology Club. p. 17.

[21] Tweedie, I. (1979) Chasm of Fire. Great Britain: Element, p. 207.

[22] Jones, F. (1972) The Knee of Listening. Los Angeles: The Dawn Horse Press, p. 126.

[23] Kennett, R. and MacPhillamy, R. (1977) How to Grow a Lotus Blossom, Mt. Shasta, CA.: Shasta Abbey, p. 263.

[24] Thornton, E. (1967) The diary of a mystic. London: George Allan & Unwin, p. 78.

[25] Op. cit., p. 104.

[26] Op. cit., p. 105.

[27] Op. cit., p. 81.

[28] Op. cit., pp. 89-90.

[29] Kennett, R. and MacPhillamy, R. (1977) Op. cit., p.111.

[30] Op. cit., p. 130.

[31] Krishna, G. (1970 rev.) Kundalini: The evolutionary energy in man, Boulder: Shambhala, p. 60.

[32] Sivananda, S. (1969) Spiritual experiences (Amrita anubhava) Himalyas, India: Divine Life Society, p. 69.

[33] Aurobindo, S. (1953) Eight Upanishads. Pondicherry: Sri Aurobindo Ashram, p. 195.

[34] Aurobindo, (1971) Op. cit., pp. 932-933.

[35] Op. cit., p. 933.

[36] Vivekananda, S. (1985) Six lessons on raja yoga. Calcutta: Union Press, p. 25.

[37] Kennett, R. and MacPhillamy, R. (1977) Op. cit., p. 3.

[38] Op. cit. p. 6.

[39] Muktananda, S. (1978) Op. cit. p. 37.

[40] Jones, F. (1978) Op. cit., p. 126.

[41] Op. cit.

[42] Op. cit.

43 Op. cit., p. 120.
44 Perry, J., (1986) Spiritual Emergence and Renewal, ReVision,8
    (2), p. 34.
45 Op. cit., p. 35.
46 Muktananda , S. (1978) Op. cit., p. xx.
47 Aurobindo, S. (1971) Op. cit., p. 944.
48 Op. cit., p. 948-968.
49 Aurobindo, S. (1977) The Life Divine. Pondicherry: Sri
    Aurobindo Ashram. p. 944.
50 Metzner, R, (1986) Opening to the Inner Light, Los Angeles: J.
    P. Tarcher, p. 85.
51 Anandamurti, S.S. (1973 Baba's grace, Los Altos, CA.: Amrit,
    p. 109.
52 Satprem (1970) Sri Aurobindo or The Adventure of Consciousness,
    Pondicherry: Sri Aurobindo Ashram Trust, p. 209.
53 Op. cit., pp. 209 --210.
54 Bhaiji (1962) Mother as revealed to me .(G. D. Gupta, trans)
    Varanasi: Shree Shree Anandamayee Sangha, p. 92.
55 Keshavadas (1976) Cosmic Shakti Kundalini: The universal
    mother, Michigan: Harlo, p. 77.
56 Tyagisananda, S. (trans) (1971) Svetasvatorophanisad, Madras:
    Sri Ramakrishna Math, p. 39.
57 Madhusudandasji, D. (1979) Op. cit. p. ii.
58 Taimni, I. K. (1961) The science of yoga, New York: the
    Theosophical Pub. House, p. 432.
    (The definitions and descriptions of samadhi are synthesized
    primarily from the writings of two yogis who have
    interpreted the Yoga Sutras of Patanjali, Taimini, and Baba
    Hari Dass (1986) The Yoga Sutras,an unpublished
    manuscript, Mt. Madonna Center: Watsonville, CA.)
59 Wilber, K. (1980) The Atman project: A transpersonal view of
    human development. Wheaton, Ill. :The Theosophical
    Publishing House.
60 Jayakar, P. (1986) Krishnamurti: The years of awakening, p. 282.

CHAPTER THREE

YOGIC VIEWS OF ENERGY, THE BODY AND THE SELF

Those who awaken Kundalini sometimes see images representing the movement of energy in their bodies that seem to them like a chart mapping the internal path that Kundalini follows. These usually show an upward movement through the spine, the awakening of various chakras, the condition of body organs, and/or variations of colored lights. Often they see the energy reach beyond the physical body and into astral dimensions they find indescribable.

> When I closed my eyes and peeped inward, I found that the whole backbone was hallowed inside and was clearly visible. There was a red-string passing through it and joining the base of the spine with the Brahma-randhra (in the crown), and in place of the cobra which was emerging out of the Brahma-randhra. . . there was an engaging figure of the blue Lord Krishna . . . B.S. Goel[1]

> While I was doing shoshuten (a Taoist practice of circulating energy in the upper part of the body), I could see the inside of the sushumna, the sahasrara and two or three other chakras shining. After I had practiced yoga for six months or a year, a   shining golden light

> began to enter and leave my body through the top of my head and I felt as if the top of my head protruded ten to twenty centimeters, in the astral, but of the physical dimension. I saw what looked like the head of Buddha, shimmering purple and blue, resting on the top of my own head. There was a golden-white light flowing in and out through the gate on top of the Buddha's crown. Gradually I lost the sensation of my body, but I held a clear awareness of consciousness, of super-consciousness....Motoyama [2]

According to Vedic scriptures Kundalini energy is the fundamental power of creation and the primary consciousness of the universe. Swami Visnu Tirtha, described it precisely in a classic volume on Kundalini, <u>Devatma Shakti (Kundalini): Divine Power</u>.

> Vedic philosophers regard the whole creation on physical and metaphysical planes as a play of different forces, all being different forms of one universal cosmic energy or Power (Shakti), which comes into manifestation from the all-pervading and all-powerful Brahman. The phenomenon may be compared with the formation of mists, clouds, lightning, thunder, rains, hail, snow and so forth from an all-pervading atmosphere of vapour. Every manifestation of the cosmic power is followed by a corresponding merger completing one cycle. The infinite cosmic Power appears in the dynamic state during the creative process and after having accomplished a particular item in hand conceals itself with its infinite potential in the static residual form at some basic center of that individual item. In this residual form it is known as Kundalini Shakti or the Coiled Power, which when it uncoils on being roused to action begins to retrace its reverse path to its parental source as is the case with electric energy.[3]

In the dynamic process of creating human life, according to the Vedas, the life force goes through a specific process of creating three bodies: the causal body (containing bliss and consciousness), the subtle body (containing potentiality for mind, ego, energy, emotion and senses) and the gross body (the material or physical body). Once this force has put into matter the patterns of personality, intellect and physiology, the residual energy coils into a point at the base of the spine, identified as the muladhara by Eastern Indians. When Kundalini awakens, the coiled energy is believed to raise like a serpent from the base, transforming the natures of the six chakras in its path, and ultimately moving through the crown of the head (the sahasrara, usually designated as a seventh chakra). This activates God-realization or enlightenment.[4]

Kundalini is a power with immense potentiallty, opening the spiritual life to the previously latent capacity for cosmic awareness and ecstatic experience, but sometimes causing major disruption to the physiologic system. Some describe her energy as moving gradually up the spine and triggering specific capacities, knowledge and samadhi experiences as each chakra is fully enlivened. It appears as if the chakras generally operate to maintain balance and energy distribution in an individual until Kundalini awakens. As their energy is accelerated the chakras appear to undergo significant changes, and when the psyche responds to these impulses a progression of personality changes, paranormal abilities and "enlightenment" experiences may occur.

In some people Kundalini energy initially springs up suddenly and erratically like blasts of a geyser, causing glimpses of awareness, snatches of bliss and disruption of physical and psychic processes. In others there is a sudden solid streaming of energy through the body which lasts a few minutes (or longer), after which experiences of energy, vision, sounds, and awareness occur periodically and an ever-increasing vibration which feels like a hum in the body is permanently established. Others experience her as a fine and steady stream coming only during meditation, bringing samadhi and bliss. Some experience only subtle shifts in energy and primarily feel shifts in consciousness, while others experience massive and continuous movements of energy or burning sensations, and many other difficult conditions.

Kundalini is nurtured and enhanced by spiritual practices (especially meditation), healthy physical habits, respect and devotion toward the divine, physical exercises, and certain body therapies. Some yogis believe the energy cannot become dormant once awakened; others advise that it must be invited daily through spiritual practices until permanent realization occurs, which happens with the piercing of the sixth or seventh chakra.

Swami Muktananda emphasized that Kundalini is always active in the body, holding the system in stasis and maintaining the energy balance, and that it is the "inner" aspect of awakening her that triggers the true beginning of the spiritual journey. He wrote "Just as through her aspect of creation we explore the outer world, through the activation of the inner aspect we are able to experience the inner, spiritual world, leading to realization of our identity with the inner Self and the understanding of God."[5]

This differentiation is useful in understanding some of the contradictory writings about Kundalini. Most yogis identify the true movement of Kundalini as the awakening of consciousness or Self, implying a "knowing" other than intellectual knowing about life, a knowing which in itself triggers transformation. Although Kundalini may be working in the body, and even generating body movements and psychic disturbances through highly charged pranic activity, until there is a shift in consciousness, one has not really activated this "inner" aspect of spiritual awakening. Conversely, because it is this inner aspect that is the essential spiritual movement, Jung was led to identify it as primarily a psychic change, failing to recognize the great physiological ramifications of this upheaval.

The Yoga of Light, a translation of the ancient Hatha Yoga Pradipika, interprets the Sanscrit text definition of Kundalini as:

> The latent force of higher potential, said to lie in three and one-half coils, like the snake in the churning of the ocean of milk, sleeping at the lowest center (muladhara chakra) at the foot of the 'tree of life', the spinal column. This serpent power, Kundalini, cannot be described fully, even by one who has succeeded in awakening it. When it awakens, it shoots through the body like an electric shock, and, trembling and amazed, the person realizes that a powerful event has taken place within him. This is only the beginning. The whole body trembles. A door seems to have been pushed open through which a flood of light flows from some unknown world, a light of incomparable radiance. After a long time the trembling body becomes calm, but the flash of light shooting through the spinal column to

the crown of the head is unforgettable. This
flash of light is not really the Kundalini,
however, it is merely a sign of its awakening.
The Kundalini itself does not shoot up, but
will later rise slowly, passing through the
stations (the chakras), each of which creates
another new and powerful experience. [6]

Here again we find a differentiation between a physical
opening, and a movement of consciousness, which reportedly follows
more slowly in one who awakens the energy.

Swami Narayanananda quoted Swami Vivekananda as saying
that when the coiled up energy of Kundalini is aroused and enters the
canal of the sushumna (within the spinal column), its action upon
the chakras causes a tremendous reaction, immensely superior to the
reaction of dream or imagination, more intense than sense
perceptions. "And when it reaches the metropolis of all sensations,
the brain, the whole brain, as it were, reacts, and the result is the full
blaze of illumination, the perception of the Self." As the force
moves through the chakras it opens up "layer after layer of the mind.
. . and this universe is perceived by the yogi in its fine or causal
form. Then alone the causes of this universe both as sensation and
reaction are known as they are, and hence comes all knowledge."[7]

Narayanananda also described a partial arising of Kundalini,
occurring often during deep devotional songs and dancing, when
emotions are very high. At these times it does not rise up fully, but
a sudden partial rising will cause devotees to weep, sing, dance and be
carried away by a sudden outburst of feeling. The danger of this is
that if it comes down again suddenly to the sexual center
(svadhisthana chakra), it may trigger "abnormal" sexual drives and
cravings. (He did not define what he meant by "abnormal".) He cited
this as a reason that some devotees who have not developed the purity
of strong will become immoral, even though they hold positive
spiritual intentions. He said one-pointed study and concentration can
also trigger a partial uprising, which leads one not to emancipation
but toward inspiration in art, poetry, literature, science or research.[8]

Prana: Energy of the Life Force

The term "prana" is used by some scholars interchangeably
with "Kundalini" but this is correct only in the most general sense,
as Kundalini is sometimes referred to in a cosmic form as all energies

in the universe, being the life force or the source of all existence. Prana is an electrical-like energy flow in the body, which is more gross and more accessible than Kundalini, and in fact, keeps the entire system in working order even while Kundalini lies asleep or dormant at the base of the spine. It could be considered a stepped-down vibration of the more powerful Kundalini force. "Prana" is the creative and active energy that flows in the body and operates it functionally and directionally. It links consciousness with the entire operating system. "Kundalini" is the dormant residual of this energy that lies coiled in the muladhara. Descriptions of "*chi*" or "*ki*" in Oriental medicine are more akin to the concept of "prana" in the yogic tradition than to Kundalini

In the Chinese system *chi* is described as the life force, present in two primary forces, yang and yin, which are polarities reflecting opposite states in continual interchange. Their interaction determines the nature of the universe and is manifest as the five essential elements which make up all things.   According to traditional Chinese medicine *chi* flows throughout the body and 12 body meridians (or channels of energy flow) in specific patterns and directions, and when this energy flow is upset or out of balance physical and emotional problems may occur. In Ayurveda, the classical Indian medicine system, the correct balancing of prana is similarly important.   Acupuncture and acupressure are among Chinese methods for balancing this energy, and yoga asana and breathing practices are among the Indian methods.

According to the yogic guru and teacher Baba Hari Dass, body jerks, vibrations and other movements sometimes identified as "Kundalini" are the reactions of prana as it moves through the system.   It appears such activity is intensified in some people after Kundalini awakens, particularly if they have not adequately prepared their energy system with proper purifications, involving cleansing processes, breathing exercises and diet.

Other explanations that have been proposed regarding this intensified kriya activity suggest that there are physical and psychological blocks, armoring, or holding in the body which prevent the direct flow of energy; that what is occurring is a mechanism of stress release; and that the sushumna or central channel through which the energy flows is not large enough to accommodate the intense energy. It is also known that disruptions of energy flow to the brain may cause body jerks and spasms as may electrical brain stimulation in laboratories, factors which will be considered further in chapter four. I have observed in therapeutic sessions that people who are very emotionally blocked and unable to express feelings, as well as people who are engaged in powerful cathartic releases, may demonstrate intense kriya activity, especially if their Kundalini energy is awakened.

Prana is used in Eastern literature to define three levels of activity -- 1) in reference to the life-force or the total of all energy residing within the universe; 2) related specifically to the energy inherent in various biological functions; and 3) synonymously with breath. It is the vital force or biological energy which links the material or physical energy to mental energy; that is, it connects the gross and the subtle bodies. According to Singh "It is not like a physical energy but is a subtle biological energy which catches the vibrations of the mind and transmits them to the nerves and plexuses and also (carries) physical vibrations to the mind. By controlling the mind one can control the prana and by controlling the prana, one can control the mind." Singh states that prana cannot be contacted or influenced directly, but only through the breath, so the word "prana" is often used to refer to breath, sometimes with the word vayu (as "prana-vayu"). Usually "prana" refers to the exhaled breath, suggestive of the manifestation of the world, and "apana" to the inhaled breath indicating the withdrawal back to the source.[9]

Prana emanates from Self, according to Tirtha, who quoted from the Prashnopanishad "As Aura or shadow is to the body so prana is within it, it pervades and dominating the mind it comes into the body."[10] Yogis learn to control the prana which flows through subtle body nerves and to focus it at the root of the spinal cord in order to awaken Kundalini. This kind of control is also the source of many of the paranormal activities and talents of advanced yogis.

The senses of perception and the organs of action perform through the influence of prana which separates into five different aspects that fulfill various body functions : (1) prana, which works in the heart and draws air into the system; (2) apana, which draws downward and throws out of the system things that are not needed, such as waste matter and urine; (3) samana, which functions in all places with the task of distributing nourishment from the food we eat and digestion; (4) vyana, carrier of movement through the entire system and responsible for blood circulation; and (5) udana, which brings life-currents upwards to the heart and brain. In addition to the major divisions, which are all considered derivations of the primary prana, there are usually five minor pranas described in yogic theory. These perform the tasks of belching, opening eyelids, sneezing, yawning, and managing the gross body. Each is governed by five vayus or nerve impulses, named the same as the five main pranas. Tirtha called prana a fine form of energy different from physical energy which is the motive force that keeps the living organism, in good working order.[11]

Tirtha wrote that prana operates the sympathetic and parasympathetic nervous systems, working both under volition and independently. Prana controls the mind and every activity of the physical and psychic bodies, and this is why by controlling prana through yogic breathing exercises the yogi can gain control and mastery of mind and emotions. Advanced yogis reportedly have the capacity to bring aspects of autonomous motor systems such as the heart beat, pulse rate, and kidneys under control, and to change temperature in their bodies, making them as hot or cold as they like. When more prana is moved consciously into the mind it is reflected as consciousness and can be conserved and focused to use for highly creative work or occult purposes. According to Tirtha, if a yogi focuses prana subjectively as reflection on the inner self it leads to samadhi.

The relationship of prana and breath is particularly significant to those who practice yoga and pranayama techniques, yogic breathing exercises designed to control and direct prana. Swami Radha indicates that these lead to emotional control, a calm mind, curing of nervous disorders, the refinement of sense perceptions, and limitation of selfish desires, preparing the mind for higher stages of yogic practice. She says pranayama increases the alpha waves in the brain, brings the vagus nerves under control and provides a relaxing effect on the heart and nervous system. Other long-term benefits include extrasensory perception and the burning up of karma. [12]

Pranayama is also practiced specifically to stimulate the awakening of Kundalini energy. Vishnudevananda says that prana-vayu is generated by inhalation, affecting the afferent system and apana vayu is generated by exhalation, affecting the efferent system. During retention of breath in pranayama the yogi unites these two impulses at the muladhara. This acts like a dynamo sending lots of energy to stimulate Kundalini, which tries to move up the sushumna, the invisible nadi or nerve channel in the center of the spine. [13]

The Siva Sutras claim that by stilling the prana through various means one may experience seven different kinds of bliss: the bliss of one's own self; transcendental bliss; supreme bliss; the bliss of the absolute; great bliss; the bliss of consciousness; and the bliss of the world. [14]

Activities such as spontaneous movements, waves of bliss, shaking or jerks of the body, sudden pains, hot and cold flashes, feelings of energy or numbness in the hands and feet, and other sensations are often observed in meditators, people doing altered-state transpersonal work and those experiencing physical release. These are pranic activities, but not necessarily indicative of Kundalini awakening. Likewise, waves of emotions and psychic upheavals can occur without Kundalini energy, although all of these phenomena may indicate one is in states preparatory to or preliminary to the awakening process. A stronger and more conscious flow of pranic energy or *chi* is commonly felt by many who practice yoga, acupressure, Tai Chi, Aikido, meditation, and other processes in which there is focus on the breath and concentration.

"Shakti" or "sakti" is another term sometimes used in Eastern references to energy, prana or Kundalini. "Shakti" is a principle most commonly found in tantric Yoga. The word comes from the root *sak*, "to have power" or "to be able". It is the universal cosmic substance that is the source of creation. Siva (or Shiva) is the god representing pure consciousness (in a formless state), who resides in the cerebrum or sahasrara chakra, and Sakti (or Shakti), his consort, is the powerful feminine energy from which creation emerges. In humans, she resides at the base of the spine, where she is known as Kundalini. The two are inseparable. Sakti is the active or the manifest form of the divine, that which is created and from whom the five elements spring. She is the beginning, the primordial universe, whose nature is bliss.

Some schools of yoga, especially Siddha Yoga, identify "shaktipat" as a primary method of awakening Kundalini. This term refers to the energy transmitted from a guru to a follower, usually as part of an initiation, that stimulates the awakening. Some classical yogic texts suggest this is the only way Kundalini can be awakened, and if it should appear to happen spontaneously this is because of a relationship with a guru in a previous life. According to the teaching of Kashmir Shaivism there are three classes of shaktipat (also identified as redemptive grace), sub-divided into nine minor sub-divisions, and the kind of experience one has with shaktipat indicates one's level of spiritual evolution. The most highly developed people experience an intense shakti which instantaneously liberates them, even if they have never followed any spiritual practices. This is a very rare experience. Moderate levels of shakti stimulate spiritual life, drawing people into spiritual practices, austerities, initiation, and ritual. Mild shakti induces a longing for spiritual knowledge, meditation, and detachment from worldly preoccupations.[15]

Tirtha describes shaktipat as an injection of shakti, or cosmic energy:

> The master injects in the astral body of the
> initiated a current of psychic power, or a dose
> of astral fluid of a high potentiality by the
> touch of his hands, by casting a look or by
> speaking out to him some word or words
> called mantras, or any one of God's holy
> names, or simply by a mere thought. When
> the Divine Power is thus transmitted She acts
> in the favoured in such a way that the dormant
> power of Kundalini is awakened, or we may
> say that the fire of Kundalini is ignited and set
> into flames throughout the nervous system.[16]

Baba Hari Dass has stated that one who is advanced by birth
and has total faith in the teacher can attain enlightenment by
shaktipat. He believes it is not the power of the guru but the power
of one's own faith and samskaras (tendencies and conditions brought
in from previous lives) that accomplishes this.

Subtle Body Theory & Kundalini

It is essential for the therapist, physician or bodyworker who
wants to understand and work effectively with Kundalini energy to
understand the spiritual-physical system that is the foundation of
yogic theory, because it is apparent that Kundalini awakening is not a
manifestation or process of the physical body as it is known through
Western medicine and biology. Westerners must overcome the
cultural bias against recognizing the relationship of spirituality to the
physical universe and the human body; yet this is paradoxically
difficult because the subtle body system appears to defy attempts of
Western science to observe it conclusively with medical or scientific
equipment yet developed. It can only be theorized from its effects on
the physiology and psyche of those who experience it.

Yogic literature generally describes the life force as creating
individuals through the manifestation of the previously identified
three bodies -- the causal, the subtle and the gross, in which are
contained five kosas, or sheaths, which form the human. The bodies
link with one another through the chakras or energy vortices, five
major and five minor pranic fields of energy, and from 72,000 to 720
million nadis (subtle lines of directional force through which prana is
distributed, the speculated number of which varies greatly in the
literature). The nadis emanate from the muladhara, the root and

support of the subtle body system, close to where the Kundalini energy lies coiled. They correspond generally to the channels of energy flow identified in the Taoist tradition, which are the basis of acupressure and acupuncture meridians, and also extend considerably beyond the physical body. All of these are components of the human system, but are too subtle to be identified or measured by Western medical techniques.

Some researchers have mistakenly identified chakras with nerve plexuses in the body, and it is certain they influence various physical organs as well as the entire system, but it is best to avoid correlating the subtle body very specifically with the gross body as this is not a material energy field. It is invisible in a state of ordinary consciousness. I think of the human body as a functional, material mechanism made of various earth-elements, activated, directed and energized through these subtle forces and structures, through which psychic, mental and emotional processes flow. The breath activates and moderates these energies and fields as they act through the physical system, and hold the system in stasis until death. I expect that when breath ceases the energy fields recede from the body and may be held in a seed form, or in another space, or reincarnate to animate another body in another lifetime.

Being part of the subtle body, the five kosas or sheaths, the chakras and nadis also form the substance of the psychological and mental being, carrying through the system propensities from previous lives, inspirations, talents, desires and motivations which form the core of the individual's life direction and personality patterns. This is truly a transpersonal system.

The causal body is called in Sanscrit the anandamaya kosa, or bliss sheath. It contains the three energies of creation (gunas)in dormant form -- harmonious consciousness,(sattva); activity or the will to create (rajas); and inertia or matter (tamas). These are the qualities of prakriti (the active creative principle) that allow form to exist in matter. We cannot directly impact the nature of the causal body but as a person brings the mind and the senses under control by following the yamas (positive actions) and niyamas (avoidance of negative actions) of yoga, and performing purifications, breathing and meditation techniques these energies become more balanced. The particular mixture of energies varies with each individual and is said to be contained with the seed of the subtle body between lives. When one achieves liberation, sattva will dominate the energy field.

The subtle or energy body contains three sheaths: vijnanamaya kosa, containing potentiality of both intellect and ego;

manomaya kosa, containing potentiality of the mind and sense organs; and pranamaya kosa, containing the vital energies.

The **gross** body is the annamaya kosha sheath, where the
24 subtle body energies are divided into mental faculties, sense
organs, organs of action, ten pranas and five elements, all of which
are used in the functioning of the human body.

In The Pancadasi, as interpreted by Mahadevan, the Atman
(or soul-essence) is said to be hidden in the cavity of these five
sheaths:

> The grossest of the sheaths is the annamaya,
> the physical body made of food; pranamaya is
> the sheath of the vital air, and is the energizer
> of the body; manomaya is the sheath of the
> mind; subtler than that is the vijnanamaya, the
> sheath of the intellect with the power of
> cognition; and the subtlest of all is the
> anandamaya, the sheath of enjoyment
> enveloped in ignorance. These five sheaths lie
> one within the other in a serial order; and that
> which is within takes on the form of that
> which is without, like mercury that is poured
> into a crucible. [17]

According to The Pancadasi, the body sheath is born of
the food assimilated by the parents, and it is sustained by food alone.
The sheath of vital airs (pranamaya) is the vitalizer of the physical
body, giving it strength, activating various senses to perform their
respective functions.   The mental sheath is that which identifies
itself with the body and considers itself to have possessions,
relationships, etc. It is subject to changing passions and passing
moods and desires.   The sheath of intellect is a reflection of the
Supreme Intelligence, but is dormant in sleep.   On awakening,"it
fills the body to the finger-tips. . . it is the doer of all deeds,
possessing the power of cognition." Anandamaya, the sheath of enjoyment, represents the mind turned inward, which is a reflection of
ananda or bliss. It is not the Self because it exists only at certain
times, and it is described in the shape of a body. It is a modification
of the bliss of Atman (the Divine Self) just as annamaya is a
modification of food.[18]

Anandamurti called the five sheaths or kosas "cells of the
mind", and also linked them with the activities of the chakras. He
wrote "The all-round perfect sadhana (spiritual practice) is the

sustained effort to identify every kosa with the Inner Self completely.
. . the more forward a sadhaka (spiritual aspirant) goes in his sadhana,
the more his chakras and propensities get controlled by the higher and
higher kosas." He stated that the controlling point of every kosa or
cell is situated at the ajna chakra (located in the center of the forehead
just above the eyes), and with the help of the crude nerves the kosas
control the different chakras as well as the propensities belonging to
them. As one increases control over the kosas through spiritual
practices, he said the organs become more docile and submissive, and
as one gains control over mind and organs, one is less affected by
external influences, vanity, inertness and superstition.[19]

In an ancient tantric text translated by Rama Prasad in 1889,
the creation of the human through kosas is described as a microcosm
of the formation of the planets and the universe through the
constellation of the five various ethers. These are: (1) akasha,
through which every form lives and comes to be and which brings the
quality of space to give room for movement in creation; (2) tejas,
which brings the luminosity and color to form, enabling it to be seen
through the reflection of light; (3) vayu, related to touch, moving in
spherical motion, giving birth to and nourishing the skin, and
bringing the quality of locomotion; (4) apas, related to taste and
bringing the quality of contraction so that various ethers move
together, and of smoothness, allowing these atomic structures to
glide over one another; and (5) prithivi, the odoriferous ether , related
to smell and having the quality of cohesive resistance which creates
bones. It is notable that the vibration of each of these ethers follows
a specific form, which is indicated symbolically by the circle,
triangle, spiral, half moon and quadrangle, respectively. These
symbols frequently emerge during altered states of awareness related
to the Kundalini experience, and are also connected with the chakras.
Prasad states that without these ethers or elements there is no adequate explanation of the phenomena of light, sound, touch, taste and
smell in the human, and he describes them in various combinations
as molecular structures.[20]

The knots or "granthis" (named Brahma, Vishnu and Rudra
or Shiva) are three aspects of subtle body theory often overlooked or
poorly defined in treatises on the subject. They refer to places along
the spinal column (in locations which vary considerably in the
scriptures) where the energy-connection or identification with creation
is especially strong and the energy must be pierced by certain yogic
practices.

According to The Siva Sutras, the Brahmagranthi is the
first point to be pierced by Kundalini before the muladhara chakra (at

the base of the spine) is pierced; the Visnugranthi is pierced between the manipura (at the abdomen) and anahata (at the heart) chakras; and the Rudragranthi is pierced between the visuddha (at the throat) and before the ajna chakra (between the eyes in the forehead). In yoga these represent three levels of consciousness, or stages of bondage which must be released. When piercing Brahmagranthi the physical level or the false identification with the body ceases, releasing identification with physical, emotional and sensate interests. One is said to become established in totality. Since this is the initial granthi to be pierced upon awakening of Kundalini, this action may carry the responsibility for the chaotic physical and emotional activities that occur in early stages of the process. When the Visnugranthi or mental knot is pierced one gains control of the subtle body, releasing identification with the mind, including desires and mental vacillations. One perceives the existence of the universal life principle. When the spiritual center or Rudragranthi is pierced one removes all ignorance and attains the Self, releasing into a permanent state of bliss.

These piercings represent major shifts in consciousness and orientation, and are correlated with the several stages of enlightenment or "kensho" described in yogic and Zen literature. They represent a reversal of consciousness, as it were. Our identification with the body as "who I am" is the last attachment we make as we come into physical form, losing touch with cosmic awareness, according to yogic cosmology; more refined is the awareness we might identify as "I am not my body, but a being of consciousness" - - an experience of subtle-body awareness, which is the level of consciousness prior to physical embodiment. Prior to this was a formless, mergent state with the infinite where there was no separation, only a potentiality. So as we seek higher and higher states of samadhi we are reaching to return into that state of no-separation. These states are well-documented in The Tibetan Book of the Dead and in Ken Wilber's The Atman Project (1980), as well as in classical Indian scriptures.

The Chakras

Chakras are probably the most commonly known elements of subtle body theory in the West, as many writers with interests in yoga, Tibetan Buddhism, Theosophy and psychic studies have provided varied descriptions and interpretations of them. Although seven stages of samadhi are referred to in the classical yoga sutras, developments of concepts about chakras probably did not emerge until tantric practices began. Some interpreters of Eastern literature relate the piercing by Kundalini of the six major chakras, and its merging into the seventh, as analogous to these stages of samadhi, and report specific conditions which follow each stage. Others do not put much emphasis on chakras, and suggest that the basic yoga practices and disciplines can transform the chakra energies so that when Kundalini awakens they are of minor importance, but simply sustain the spiritual opening.

Often I have observed repeated kriyas (that is, shaking, jerking, twisting or vibrations) occurring in chakra areas in someone who is doing body therapy, or experiencing emotional or physical stress. It appears as if there is a blockage so that energy is not moving through the body smoothly at that point. It is possible that unresolved issues or mental conditions related to the chakras cause such blockages.   It is also possible that some of the physical problems associated with spontaneous Kundalini awakenings are due to the impact of Kundalini energy on chakras relevant to the affected body organs, as most chakras control the functioning of certain organs.

Other phenomena that may be associated with chakra energies are the spontaneous emergence of specific images, sounds, and symbols which the tantric cosmology has associated with each chakra. Their emergence during times of crisis may provide information pertinent to the kinds of issues one needs to resolve, or point to the area of the body where specific attention can most effectively be focused. For these reasons it is helpful to have some understanding of the chakra system. Since many books are available on this subject the following remarks provide only a slight overview.

Chakras have been called such things as neurohormonal mechanisms governing zones of the body (Mishra); multidimensional entities through which formative forces flow between the three bodies (Scott); centers of the body's energy system (Pandit); energy vortices; intermediaries which convey energy from one dimension into another; "interdimensional transducing systems capable of being directed by thought and converting matter into energy "(Joy); centers of subtle forces, cosmic consciousness and the generation of prana; openings on the macrocosm; and springs which release into action several powers and energies that are centered in them.

As atoms are to the field of matter, so the "bindu" of the chakra is to the pranic energy field, according to Goswami, writing on Layayoga. He says "the motional or active state of pranic force concentrates and centralises to form petaline bindus at various points of the body, termed by the yogis chakras or lotuses. This development begins with the sahasrara chakra, and develops progressively downward as the human consciousness and material body is formed. All this is invisible to the naked eye. Chakras function supramaterially."[21]

Generally chakras are considered the links between all the activities of the causal, subtle and gross bodies. Vrittis (thought waves) emanate from them, as well as other energies which are distributed throughout the body. That is why specific emotions and characteristics have been ascribed to each of them. If we accept a view of chakras as the main transducers of energy between these bodies, it is understandable that the intensification of consciousness and energy associated with Kundalini awakening would put powerful extra stresses on the chakra system. Often they are described as lotuses which move from downward to upward positions as Kundalini rises through them. It is possible that this is symbolic of a gradual process, nowhere near as dramatic and rapid as the mind can imagine, and that much of the physical and emotional turmoil which some people experience with Kundalini is concurrent with the readjustment of the chakra which is changing to serve a different level of consciousness and energy than that to which the body was normally accustomed.

The difficulties of shifting one's essential way of being in the world can be enormous for those who have little previous experience with self-discipline or mastery of the emotions. The lengthy preliminary practices and disciplines of yogic and tantric initiates, including years of ego-deflating practices and subservience to a teacher, are in part an effort to accomplish mastery of the personality before Kundalini awakens, in which case the movement of energy through the chakras could proceed in a relatively unobstructed manner. These chakras are holding all the knots and problems of one's personal and emotional lives and during spiritual transformation they may be turning toward the integration of a more unitive and less self-involved form of consciousness.

There are seven major chakras and 43 less significant ones, with many characteristics ascribed to them in a variety of texts. Prana is said to dominate in various chakras following a sixty-minute pattern throughout the day. Several kinds of symbols are associated with each of the major chakras. These include an animal, representing subtle forces which rule the chakra; a god, who signifies one of the divine forces of manifestation; and a goddess, who demonstrates the kind of energy localized at this point. Other symbols indicate the dominant element and the sensate capacity connected with the chakra. Meditation on each chakra is said to awaken the energy of the respective goddess contained there, who will lead one into a unique divine potential. The lotus petals represent various qualities, emotional tendencies and capacities. The following brief descriptions, provide information which may be relevant to those who are experiencing Kundalini, and are impacted by specific emotional problems, visions, sounds, occult responses and other events associated with the chakras.[22]

Muladhara

Located almost at the bottom of the backbone, adjoining the anus and the testicles or cervix, this chakra is identified as a four-petaled lotus, with the petals representing supreme happiness, innate bliss, the bliss of union, and the bliss of bravery, strength or power. It is said to be a reflection on a gross level of the crown chakra, and this is why the petals carry bliss. The nature of this chakra is identical with Brahman, the creative principle of the universe. We might think of it as holding the body in its material form, thus forming creation; and that within it's essence lies the primordial history and potentiality of human evolution. It is the foundation and support of the system, and its proper functioning is associated with issues of security and self-preservation, the element earth, the colors orange-red and the tanmatra (or sense) of smell. An elephant with a black strip around its neck is its symbol, standing for the terrestrial qualities of strength, firmness, balance and support, as does a yellow square contained within a circle in the yantra or mandala depicting this chakra. It also holds a triangle, called tripura, representing will, knowledge and action.

The muladhara influences the rectum, kidneys, accumulation of sperm and the sexual organs, and also the bones, skin, flesh, nerves and hair. Specific physical conditions such as hemorrhoids, constipation, sciatica and prostate problems have been associated with it. It is connected to the sense of smell, and its vibrations bring about expansion and contraction of the lungs.

Mishra writes that anger, lust and greed are controlled by practicing pratyahara (the withdrawal of sense-awareness) on this chakra. Grief and depression have also been considered symptoms of imbalance. Meditation on it is also said to bring control of attachment to luxury, deception, pride, envy and selfishness. Pandit said the muladhara governs physical or subconscious movements or impulses. Within the yantra (a symbolic representation of the chakra) is a blood-red triangular zone of fire which blows kandarpa vayu which is the cause of sexual excitement, essential for procreation. Motoyama wrote that when this chakra awakens it releases repressed emotion in an explosive manner that may lead one to feel extremely irritable and psychologically unstable, follow erratic sleeping patterns, and become passionate, overly-talkative or easily enraged. Meditating on the god at this chakra, the Sayambhulinga Mahadeva, who is seated with his face turned backwards, is said to free one from sins. Brahma, the god of absolute creative force, also empowers this chakra with the goddess Dakini Sakti, the energy of creation. Saying the "mula mantra" with a placid mind and devotion, while focusing here, is said to awaken her energy. In yogic cosmology Kundalini energy is coiled three and a half times just below this chakra. Here it is that yogis consider to be the confluence in the body of the sushumna (a nadi carrying life current); Bajra Nadi (a nadi carrying electric current) and Brahma Nadi (sound current or spirit current). This explains how it is that three specific practices can awaken Kundalini -- using the breath (life current) and controlling its flow through the sushumna; withdrawal of sense-awareness (pratyahara), which is a withdrawal of prana, and concentrating it at the base of the spine which would impact the electrical current; and recitation of mantra or repetition of certain sounds, impacting sound current. It also explains the interrelationship of several Kundalini symptoms -- experiencing of certain energies which feel electrical; pranic energy releases; and emission of certain spontaneous sounds.

Svadhisthana

Located a little above the muladhara and at the root of the genital organ, or in the center of the lumbar region, this chakra is associated with conquest of the element water, symbolized by a half-moon, and with the god Vishnu, the sustaining principle of the universe. Its color is usually identified as red or vermillion, sometimes as white. Rakini Sakti, in dark blue, with three red eyes, a bleeding nostril, and four arms, is the goddess who carries this energy. She holds a trident, lotus, drum and chisel. A light gray or green sea-monster which looks similar to a crocodile is the animal symbol, representing dominion over the sea, and indicating an association with the unconscious. Meditation on it is said to bring victory over the elements.

It has six petals which carry the mental conditions of neglect, insensitivity, credulity, suspicion, destructiveness and cruelty and also represent six nerves associated with the large intestines, rectum, kidney, bladder, sexual organ and testes. The circulation of the fluid substances in the body, their preservation and sustenance, is helped by this chakra, which has also been considered to be the center of heterosexual attachment.   Mishra wrote that this chakra controls, governs and nourishes the legs.   One feels magnetic pulsation, magnetic circulation and magnetic vibration by focusing here, and can remove all pains, aches, and diseases from the legs. Other physical conditions related to it include sexual problems, diabetes, kidney and bladder problems. By meditating on it one is relieved of egoistic feelings, petty impulses and desires.   Qualities of equanimity and placidity of mind are developed.   Self-confidence and well-being are attributed to svadhisthana's proper functioning, while frustration, attachment and anxiety are associated with dysfunction.   It is also associated with the sense of taste and the tongue. According to some of the tantras, to master it one must bring the tongue under control in such a way that the mind can think of nothing other than God and the tongue can utter nothing but references to the glories of God. Specific practices to control the tongue, pulling it into the back of the throat, often cutting it slightly over an extended period of time, are taught in some Tantric cults.

Manipura
Located above the svadhisthana opposite to the naval, the manipura is associated with Rudra, a god who grants boons and generates fear, representing the destructive principle of the universe (the world of mind). The goddess Lakini Sakti, clothed in yellow, is called the universal benefactress, and in one text is described as loving the flesh of animals, having a breast covered with blood, and with fat dripping from her mouth. The animal symbol is the ram, a sacrificial animal, implying the need to sacrifice passions, impulsiveness and other strong emotions.
Concentration on manipura is said to bring realization regarding kala, or eternal time. It may be to this level of opening we can attribute memories of other lives, or experiences which carry people out of awareness of boundaries created by time. It is also associated with control of the element heat, and presides over agni, the fire-state, believed to govern the expansive movements of the being, and rule the digestive system.   It controls the abdominal organs, particularly the functioning of stomach, liver and large intestine, and is related to the central nervous system, above the lumbar region. Focusing here is said by some to cure abdominal disease, especially if one meditates on the red color within it.   Mastery of it means mastery of the subtle elements.

Ten petals, which carry the mental conditions of shame, treachery, jealousy, desire, drowsiness, despondency, worldliness, delusion, aversion and fear are identified with this chakra. However a yogi reportedly meditating on this chakra and uttering the Mula Mantra remains always in a happy mood, according to one tantric text and diseases cannot enter his/her body. Such a yogi can enter into the bodies of others and can see the siddhas (yogis saints and masters), can know at sight the qualities of material objects and see articles within the earth. It is clear why the chakra is so commonly associated with issues of power, and the capacity to assert oneself effectively in the world. This is also the area of the hara, where attention is focused in certain Zen meditation practices. Such concentration accomplishes a sense of stability and centeredness in the being, as the above mentioned qualities are acknowledged, mastered and transcended.

Opening of this chakra is said to require the help of eyes, controlling their movements in such a way that they do not deflect even for a moment from the center located between the two eyebrows.

Anahata

The heart chakra is usually described as located opposite to the central line in between the two nipples, but sometimes placed slightly to the right of the sternum rather than directly over the heart. It is associated with conquest of the air element, as well as the heart and with nada, the sound of cosmic consciousness. When one focuses on meditation here energy can sometimes be felt flowing throughout the entire nervous system, as if it is full of magnetism. Many spiritual traditions emphasize the heart chakra as the primary chakra necessary to awaken in order to experience spiritual awakening, as this is where energies from lower and upper levels of consciousness merge, symbolized by two intersecting triangles. In addition to linking the energies of the chakras, it links left and right sides of the body, yin and yang characteristics. These two interlinking forms create a cross which symbolically represents integration of these polarities.

Isha is the god of this chakra, seated on a black antelope or a gazelle, which symbolizes swiftness and the lightness of air. Isha is the supreme God endowed with complete yogic power, omniscient and omnipresent. He is white, symbolizing purity, and he has three eyes, the third representing samadhi-knowledge. When his form appears in meditation, fear vanishes and concentration is strengthened.

Images in the yantra for the heart chakra include intersected triangles holding within a bright gold-colored being and a lightning-colored Kakini Sakti radiant with light and joy. Kakini is called the door-keeper of the anahata, and it is through concentration on her one learns to stabilize the prana and remove all obstacles to Isha. When she is red it indicates that her power is being utilized in the control of pranic energy; when she is white she is Isha-consciousness.

Twelve petals the color of vermillion are associated with anahata, representing the mental conditions of expectation, anxiety, endeavor, attachment, hypocrisy, infirmity, egoism, discretion, covetousness, fraudulence, indecision and regret. Meditation on this chakra is said to bring mastery of sound and using mula mantra with it is said to make one fit for God-realization, as one becomes capable of controlling the senses by restricting the sensation of touch. It is said no desire will then remain unfulfilled -- one will then always maintain a state of bliss.

Another way to view this is to consider that through releasing attachment to all of the things the "heart" desires (as evidenced by the mental conditions) one becomes capable of withdrawing the senses from worldly things, and thus is enabled to contact the experience of bliss, perhaps at first only for short periods, but ultimately in a permanent way. I am convinced from my work with Kundalini that it is just these desires and attachments, the expectations and emotions of the heart, that shut off the natural flow of bliss once it has awakened, and the ups and downs which often accompany this experience emotionally may be related primarily to the issues of this chakra.

Qualities of compassion, acceptance and unconditional love are said to indicate a balanced functioning of the heart chakra; insensitivity, passivity and sorrow indicate an imbalance. Some writers have associated arthritis and respiratory problems, as well as cardiovascular and hypertensive illness with issues of the heart chakra.

Realization of the chakra is believed to require the help of skin, that is to transcend the sense of touch, which is done by bringing the power of sense perception under control through kumbhaka (breath retention). It is also common to focus meditation on the heart chakra, imaging a light, or following the breath in and out of it, as ways of opening its energy. Pains and unfamiliar energy moving through the heart area are commonly reported by people who have awakened Kundalini energy.

Visuddha

Located opposite to the throat, in the neck, the lotus of visuddha is gray or silver (or sometimes smoky-purple) and its lotus has 16 petals. These are said to contain seven notes of the musical scale, poison and nectar, and seven"calls" used for purposes of exorcism, sacrifice, fire ceremonies, self-determination, blessings and exaltations. This suggests the beginning of priestly or occult powers, associated with the power of projection, or expression. The chakra is also associated with conquest of the etherial state of matter (space) which governs the expressive mind.The expression of creative activity and inspiration are commonly connected with this chakra, along with the capacity to receive nurturing, especially the contact with the inner unlimited source of "grace". One begins to experience that the inner giver and receiver are one. Energizing this chakra may involve devotional practices such as ritual, prayer, chanting and using sound vibration, and creative expression.

The god of this chakra is Siva in a half-male, half-female form (Adrhanariswara) sitting on a white elephant accompanied by the yellow-colored Sakini Sakti (goddess) with four hands. He has mastered diverse knowledge. She reigns in the lunar region, over the minor mysteries.

The visuddha controls both arms and is the center of pratyahara, or sense-withdrawal. As one concentrates here one loses sensitivity to heat, cold, pain, pressure, touch and temperature in the arms. The tantras say its instrument is the ears, used in such a way that the sounds of the world are not distracting and only one sound is heard, either nada (a less intense sound of Om) or the name of god. Meditating on this chakra reportedly brings one to the threshold of great liberation.

Ajna

Located at the base of the nose between the two eyebrows, ajna is the source of two nervous flows, one through the eyes and the other through the mid-brain. Here the three principal nadis (sushumna, ida, and pingala) meet. Creativity and accomplishments are generated from the thought waves of this point. This chakra governs inner vision and the dynamic activities of will and knowledge. This "third eye" has been associated in many cultures with light, inner knowing, intuitive and psychic abilities. Opening to these capacities involves integration of both intellectual and emotional poles. According to Layayoga, it is when aroused Kundalini reaches this chakra that consciousness transforms.

The goddess of ajna is Hakini Shakti, who has six faces and six arms, representing the five principles centered in the lower chakras and the gifts of the ajna chakra. When she is depicted as red this indicates Kundalini knowledge is fully awakened; when white she represents a state of calm; when dark-blue she is about to proceed into a formless state. If seen as a mixture of white, red and black she is demonstrating a blending of the three gunas -- sattva (harmonious consciousness), rajas (activity) and tamas (inertia). Meditating on this center is said to bring visions of the highest truth as well as yogic powers, relief of all sanskaras, and ultimately the wisdom of the Self, the highest knowledge. This is the center of individual consciousness, which through pratyahara may be expanded into universal consciousness. It is often referred to as the governing chakra for all of the others, and some yogis recommend concentration only at the ajna, or initially there, before awakening the energies of other chakras. It can impact the development of the qualities inherent in all of the preceding chakras, and enable an aspirant to reach a state of non-dual awareness. Complete mastery of the lower chakras is believed to be impossible until ajna is pierced.

Sahasrara

According to some scriptures the sahasrara is located at the crown of the head in the cerebrum; in others it is considered above the physical body, and is identical with Parambrahma, the supreme creator. Its lotus contains a thousand petals, of which five represent all the letters of the Sanscrit alphabet. Samadhi as it is experienced through this chakra is the sense of merging completely into existence, with no boundaries of "I" consciousness in the body. (Although there are yogic systems with additional levels of chakras, extending further beyond the physical body and this first level of higher consciousness.)

Parambrahma rules this center, symbolized by the triangle of consciousness (called Veeja), another name of the divine essences of sat, chit and ananda This represents the overcoming of the obstacles, and merging into the void, or the supreme light beyond form, an experience beyond one's capacity to describe, according to most yogic scriptures and saints.

By meditating here, according to Bose and Haldor, one crosses the boundaries of creation, preservation and destruction and can taste a sweet nectar (amrita) that flows in a constant stream from the sahasrara. One is emancipated and all sanskaras are destroyed, so one is no longer subjected to birth nor to death. At this state of awakening, individual identity disappears forever and one identifies with supreme consciousness. (It is useful to remember that when yogis talk of a deathless state they do not usually mean one will literally never leave the body, but rather that conscious merging with the infinite is achieved as a permanent state which will not be disrupted by the body's dying.)[23]

Development and Expansion of Chakra Energies

When Kundalini is awakened through all the chakras yogis are said to acquire certain occult abilities called "siddhis". These reportedly include the power of making one's body as minute as an atom, the power of increasing the weight or size of one's body at will, the power of making the body exceedingly light, the power of creating what one desires, the power of winning or hypnotizing others, occasional God-realization, and God-vision at desire. According to Motoyama, a Japanese parapsychologist and yogi, "These powers are automatically acquired by all good souls who can systematically concentrate on the life-force or Atman. The acquisition of these powers often operate as great stumbling blocks in the path of Self or God-realization, particularly when they are employed for personal glorification in any way."[2]

There are tales of Tantric adepts who acquire the ability to penetrate into the body of a dead person and animate it in its place, and who become invisible, to fly in the sky and walk on water. These indicate mastery over the planes of creation, according to scripture. On the whole these extreme claims are not observed in Westerners who experience Kundalini, although one occasionally hears stories of a modern spiritual teacher, such as Sai Baba, who performs some of them (i.e. materializing objects and transporting his body to distant places). They are interesting to note however, because similar themes may appear in the dreams and fantasies of someone in this process.

Motoyama summarizes the significance of chakras as the centers of the body's energy system, existing in three different dimensions: physical, astral and causal, acting as intermediaries between these dimensions and capable of converting the energy of one dimension into that of another. Each chakra has its own sounds (nada and mantra) and geometrical figure (yantra), which can be perceived extrasensorily. The aura of an awakened chakra is brighter and larger than that of a dormant chakra, and emits more energy. Motoyama believes the chakra most easily awakened through yoga practice depends on karma and on the person's nature and is usually the one which is working most actively due to these two factors. He sees the awakening of chakras as of extreme importance in spiritual advancement, and states that overuse of one chakra is dangerous and can cause disease and even death.

Brugh Joy, a Western physician and spiritual teacher, wrote that in working with chakra energy he noticed a field of energy radiating nd extending as far as 20 feet away from the body of some people, and that he has located 40 such fields radiating form the body surface in the normal individual. He identifies 16 major points of energy, including the seven chakras commonly identified in the yogic system. He correlates certain physical and emotional problems with strong or weak energy flows in various chakras. He believes "tentatively" that the "chakra system is an interdimensional transducing system capable of being directed by thought and capable of converting matter into various forms of energy, and vice versa, transcending the constraints of time and space."[25]

Joy distinguishes between active chakras and awakened chakras: "Even in the most unawakened individual all the chakras in the human being are active, but in most people, they function primarily in relation to the physical body in the physical manifest plane and in the more subtle manifest plane, to the etheric (subtle) body. These chakras are in what is called a dormant or resting state of activity. Despite the terminology, energy activity from these dormant or resting chakras is readily felt with the scanning technique. An awakened chakra not only feels different in scanning, it looks different to clairvoyant vision."[26]

Joy teaches practices in which one works with the chakra energy fields or light body touch to heal physical and psychological imbalances. His work demonstrates the possibility of sensing and affecting the energy through bodywork, an experience often reported by body therapists and psychics. Some healers focus on balancing the energy of the chakras, which seem to change in intensity as they hold their hands over someone's body. It is possible then to feel when the energy is emitting approximately equal intensity.

Acupressure flows may also affect the distribution of pranic energies through the chakra system. People feel these movements and shifts while they are being worked on and often show remarkable changes in energy and well-being following treatments. Theoretically, treatments of the spleen and the liver meridians should help to balance the distribution of energy and reduce extremes of heat or cold in the body, and acupressure flows for the heart or stomach meridians should help to ease problems that clients experience with Kundalini in those areas. I have found this effective in several cases. The usefulness of acupressure with Kundalini is basically untested, however, because few people are available with similar symptoms who are aware of the possibilities for help with this system.

The Nadis & Prana

"The human body may look like a lump of flesh, but that's not really what it is" said Muktananda.

> In fact, it is a wonderful creation, composed of 72,000 nadis, or channels. These nadis, together with the six chakras and nine openings, form a sort of house. It is also sometimes called a twon, composed of seven elements. Of the 72,000 nadis, a hundred are important; and of these hundred, three are most important; and of these three, the central channel, called the sushumna, is supreme. All activities of life are carried out by the sushumna, which extends unbroken from the dwelling place of Parashiva in the sahasrara (the crown) to the side of the Kundalini in muladhara (the base of the spine).[27]

When the nadis are purified prana and the four psychic bodies (the physical and the three kosas of the subtle body) also become pure, and the level of meditation improves. To do this purification Muktananda advised one to sit in the lotus posture for three hours. Yogic breathing practices also purify this complex structure, and are often considered essential to Kundalini awakening.

The three principal nadis (ida, pingala and sushumna), are considered the principle channels of spiritual force in the human system. Pandit described how to awaken Kundalini after one has followed the precepts and preparatory disciplines of yoga by withdrawing prana from the ida and pingala nadis, contracting the anus and collecting energy at the base of the spine until the body is devitalized and all the energy is drawn upward through the sushumna.

> . . . one then would practice opening the Kundalini by sitting in the prescribed asana, palms upward in the lap, with the focus of attention between the eyebrows. Air is inhaled and retained. The upper body is contracted and the upward breath checked, so that air is prevented from going upward and rushes downward. To prevent escape the lower body is

contracted (the anus). The vayu (prana or air)
thus collected goes directly to the muladhara
and the mind and will concentrate on it with
the result that the frictional pressure of prana
and apana held tight together will generate
intense heat, which arouses Kundalini,which
moves upward.The initiate should concentrate
on the mantra and the heart jigatma then
moves down to unite with awakened shakti.
This opens the mouth of the sushumna.[28]

Some texts say the sushumna arises at the base of the spine,
above the anus, and ends at the crown, and others say it ends at the
sixth chakra, the ajna, between the eyebrows. The nadis ida and
pingala also begin from the muladhara and rise towards the spot in
the forehead between the two eyebrows but in a serpentine movement
from left to right in the case of the ida, and inversely from right to
left in the case of the pingala. Many yogis describe these as rising in
a circular path surrounding each chakra but without actually passing
through it in the way the sushumna does. After meeting at the spot
between the eyebrows they separate again. The ida then penetrates
the left nostril, the pingala penetrates the right nostril. These nadis
are subtle and invisible and are only seen through the psychic sense.

Three finer nadis are located inside the sushumna: the vajra,
which regulates electrical energy flow; chitrini, the source of the
sound of the universe; and brahma, which regulates the most subtle
flow and is sometimes identified as the source of libido. Scholar
Mary Scott claims the vajra and chitrini nadis act upon the chakras
more directly than ida or pingala. Chitrini is downward-flowing like
ida, and vajra upward like pingala, both carriers of active pranic
currents. She believes "The sushumna. . . appears mainly to
mediate those stabilizing energies which keep activities in balance
and prevent the too-rapid emergence of consciousness relative to the
body's ability to meet it's demands."[29]

According to Scott's research the flow of prana circulated
through the chitrini supplies the brain and voluntary nerves with
energies from the higher levels of mental matter, and is influenced by
the balance of tamas, rajas and sattva gunas in the system as a whole.
She states that chitrini energy is sattvic, and tends to stimulate
tamas and quiet rajas, thus it is important in stabilizing the system as
Kundalini arises, and it assists in the evolution of the nervous and
glandular systems towards the goal of liberation.

Contributions of Subtle Body Theory

Yogic and tantric literature provides a comprehensive framework with which to explore the nature of pranic energy and its distribution through the body, the powerful effects of breathing techniques on this system, and the potential impact of Kundalini awakening. It demonstrates significant links between the body, the mind and universal consciousness which go far beyond the capacity of models available in Western medicine to explain the experience of Kundalini. It shows specific correlations between various energy centers and emotional problems, and suggests the value of mental discipline and the relationship of psychological health to the activity of Kundalini arising. It describes Kundalini both as the stabilizing force in the normal physical system and a transformative force for those who are adequately prepared. It has provided a framework for the development of a number of healing modalities which work directly with the subtle body and the distribution of prana through the nadis. All of these factors help the therapist or physician to interpret Kundalini symptoms.

Whether or not one seeks a literal understanding of this metaphysical system, as a model it works like a mathematical formula. It is challenging to the mind to accept the presumption of a "mystical' body, yet no more difficult perhaps, than the challenge of modern day physicists to unravel the paradoxes of the submicroscopic phenomena of non-material reality. Physicist Fritjof Capra writes that since the 1920's physicists have had to wrestle with the awareness that the universe is not "a collection of separate objects but rather appears as a web of relations between the various parts of a unified whole", and Capra's explorations have led him to point out strong correlations between Vedantic and Buddhist teachings and the discoveries of quantum physics.[30]

Despite the popular notion that there are basic building blocks in material reality, submicroscopic research serves to invalidate the assumptions about the nature of that basic building block and leave scientists with a roaming particle-wave entity that inconsistently changes form from one to the other. Perhaps the realities of the "material" universe are elusive because they do not exist independently of the thought waves of cosmic creation, just as our physical body may be held together by a web of energies and thought waves in the subtle body, predetermined by an even more elusive potentiality emerging from the causal body. I find subtle body theory very useful as a model with which to map and interpret these elusive waves and processes of the Kundalini experience.

References: Chapter 3

1 Goel, B.S. (1985) Third eye and Kundalini. India: Third Eye Fd., p. 86.
2 Motoyama, H. (1981) Theories of the chakras: Bridge to higher consciousness. Wheaton, Ill: Theosophical Publishing House, p. 241.
3 Tirtha, V. Devatma shakti (Kundalini): Divine power. India: Yoga Shri Peeth Trust, p. xix.
4 Bharati, A. (1982) The tantric tradition. New York: Anchor, Hari Dass, B.(1985) Liberation (unpublished manuscript); Madhusudandasji, D. (1979) Shakti: Hidden treasure of power vol. 1, Pasadena: Dyanyoga Center; Pandit, M. P. (1985) More on tantras.new Delhi: Sterling, and (1979) Kundalini yoga (1979) Pomona, CA: Atmaniketan Ashram.; Tirtha,V. (1948) Op. cit.
      (There are actually 50 other chakras or energy vortices in the body, according to Baba Hari Dass (personal communication), but these six or seven are the ones most commonly identified in Eastern scriptures and are the most significant in relation ship to Kundalini movement.)
5 Muktananda, S. (1979) Kundalini: the Secret of Life. S. Fallsburg, N.Y.: SYDA Fd. p. 16-17.
6 Rieker (1971) The yoga of light: The classic esoteric handbook of Kundalini yoga. Clearlake, CA.: The Dawn Horse. p. 49.
7 Narayanananda, S. (1950). The primal power in Man or the Kundalini Shakti. Gylling, Denmark: N.U.Yoga Trust & Ashrams, p. 19-20.
8 Op. cit,. p. 80-81.
9 Singh, J. (trans) (1979) Vijnanbhairava or Divine consciousness. Delhi: Montilal Banarsidass. p. xv.& (1979) Siva Sutras: the yoga of supreme identity, p. 117.
10 Tirtha, V. Op. cit. p. 55.
11 Op. cit. p. 76.
12 Radha, S. Op. cit., p. 213.
13 Visnudevananda, S. (1960) The complete illustrated book of yoga. New York: Julian, p. 250.
14 Singh, J. (1979) Op. cit., p. 89.
15 Tejomayananda, S. (1977) Introduction to Kashmir Shaivism,

Fallsburg, N.Y. S.Y.D.A. Fd.

16 Tirtha, S. Op. cit., pp 77-78.

17 Mahadevan,T.M.P. (1969) The Pancadasi of Bharatirtha-Vidyaranya,
    Madras: Center for Advanced Study in Philosophy. p. 29.

18 Op. cit., p. 30-32.

19 Anandamurti, S. S. (1971) Subhasita samgraha. India: Accirananda
    Avadhuta p. 90-91.

20 Prasad, R. (trans.) (1889) "The science of breath". Nature's finer
    forces. London: H.P.B. Press. pp. 23-29. (Republished in 1969 by
    Health Research, Mokelumne Hill, CA.)

21 Goswami, S.S. (1980) Layayoga: An advanced method of concentration
    London: Routledge & Kegan Paul, p. 143.

22 Information on chakras and their symbols are compiled primarily from:
    Bose, D. N. and Haldor, H. (1956rev.) Tantras: Their philosophy
    and occult secrets. Calcutta: firma KLM; Goswami, S. S. (1980)
    Op. cit.; Motoyama, (1981) Op. cit.; and Hari Dass, B. (1984)
    Ashtanga yoga teacher's training course 11:Student handbook.
    Watsonville, CA.: Mt. Madonna Center.

23 Information on chakras and their symbols are compiled primarily from:
    Bose, D. N. and Haldor, H. (1956rev.) Tantras: Their philosophy
    and occult secrets. Calcutta: firma KLM; Goswami, S. S. (1980)
    Op. cit.; Motoyama, (1981) Op. cit.; and Hari Dass, B. (1984)
    Ashtanga yoga teacher's training course 11:Student handbook.
    Watsonville, CA.: Mt. Madonna Center.

24 Motoyama, H. (1981) Op. cit., pp. 282--283.

25 Joy, B. (1979) Joy's way: A map for the transformational journey.
    Los Angeles: J. P. Tarcher. p. 159.

26 Op. cit., p. 196.

27 Muktananda, S. (1978) Play of consciousness. Ganeshpuri, India:
    Gurudev Siddha Peeth. p. 31.

28 Pandit, M. P. (1979) Op. cit., p. 52.

29 Scott, M. (1983) Op. cit., p. 178.

30 Capra, F. (1985) Uncommon wisdom, p. 20.

CHAPTER FOUR

WESTERN PHYSIOLOGY: PLEASURE AND PAIN IN THE BRAIN

I felt energy in my head, starting with a
bursting in the throat which felt enormous,
like a goiter, heavy and pulsating; then I would
get shooting pains to the right of the third eye,
and through the middle and back of the head,
accompanied by yellow and white lights. . . .
subject, Jayne

All that we experience as conscious beings happens through
our bodies. We are the producers of our own lives, living within a
vehicle designed to experience and process an infinite range of
phenomena. Our movements, sounds, impulses, emotions,
memories, pleasures, pains, insights, and intelligence spring from
within us and are the resources available to the Self. This Self is
temporarily identified with a particular set of circumstances,
contracted in such a way as to live out who we are. Although the
Kundalini process may be initiated in the subtle body, the physical
body must ultimately carry the impact of it.

It is necessary to explore responses of the physical body to
Kundalini if we are to learn to differentiate between these responses
and illness such as epilepsy, Parkinson's disease, Tourette's
syndrome, brain tumors and other problems that typically produce
similar symptoms, namely jerks and spontaneous random
movements, trance-states, visions, inner sounds, irrational mood
swings, seeing intense lights, euphoria, the sudden reliving of early

memories and many other phenomena. Recent research into patterns that accompany right-brain and temporal-lobe trauma suggests many ways in which brain stimulation by electrical disturbance or chemical interaction can produce Kundalini-like symptoms. These correlations indicate several possibilities:

1. Increased pranic activity and breathing irregularly increases the levels of energy pumped into the brain, or changes brain chemicals and people respond in patterns that correlate with those areas of the brain which are being stimulated -- these may produce vision, sound, memory, movement, emotion and lights.

2. Some spiritual practices stimulate the production of certain brain chemicals that produce emotional swings from ecstasy to depression.

3. Certain states of consciousness promote waves of movement through the brain that set off patterns of physiological and emotional response.

4. As we learn new practices we create expanded neuron networks and interconnections in the brain. If we do nonlinear practices that particularly stimulate the right brain (such as visualization, concentration on lights, chanting and the like) we undoubtedly increase the possibility for greater varieties of right-brained activity, such as creativity, vision, dreams, merging into sound or space, etc.

5. Is it possible there is a part of the brain pre-wired for the unitive experience? The trance-state of some epileptics plunges them into a black void in which they are aware they exist but have no input or capacity to act. How similar is this state to the Buddhist void? Is there a deeper experience where unitive oneness is inevitable? Are yoga practices, shamanic rituals and breathwork simply ways of activating chemicals or stimulating sections in the brain that produce this experience? Would spiritual awakening be any less real just because it was an innate brain process? The brain must also be stimulated when one "falls in love" or writes inspired poetry but these responses are not considered "unreal".

All individuals have unique brains that contain over 15 billion neurons, encoded with many possibilities, according to the genetics of our species, and developed and altered according to our experiences. Learning takes place because neuron pathways develop and link with one another in response to experiences, so that in time great networks interact. Nerve cells communicate through electrical signals that travel along fine extensions, forming millions of cells in complex circuits. It is inappropriate electrical activity, producing irregular or disorganized electrical charges, especially in the superficial areas of the brain, that triggers epileptic seizures and other symptoms of psychomotor disorder. These problems can be hereditary or occur in response to accidents or trauma. Some symptoms of psychomotor epilepsy, which may occur without ever demonstrating a grand mal seizure of the kind the public usually identifies with this illness, are remarkably similar to Kundalini symptoms. These include falling into a trance or fugue-like state; loss of consciousness; visual or auditory hallucination; changes in vision, hearing, smell and taste; the appearance of lights; localized numbness; deja-vu (familiarity, as if one has been there before); and jamais-vu (a sense that a well-known place is foreign to one).

Factors known to trigger seizures in epileptics include starvation, dehydration, exhaustion, seeing a flashing light, infections, drug or alcohol abuse, dental problems, foot infections, viral syndromes and gum infections. A few of these factors are reflected in certain spiritual practices such as fasting, staring at a candle, and meditating long hours. Early warning signs of epilepsy include staring spells, bedwetting, memory gaps, wandering aimlessly, nocturnal tongue-biting, and having violent muscle spasms in sleep. Sometimes meditators fall into trances, experience short-term mental confusion, wander aimlessly and wake up with muscle spasms. We need to be able to differentiate qualitatively and quantitatively between the two experiences if one is not to be misinterpreted as the other. It is as unfortunate for someone with Kundalini symptoms to believe they are neurologically ill as it is for one with epilepsy to go untreated.

It is important not to ignore the possible diagnosis of psychomotor epilepsy, or another disease that triggers epileptic symptoms, when there is pervasive evidence of these symptoms, especially if there are indications of a prior history, family hereditary factors, or a recent accident which might have triggered it. This does not mean one needs to discount any spiritual components of the process should this seem significant to the individual involved, for there is no reason that epilepsy would preclude an experience of spiritual awakening. However, if someone has many of these symptoms, and is unable to gain any control over them, it will be appropriate to place them in the hands of a competent neurologist for an evaluation, especially if the trance states are dark and uncomfortable, and spontaneous rather than correlated with meditation.

Understanding brain physiology need not reduce mystical experience to a quasi-epileptic phenomenon. It could lay a foundation to support Eastern theories that emphasize the developmental steps of spiritual awakening. Since learning takes place through the growth and interweaving of neuron patterns, it may be that unique practices such as yoga, meditation, visualization, breathwork, etc. may weave new strengths and possibilities in parts of the brain that would otherwise lay fallow, most likely the right-side of the brain. Artists, musicians and others with creative genius show evidence of greater right-brained development than people who pursue more intellectual and rational studies. If spiritual processes develop more of the right brain, this would explain the sudden surge of creative activity in many who have spiritual awakenings. It may also explain the capacities for healing and psychic insight that emerge spontaneously, sometimes after accidents that damage the right brain, as well as in the context of spiritual growth.

A Few Brain Functions

The following is a very simple description of some of the functions of the brain, and indicates how various patterns and processes occur which may have some bearing on the response of the brain during the Kundalini process. It is interesting to speculate on the interaction between the natural and "normal" functioning of the brain and the radical changes that may be occurring with Kundalini.

There are three distinguishable subdivisions of brain development, informally labeled reptilian (a depository for unlearned preprogrammed behavior, deeply buried beneath the surface); the old mammalian or paleomammalian (the limbic system's headquarters for emotions, survival and preservation concerns, pleasure and pain); and the neomammalian or neocortex (connected with the most recently developed capacities of civilized humans -- invention, abstract thought, and insight). Paul MacLean, creator of this triune brain theory, states that these three in one operate like "three interconnected biological computers, (each) with its own special intelligence, its own subjectivity, its own sense of time and space and its own memory."[1]

The Cortex

The cortex wraps around the brain in seven layers, contains 70% of the neurons of the central nervous system, and creates our capacities for speech, sight and sense capability. Each layer has varying numbers and kinds of cells. Firing between neurons sets up circuits in the brain called cell assemblies or neural nets, which interact and branch together in response to sensory stimuli. The largest number of cells in the brain are called "glial" (which means glue). Scientist and physician Richard Restak (The Brain: The Last Frontier) describes these as having a nutrient function, and indicates they have a relationship to the initiation and termination of seizures. There is some evidence they have their own communicating network.

Dr. Marion Diamond, a professor and scientist at UC/ Berkeley found in her research with rats that when they were stimulated by living in enriched environments their brain chemistry changed and their cerebral cortices thickened by an average of 7%. Nerve cells grew larger and glial cells multiplied, chemical connection between the cells improved, and the dendrites lengthened and added new spines. [2] She discovered the brain's capacity to change and grow, a revolutionary idea in the 60's.

The Brain Stem

This is the major connecting source for sensory and motor signals between the spinal cord and the brain. It maintains consciousness through the mechanisms for breathing, heartbeat, sleeping and waking.It includes the reticular activating system, which keeps the brain awake even while sleeping and spreads alertness through excitation of the brain in response to stimuli; and the pons, which controls dreaming and waking. Just above the brain stem is the diencephalon, which is dominated by the thalamus. All signals of the eyes, ears and sense organ pass through this organ on the way to the cortex. Next to this is the hypothalamus, which signals the release of hormones from the glands, and to which all parts of the limbic system are linked bidirectionally. These hormones regulate blood pressure, body temperature and appetite control centers. Damages to various parts of the hypothalamus will cause animals to stop eating or trigger gorging to the death. Electrical stimulation to parts of the hypothalamus triggers panic, rage and fear. Irregularities in eating patterns, heat and cold flashes, raised blood pressure and inexplicable emotional states occurring in Kundalini could therefore be responses of the hypothalamus to chemical or energetic changes.

The Cerebellum

Attached to the brain stem at the back of the skull, the cerebellum processes input from muscles, joints and tendons, and controls postures, equilibrium and movement. It contains movements within reasonable boundaries so that arms do not flail wildly when one is trying to engage in activity. It is likely a reaction in the cerebellum that causes arms or legs to flail out randomly during a Kundalini episode. The paleocerebellum governs proprioception -- our sense of ourselves as a body, which affects our balance and the ability to move. It holds a pattern in a giant feedback loop through the septum, hippocampus and amygdala, which carries electrical input from muscles, joints and tendons. Experiences of feeling weightless, out-of-the body, bigger than the body, or unable to control the body and depersonalization (lack of identification with the body or with parts of the body/ not knowing who one is) are connected to inadequate functioning of the cerebellum or cerebellar-limbic nerve connections.

Researcher and psychologist James Prescott says "to experience profound states of consciousness you've got to have the neural equipment. Sensory experience must be integrated into higher brain centers and that requires a cerebellar-limbic-neocortex connection." He says many people in our culture cannot experience this connection because our cultural preoccupation with anhedonia (joylessness) has stunted our neural pleasure systems. He believes women have neurocircuitry better suited to real spirituality because of the rich nerve connections between the cerebellum and the higher brain centers. He suggests that the difference in the cerebellum is responsible for floating, out-of-body sensations and the feeling of union in female orgasms.[3]

The Cerebrum

This is the newest development of the brain, covering 2/3 of its content, divided into two almost mirror-like hemispheres, the right, which controls the left side of the body, and the left, which controls the right side of the body. Visual perception is crossed correspondingly. The left side of the brain is oriented to time, analysis and logic. It seeks reason and explanation. The right side is oriented to space. When spontaneous activities are elicited through right-brain stimulation in the laboratory, the left-brain will construct a theory to explain it. There are kinds of brain damage in which it appears that the brain is split in such a way that one side has no awareness at all of what the other side does, and some scientists have speculated that problems such as split personality derive from this kind of brain dysfunction. (Psychologists might well argue this, as split personality can be healed through psychotherapy.)

It is interesting to speculate about the ways in which the struggle develops between the spiritual side, the creative or the Taoistic flowing aspects of human nature, and the more rigid, concretized and security-minded self during processes of individuation and spiritual awakening. The right side of the brain may hold the template of spiritual experience, activated through spiritual practices, while the left-brain holds the template for management of the civilized material world. The flow of ida and pingala nadis may represent at the subtle level the need to bring into balance and order the activities of these two sides.

The Limbic System

Located in the depths of the cerebrum, this part of the brain is a lobe which surrounds the brain stem and has extensive connections with the olfactory structures, drives and emotional responses and the storage of memory. It occupies the lower one-fifth of the brain. Experiments in stimulating the limbic system indicate that certain cells hold rage, joy or fear, but that which cells do what seems to vary among individuals and from day to day.

Psychiatrist Daniel Weinberger states "Electrodes in this area produce schizophrenialike phenomena, such as 'forced thinking', bodily illusions, fear, ineffable somological experiences, paranoia. If the connections between the limbic forebrain and the frontal lobe are disordered, you've lost one of the highest integrative systems in the brain."[4]   All of these symptoms sound precisely like some of the core vulnerabilities during Kundalini awakening -- unpredictable thoughts and images, body sensations and movements, and fears. Theoretically, spiritual awakening launches a direct assault against the drives and emotions, challenging one to move beyond instinctual responses. Such energy may produce confusion and unbalance the integrative capacities. This would explain in theory why there is value in the long disciplined apprenticeship designed to precede awakening, which helps one establish habits and perspectives beyond the range of ordinary responses to drives and emotions.

The Lobes

There are four set of lobes. The temporal lobes are above the ears on either side of the head, and connect to the limbic system. They appear to function like memory and storage systems, and long-term memory is damaged if they are injured. Electrical stimulation to this area triggers out-of-context emotions, weird reveries or dreamy states, deja-vu (a sense of familiarity) and jamais-vu (the familiar seems foreign). People with temporal-lobe epilepsy (which is an infusion of chaotic energy) may have none of the seizures commonly thought to be epileptic, and instead have these primary symptoms.

Electrical probes in this area produce sudden flashes of the past, including all the emotions, sounds and smells of the event.

Neurologist Oliver Sachs attributes the experience of powerful imagery, mystical experiences such as those of Hildegarde of Bergin, and the feeling of being transported in time and space, to abnormal stimulation of the temporal lobes and limbic system. He considers the possibility that such experiences, even if induced by epilepsy, may be "portals to the beyond or the unknown."[5]

Stanford neuro-physiologist Karl Pribram has reported that "A lesion in the temporal lobe near the amygdala can produce something akin to mysticism.   There is a disruption in self-awareness. There is a kind of consciousness-without-content, like the oceanic consciousness of the mystical state. The distinction between the self and the other disappear."[6] Paul MacLean reports that during temporal-lobe seizures people may have "this Eureka feeling all out of context -- feelings of revelation, that this is the truth, the absolute truth, and nothing but the truth."[7]

Arnold Mandell, physician, philosopher and professor at U.C. San Diego, says that temporal-lobe epileptics may experience "long-lasting beatific states, permanent personality changes, and religious conversions."[8] He thinks mystical revelations spring from a state similar to epilepsy, which he likens to a raging electrical storm in part of the brain. Ordinarily the cells of the hippocampus, a brain structure shaped like a sea-horse which is critical to memory formation, are inhibited by a chemical called serotonin. When this is deficient they fire in over-excited kindlinglike fashion. The hippocampus ordinarily modulates information between inner and outer environments, seems to generate a movement toward novelty (exploring something new), and adjusts moods and emotions to incoming data. When this electrical storm overpowers its function the inner reality becomes dominant. Hallucinogenic drugs dampen serotonin in order to create their psychedelic affect. So do long-distance running and meditation.[9]

The parietal lobes stretch over the cortex of the brain, and hold maps covering every inch of both motor and tactile regions of the body. This is the area identified by Itzhak Bentov and Lee Sannella as the site of a speculated progressive sensory-motor cortex syndrome -- the physio-kundalini complex. A sequence of points (distributed roughly in the shape of a man) correlate sequentially to a pattern of symptoms the two had identified as a typical response to Kundalini awakening. That is if each of these points were stimulated sequentially they would follow a pattern of symptoms often reported with Kundalini that begin with the left toe, (further described later in this chapter). Bentov stated that in epileptic conditions the sequence of symptoms moved in the direction opposite from that of Kundalini, beginning with lips and face and ending in the feet. He therefore speculated that Kundalini could be a potential antidote for epilepsy and suggested that meditation, which could trigger it, might reverse the pattern of the disease.

The frontal lobes are in the front of the brain, behind the forehead (the area of the third eye, and the sixth chakra), the section of brain once commonly lobotomized to cure violent and distractable behavior. Originally brain scientists felt it was not an important area for overall functioning. But lesions (and lobotomies) here cause great distractability, the inability to carry out complex actions, listlessness, shallowness in thought and feeling, insensitivity, and poor organization of intellectual activity. Some researchers have concluded that this area probably controls awareness, self-awareness and the quality of empathy.[10]

The occipital lobe, containing the primary visual area, is located at the back of the head. Damage here causes loss of the visual field, or blindness.

Chemical Correlations

It was not until the discoveries of the chemists in the 1960's that the potential existed for creating laboratory chemicals that duplicated chemicals in the human body, which made possible their ingestion to adjust body chemistry, and stimulated wide-ranging research. All moods, compulsions, emotions and behaviors involve a complicated interaction of chemicals labeled by brain scientists as neurotransmitters, precurser enzymes, metabolizing enzymes and neuropeptides (brain-hormones). Until the 1970's only six neurotransmitters were identified, but now it is known there are at least 100 to 200 others waiting to be defined and understood. Receptors in the brain are custom-designed to respond to these chemicals, and other chemicals may block their receptivity.

For example there are natural opiates in the brain and specific receptors to receive them. Although they have a variety of Latin names they are commonly called endorphins, short for "endogenous morphine." These are potent painkillers and there is evidence they are the reasons certain analgesics work -- acupuncture, electrical brain stimulation and the placebo effect. Compulsive runners have been found to have elevated beta-endorphin levels as do anorexics, schizophrenics and meditators.[11]

Following research showing that baby guinea pigs, puppies and chicks stopped crying for their mother when given low levels of endorphins, Scientist Jack Panksepp surmised that "Perhaps brain opiate systems can create feelings of belonging, so people who are lonely and isolated can use narcotics as a substitute for interpersonal bonds."[12]

Long-distance runners have long credited production of endorphins for the euphoria that follows a race. Other activities that naturally trigger endorphin release are eating, music, pleasurable events, massage, meditation -- all the natural highs! It is clear that this chemical stimulates a strong sense of well-being. Laboratory rats, when given the option of self-administering endorphins, will self-stimulate to the point of starvation and exhaustion.

The brain receptors that receive opiates (endorphins) are in a recently evolved area of the brain, and parts of the brain are crowded with them. Their function appears to be to receive information from the environment, and communicate and interpret it so the brain can decide what to pay attention to. In other words they acknowledge pleasure and encourage the brain to notice it.

Although extremely seductive for drug-users, research shows that the use of opiates will not induce a permanent euphoria. Long-term use of cocaine, heroin and other street drugs cause depression, apathy and withdrawal conditions. These are concomitant conditions for some meditative experiences, and those who follow spiritual practices are amazed to discover that following a blissful meditative hour, they are sometimes irritable.   It is possible that when one breaks through from the "disciplined" meditation into the stage of feeling peace and pleasure consistently in meditation, they have triggered the endorphin system through deep concentration. (Similarly to the hybernating animal, who also has high endorphin levels and is oblivious to cold weather and activity outside itself.)

Flashes of visions (or makyo, as this is labeled in Zazen), body numbness, involuntary movements and jerks, reduced sexual interest (or spontaneous sexual arousal), and reduced appetite are all responses that some people experience in meditation which may well correlate with increased endorphin levels.   The released opiates produced are sending messages to the brain that are interpreted as positive and one experiences spontaneous pleasure and contentment with what is. The capacity of yogis to detach from home, family and emotional relationships may also be a correlate of endorphin flooding. Endorphins undoubtedly account in part for the emotional ups and down that accompany awakening spiritual energy. It may be that when spiritual seekers stabilize their energy what is happening is that a steady stream of endorphins are being released in the body. There is also evidence that when endorphin levels increase in the brain, they are reduced in the spine. So it may be that certain yogic breathing and visual practices, or activities like kriya yoga, where concentration is focused on moving energy up the spine, may be moving endorphins from the spine into the brain receptors until high level of pleasures are produced.

In the 1950's scientists discovered that the reduction of another brain chemical, dopamine, decreased the hallucinations experienced by schizophrenics, and believed the disease was due to dopamine imbalances complicated by varieties of neurochemical system disturbances. Other researchers identified dopamine as an amplifier for all sensory input, and said the real disturbance had to do with the way sensory input affected the brain. Various studies have promoted a variety of conclusions regarding the parts of the brain which must be "damaged" or "abnormal' to produce such input.

Dopamine receptors appear to decrease with age, the male brain losing about 40% and the female about 25%. This has an impact on psychomotor coordination. A deficiency of dopamine in some brain pathways is also known to trigger shaking limbs, rigid musculature and the blank stare that accompanies Parkinson's disease. The drug levodopa (L-dopa) brought many people who suffered Parkinson's back to life after spending years in the back wards of hospitals. However its side-effects included hallucinations, delirium, murderous rages, involuntary movements, delusions, ticks and compulsive growling.[13] (Many of these symptoms are occasionally reported in stories of Kundalini arousal, so perhaps dopamine levels rise at times in this process.)

Another natural chemical transmitter, acetylcholine, when injected into the septal area of the brain, causes vigorous activity including multiple sexual orgasms, lasting as long as 30 minutes. Spontaneous orgasms are also frequently reported in people who experience Kundalini awakening.

It is clear that various chemical receptors respond to increases and decreases of chemicals in the brain by creating dramatic emotional, visual and physiological phenomena. Activities which utilize breath, energy, visualization and other kinds of sensory input may impact the stimulation of such chemicals. Much is left to be identified and understood about brain chemistry in general (only a fraction of chemicals has even been identified), and it is impossible to do any more than speculate about the correlations between chemically-produced imbalances and sensorily-stimulated activities, although correlations between drug experiences and mystic experiences have consistently been noted in the literature.

Arnold Mandell has produced some of the most substantive research exploring links between brain chemistry and transcendent experience, reported in a paper titled "Toward a Psychology of Transcendence: God in the Brain", included in a book exploring consciousness and biology, The Psychobiology of Consciousness (1980). In it he theorizes "there is a biogenic aminetemporal-limbic neurology for transformed consciousness" and "Western man turning inward for metaphysical solutions has biological mechanisms with which to rationalize the journey."[14] He develops his theories based on biological psychiatry related to what is called the pharmacological bridge, and the mechanisms which control the system of forebrain limbic excitation, and credits William James for introducing "the proposition that transcendental experience was similar wherever he examined it and that the most commonly evoked source, God, was in the brain."[15]

Mandell cites numerous research efforts which present a startling case for the concept of "God in the brain." He hypothesizes that it is possible that a decrease and/or release of seratonin (which can be caused by the use of amphetamines, cocaine and hallucinogens as well as meditation or running) inhibits the regulation of hippocampal pyramidal cells, leading to their hyperexcitability and the loss of the cell's " gating" tendency (a tendency to match external events with internal responses). This leads to unitive experience and a sense of having found "truth", as one is no longer using the comparative and evaluative function of the brain. In addition, "Increased excitability in temporal lobe limbic structures as reflected in synchronous discharges from the region are associated with personality changes similar to those seen with religious conversion."[16] This appears to occur because the cells in the hippocampus overexcite themselves and die, creating a neurological state of transcendent consciousness, and an experience of emotional flooding called ecstasy. He believes this cell death may account for the permanent and positive changes reported in personality following an experience of religious transcendence. A number of researchers have found that these cells are dead in the brains of psychomotor epileptics who report experiencing religious conversion, hyposexuality, transcendent consciousness, good nature and emotional deepening. He speculates that "repeated or overwhelming episodes of loss of serotonin inhibition" may occur in those who follow prolonged running, meditation or the use of hallucinogens, thus duplicating the kinds of personality changes attributed to transcendent experience.[17]

What is clear from the scores of papers collected and synthesized by Mandell is that biochemical reactions can produce symptoms or phenomena closely akin to some of those demonstrated by people during a Kundalini process or a spiritual awakening. This includes reported ecstasy, unitive awareness, interest in spiritual matters, compulsive writing, a conviction of insight and long-term positive personality changes. But many questions must be raised when we pursue this line of research, which presently omits any study of people clearly identified as Kundalini-awakened or mystics. Mandell has merged many terms under the heading transcendent experience, as varied as St. Paul"s "peace that passeth understanding", Maslow's "peak experience", Jung's "individuation", Lao Tse's "the absolute Tao", satori, samadhi, Gopi Krishna's Kundalini awakening, and terms such as "divine spirit" and "intensity experience".[18] It is a safe conjecture that many of these experiences, subjectively described, vary from one another substantially, to say nothing of their variations from the experiences of those having a seizure, taking a drug, or being poked with an electrical probe in a laboratory. All extraordinary experiences are not the same, nor are they likely to share a single cause.

However there are enough correlates that it is reasonable to assume that meditation, breathing practices and the awakened Kundalini may have an impact on brain chemistry or electrical function. In fact some Eastern teachers have indicated that the Kundalini process entirely redesigns the structure of the cells, and others see the restructuring of the human brain as an evolutionary necessity made possible by Kundalini awakening.

But there are dangers in using Mandell's "biogenic aminetemporal lobe limbic neurology" as a catch-all description of the brain's response to ecstatic, unitive and transcendental states. Do we then assume all mystics suffer temporal-lobe epilepsy, or that all epileptic seizures are spontaneous efforts toward mysticism? Do we give the brain complete credit for all aspects of consciousness, eliminating in one stroke thousands of years of mystical teachings? Or are such teachings only a response to an instinctive move toward brain evolution, nudging us toward a destiny of living in attunement with the temporal lobes as their cells are dying and slower waves are wafting through the brain?

This approach implies that years of spiritual practices and the greatest teaching of saints are simply a result of biochemical changes which could as easily be gained through drugs or an electrical probe in the brain. Such a quick fix appeals greatly to Western egos, If it is so clearly possible to turn sinners into saints, antagonism into love, and rage into peace with a pill or a probe perhaps we should engage these techniques on populations of hard-core criminals, turning them into the likes of Anandamayi Ma, Krishnamurti, Yogananda and similar loving and wise presences. If drugs created true mystics we would have no concern about their proliferation in ghettos, schools and corporations, and would anticipate enlightenment from those we currently treat for addiction, abuse and drug-related crimes.

Another danger is that of reducing what is a powerful healing and transformative event to a biochemical malfunction of the brain. The brain may be designed to be ultimately opened to transcendent and unitive experiences, ecstasy and insight, but it is hardly an illness should this occur. As the brain is attuned and develops a capacity to withstand stepped-up pranic energies and divine intuitions it can perhaps open more to dimensions beyond the range of Western science and glimpse a consciousness existing far beyond itself. Perhaps a transformed temporal lobe is the nub of the future brain, the next step in evolution. Perhaps the slower rhythms engaged in a transcendent experience are a correlate to those sattwic (harmonious) qualities of the causal body, which as they permeate human consciousness make possible liberation. However it occurs we may hope for an evolutionary process which gives us greater access to wisdom, harmony and creativity.

Mandell's theories suggest some interesting potentials for research into the nature of the changes triggered by Kundalini awakening and other mystical experiences if they can be used as a two-way door -- not to reduce the mystical experience to a simple (or even a complex) brain function, but to open consideration of brain function in relationship to cosmic awareness, to see the temporal lobe (or the unexamined frontal lobes, the location of the third eye) as points from which to expand into a range of wisdom beyond intellectually-dominated dualistic thinking. At this point cosmology and biology may begin to merge.

Brain-Wave Theories

Itzhak Bentov, a creative inventor of biomedical equipment who did much research with the human nervous system, and reportedly had personal experiences with Kundalini energy, defined what he labeled the physio-kundalini syndrome, following his work using ballistocardiography to study physiological changes which occurred in the bodies of meditators. This syndrome was later described in the work of physician Lee Sannella, and has been used as a model for describing the Kundalini process to physicians.

Bentov observed that certain mechanical vibrations, electromagnetic waves or sounds could trigger in a laboratory a response in non-meditators that was similar to waves produced in the brain through meditation. He rigged up a biofeedback system using a pulsating magnetic field around the head that stimulated such waves. In an effort to explain spontaneous Kundalini awakening he suggested that people with particularly sensitive nervous systems might react spontaneously to exposure to similar frequencies for prolonged periods of time, such as by riding in a car whose suspension and seat combination produce that range of vibration, or by sitting for long periods next to an air-conditioning duct.

Bentov related the mildness or severity of symptoms to the amount of stress held in the body, and emphasized that only when Kundalini reaches these areas of stress do symptoms become troublesome. He cited researcher Hans Selye's work with stress to support the fact that the nervous system can be so busy handling stresses that its potential for attaining higher states of consciousness is very limited. He believed that this was why all schools of meditation emphasize the importance of calming down the body. These stresses are actually energy patterns, that must be converted and eliminated, and this usually occurs involuntarily through body movements, unexpected emotional releases, or inexplicable pains in some area of the body. He recommended meditation with light body-toning exercises, such as some hatha yoga postures, and mild breathing exercises, as the most effective, inexpensive and fastest system for the removal of stress from the body. Bentov identified the physio-kundalini syndrome as:

> A sequence of bodily symptoms (which) usually starts at the left foot or toes, either as a mild tingling stimulus or as cramps. The stimulus continues up the left leg to the hip. In extreme cases, there is a paralysis of the foot and of the whole leg. Loss of sensation in large areas of the skin of the leg may occur. From the hip the stimulus moves up the spine to the head. Here sometimes severe headaches (pressure-like) may develop. In case of prolonged and severe pressures in the head,

degeneration of the optical nerve may set in,
with accompanying visual impairment, loss
of memory and general disorientation. [19]

Bentov identified this progressive sensory-motor cortex
syndrome with the physiology of Kundalini, but he emphasized that
this concept is larger than physiology because planetary and spiritual
forces also come into play. In his physiological model meditators
produce acoustical standing waves in the cerebral ventricles which
trigger heart sounds that cause vibrations in the walls of ventricles
(fluid-filled cavities in the brain). These vibrations will stimulate and
eventually "polarize" the cortex in such a way that it will tend to
conduct a signal along the homunculus in a closed-loop pattern, starting from the toes up, which is in contrast to the way the brain
normally handles a signal. He tried to show that the layout of points
corresponds closely to the path the Kundalini takes in the body, as
described in esoteric literature. He felt the states of bliss obtained by
those who experience this closed loop of energy may occur as a self-
stimulation of the pleasure centers in the brain, caused by the
circulation of a "current" along the sensory cortex.

Bentov described most of the symptoms as occurring on the
left side of the body, and therefore termed it mostly a development
occurring in the right hemisphere, which he said follows logic, since
we are using our reasoning, rational, logical, linear thinking left
hemisphere all the time, while meditation tends to stimulate the
nonverbal, feeling, intuitive right hemisphere.

Dr. Sannella, a psychiatrist and ophthalmologist, drew on
Bentov's theories when he published a brief but significant study of
the Kundalini process, Kundalini --Psychosis or Transcendence, (later
expanded and updated as The Kundalini Experience) and he also
addressed the similarity of some psychotic symptoms to Kundalini
symptoms, saying that people were inappropriately diagnosed and
treated due to the inability of the medical profession to identify this
experience. He included 11 cases of subjects with physical and
emotional symptoms related to Kundalini, and differentiated the
characteristics that distinguish Kundalini from psychosis.

He wrote that people with Kundalini symptoms often
experience hearing voices, seeing visions, and moving in patterns
that seem irrational to the uninitiated, so are sometimes subjected to
medication and confinement in institutions. But they are different
from psychotics in that they are rarely inclined to act out if feeling
hostile or angry, are more objective about themselves and interested
in sharing what is going on in them, and are more likely to

experience sensations of heat, vibrations, tinglings and itches that move in definite patterns over the body. They may see bright lights internally, experience pains in their heads, demonstrate unusual breathing patterns or spontaneous movements, and hear chirping or whistling sounds. Voices are heard, but these are perceived to come from within and are not mistaken for other realities. He stated that the outcome of Kundalini awakening, when handled appropriately, was generally positive and creative, with the subjects reporting less stress, more fulfillment, and more inner peace.[20]

Sannella also said that in some cases a schizophrenic-like condition can result if the person receives negative feedback from others, or feels resistance to interpretation regarding the Kundalini experiences. He speculated that people who were psychic were most susceptible to awakening Kundalini and most likely to find the process violent and disturbing, because they had especially sensitive nervous systems. Many of his subjects had some psychic experience prior to awakening. He suggested that there may be three categories of responses to spiritual practices -- visionary, psychic and Kundalini experiences.

Comments of Dr. Sannella's, given in a talk at the U.C. Medical School in San Francisco in the Spring of 1981, have been circulated in a California hospital to inform physicians of Kundalini symptoms. In this memo Kundalini is presented as an unusual neurological complex or syndrome appearing among some meditators. It describes the following signs:

> Its motor signs are swaying, shaking, jump-
> ing, twitching, posturing, grimacing, crying
> out, and unusual patterns of breathing. The
> sensory experiences are the seeing or sensing
> of internal lights and hearing internal sounds,
> very hot and cold areas on or inside the body,
> tingling, numbness, pain, partial paralysis,
> ecstasy, fear, and entrancement. The amount of
> energy involved seems inexplicable in normal
> metabolic terms. When the process ends nat-
> urally, the disturbances abate and the per-
> sonality may be permanently changed. . . .The
> symptoms suggest internal stimulation or
> hypersensitivity of the sensory-motor cortex
> and deeper underlying and adjoining structures
> of the brain. A neuro-physiological model
> based on resonances generated in the meditator

has been formulated by Itzhak Bentov to explain this phenomenon. It has been partially confirmed by measurements of sounds heard and of changes in the body's micromotions during meditation.[21]

Dr. Sannella's acceptance in medical circles allows him to make a significant contribution towards alleviating the misdiagnosis of the Kundalini experience, and he is able to use Bentov's neurophysiological model aligned with medical terminology in a way that makes it understandable to the medical field. The majority of therapists and physicians who have any awareness of Kundalini have likely obtained it based on Bentov's and Sannella's theories.

It is questionable, however, whether Bentov's work is related to Kundalini so much as to pranic releases. Since he writes of simulating these conditions in the laboratory, there seems to be an absence of samadhi-like states, and the outcome of releasing the stressors appears to be primarily relaxation, it is likely the subjects are not experiencing a true Kundalini awakening.

Mary Scott, who spent years in India researching the nature of Kundalini energy, wrote that Bentov's and Sannella's work is ingenious and well-reasoned and makes out a good case for a definite physiological mechanism. She added "Whether this mechanism or the cycle have any direct connection with Kundalini as this shakti is understood in tantra is, however, far from clear. . ." And she theorized that the complex Bentov identified may be more related to locked-in brain waves correlated with deep relaxation states achieved in meditation; to stress patterns caused by conflicts between interference with the natural patterns of the psyche; or to splits between the surface and subliminal levels of the self.

Scott pointed out the disruptive nature of taking on the change of orientation that accompanies many who adopt meditation practices and the pressures on the ego when an emergent subliminal system pushes to remove it from the center stage of the psyche, and impulses are coming from two centers of control, the ego and the Self. She theorized that movement and distribution of energy in the two subtle bodies would create excess stress at the root of the sushumna, from which all the nadis rise, which might then trigger the physio-kundalini syndrome.[22]

It seems to me that recognition of the physio-kundalini syndrome need not prove or disprove the awakening of Kundalini, but is descriptive of the pranic symptoms that meditators may experience. It may be a sign of an inner conflict between ego and Self, as Scott suggests, or a symptom related to certain blockages in the subtle body that one taps into during altered states, or it could be a response triggered by stimulation to the brain.

Fire & the Big Toe

Bentov's observation of activity in the left toe has an interesting correlate with a yogic practice of reflection on the right toe in order to raise fire in the body. This stirring of activity in the toes of the uninitiated may be a spontaneous response, like a kriya, because it mirrors an ancient yogic sakti practice. In the 4th sutra of the Siva Sutras a method of contemplation is taught that is said to bring about the dissolution of identification of the gross, subtle and causal bodies by using the image of burning up successively the entire subtle body system. The initiate does this through contemplation on the right toe, in which the deity of burning light, Kalagni Rudra, is housed. The aspirant focuses on this burning imagery, allowing it to rise throughout the system until complete absorption into divine consciousness is experienced. This practice is called *dahabhavana*.[23]

This practice is also notable because of rumors that many people hear about yogis who "burn up" or disappear in a blaze of spontaneous combustion. This may well be linked to a literal interpretation of this ancient practice of Kashmir Saivism. It is certainly possible for over-zealous manipulation of heat and prana to "burn out" or damage the physical and subtle body systems, just as drug use and other kinds of abuse can do. But the only concrete evidence I have come across that such a thing might occur literally is in the remarkable story of St. Catherine of Genoa, a Christian mystic who seems to have burned to death internally.

St. Catherine was a 15th century Italian, a married noblewoman who led a life of social action, self-sacrifice, austerity and contemplation. She frequently reported unbearable heat as well as ecstasy and she endured long periods unable to eat. During the four months before her death at age 63, she underwent an illness so intense that not a part of her body was free from a torment by fire, including much internal bleeding, and vomiting gallons of blood so hot that it boiled. Numerous doctors studied this phenomena and labeled it supernatural. During this period she experienced visions of God and for two days she was in a trance where she saw a vision of herself without body and without soul, with her spirit "completely in

God, and having lost sight of heaven and earth, as if she no longer existed."[24] This is clearly the "dissolution" the sutras describe.

On another day she felt a nail driven into her heart, which caused great pain for ten hours. The next day she felt great joy and "saw a ray of divine love that was almost unbearable and burned up her humanity" and "saw a ladder of flame and felt herself drawn upwards, experiencing great joy therein". Because of the internal heat she asked if the world was on fire, and all were amazed that she could stay alive at all given the intensity of the fire, and the fact she was unable to take any food or water. Her body turned completely yellow, and remained so after death, when it appeared dried up but showed no other signs of deterioration. It still exists intact in a crystal casket in the Pammatone Hospital chapel in Genoa.[25]

Whether or not Catherine's fire began in the big toe, it clearly affected the blood. In the acupressure system the big toe is the source point of the spleen meridian which stores blood and destroys old blood cells, produces plasma cells which make antibodies, and is tied to the immunologic system. It modulates energy in the body and affects the connective tissue, the blood, mouth, tongue and taste sense. It is said to have peculiar affinity for certain aspects of sexual maturing and creative processes, and acupuncturist Mary Austin wrote it may "impact tardy developments and intellectual blockages" and "nurture higher psychological states", as well as figure "prominently in treatment of genitalia malfunctions, both male and female."[26] This suggests that intense energy through it might impact sexuality, psychological states and mental clarity. It may be that meditation or laboratory experiments with energy may send an overload of energy through this meridian, which contributes to problems from the toe upwards, and accounts for some of the symptoms. Excessive heat focused on the toe would impact and heat the blood and thus could easily bring a sensation of fire flashing through the entire body.

Bliss & the Brain

While judging from the easy addiction of laboratory rats it is quite likely that something akin to blissful experiences can be triggered by the stimulation of a certain pleasure center in the brain, there does not appear to be only one kind of bliss associated with Kundalini, nor does Kundalini need to be awakened in order to experience stimulation of this pleasure center. Experiments with laboratory rats indicate that if this point is stimulated they will become so addicted to it they will no longer bother to eat, and I would surmise this does not indicate they have awakened Kundalini, which brings with it a capacity for higher consciousness. In humans who are not being manipulated by electric probes the bliss of the reactive pleasure center is more likely the consequence of a deeply relaxed state of consciousness that redistributes, reorganizes or increases pranic activity so that it will stimulate this point.

There are scriptures that state 27 kinds of bliss accompany awakening, and I have recorded a wide range of these, ranging from bliss isolated in particular body parts such as the legs or jaw, or along one side of the body only, to feeling completely disengaged with the body and being dissolved into another field entirely, to being seized with ecstatic energy rolling down the shoulders or up the spine when doing activities totally unrelated to meditation or relaxation (like walking down the street). Bliss can occur as intense uncontrollable heart energy radiating outward, or as a sensation like melting when two people merge their energetic fields. It can vibrate the body the way a harpist plucks the strings, sending delicious rivulets of energy throughout. It can feel like firecrackers going off inside. It can be an utter, indescribable sinking into peace and understanding. It can be a flash, or it can last for days. The intensity and quality vary incredibly, and it does not seem possible to me that all of it is generated by the same isolated flow of energy identified by Bentov, or one simple pleasure center in the brain, nor to the decreased seratonin described by Mandell.

References: Chapter 4
1   Hooper, J. and Teresi, D. (1986) The 3-pound universe, N.Y.: Dell, p.43.
2   Cohen, Susan, "The real brain" West magazine , S.J. Mercury News, Jan. 7, 1990, p. 6-11.
3   Hooper, J, and Teresi, D. Op. cit., p. 179.
4   Op. cit., p. 114.
5   Sacks, O. (1985) The man who mistook his wife for a hat, New York: Harper and Row, pp. 30- 131.
6   Hooper, J. and Teresi, D. Op. cit. p. 48.
7   Op. cit.
8   Op. cit., p. 330.

9 Op. cit., p. 331.

10 Op. cit., p. 40-41.

11 Op. cit., p. 80.

12 Op. cit., p. 81.

13 Op. cit., p. 75.

14 Davidson, J. and Davidson, R.(Eds.) (1980) The psychobiology of consciousness, New York: Plenum Press, pp. 379-464.

15 Op. cit. p 381-382.

16 Op. cit. p. 400.

17 Op. cit.

18 Op. cit. p. 439.

19 Bentov, I. (1977) Stalking the wild pendulum. New York: Bantam. p. 213.

20 Sannella, L. (1976) Kundalini -- psychosis or transcendence. San Francisco: H. S. Dakin; Sannella, L.(1987) The Kundalini experience. Lower Lake, CA. : Integral Pub.

21 Sannella, L. (1981, October) A new sensory motor phenomenon with changes in consciousness. (Memo prepared from a talk at U.C. Medical School Lecture), Kaiser Hospital, Oakland.

22 Scott, M. (1983) Kundalini in the physical world. London: Routledge & Kegan Paul., p. 193.

2323 Singh, J. , (1979) Siva Sutras: the yoga of supreme identity, Delhi: Motilal Banarsidass, p. li and. pp. 135-136.

24 Hughes, S (trans.) (1979) Catherine of Genoa: Purgation and purgatory, the spiritual dialogue New York: Paulist Press. p. 143.

25 Op. cit. p. 145.

26 Austin, M. (1972) Acupuncture therapy, p. 225.

CHAPTER FIVE

EXPRESSING THE INEXPRESSIBLE: LITERATURE OF SPIRITUAL AWAKENING

Understanding the parameters of the Kundalini process makes reading the works of prophets, poets and biographers a new adventure, for it becomes possible to read between the lines and into the spiritual experiences alluded to in philosophy, biography, literature and poetry. It is clear such experiences have not occurred only among acknowledged mystics and saints.

Richard Bucke, a prominent psychiatrist who in 1901 wrote Cosmic Consciousness, a treatise on spiritual illumination, described the experience as consciousness of the life and order of the universe. He believed this awareness brings with it:

> An intellectual enlightenment or illumination which alone would place the individual on a new plane of existence -- would make him almost a member of a new species. To this is added a state of moral exaltation, an indescribable feeling of elevation, elation and joyousness, and a quickening of the moral sense, which is fully as striking and more important both to the individual and to the race than is the enhanced intellectual power. With these come, what may be called a sense of immor-

tality, a consciousness of eternal life, not a
conviction that he shall have this, but the
consciousness that he has it already.[1]

Bucke predicted a psychic revolution that would lead to the
"melt-down" of all religions, and the "revolutionizing of the human
soul", so that a new kind of religion would dominate the world. He
expected immortality and glory would exist in the here and now, and
evidence of it would live in every heart. Doubt of God and eternal
life would become impossible. Such consciousness would replace the
self-consciousness presently governing humankind, and this shift
would be as major as the shift from unconsciousness to self-
consciousness when it occurred at the dawn of civilization. Clearly
this was no ordinary psychiatrist of the Victorian era!

Bucke was a distinguished scientist and physician, who
during his career was Superintendent of the Provincial Asylum for the
Insane at two major hospitals in Ontario. Later he became Professor
of Mental and Nervous Diseases at Western University in London,
Ontario, and President of the Psychological Section of the British
Medical Association and the American Medico-Psychological
Association. In 1867, at age 35, he experienced a major shift in his
awareness through reading the works of Walt Whitman In 1872,
while visiting in London, he experienced what he termed
"Illumination", while riding in the back of a cab returning from an
intense evening of reading with friends the writings of Wordsworth,
Shelley, Keats,Browning, and Whitman. He described his mental
state as calm and peaceful, with his mind under the influence of the
"ideas, images and emotions called up by the reading and talk of the
evening." As recorded in the foreward of Cosmic Consciousness:

All at once, without warning of any kind, he
found himself wrapped around, as it were, by a
flame-coloured cloud. For an instant he
thought of fire -- some sudden conflagration in
the great city. The next (instant) he knew that
the light was within himself. Directly after
there came upon him a sense of exultation, of
immense joyousness, accompanied or immediately followed by an intellectual illumination, quite impossible to describe. Into
his brain streamed one momentary lightning-
flash of the Brahmic splendor which ever since
lightened his life. Upon his heart fell one drop

of the Brahmic bliss, leaving thence-forward
for always an aftertaste of heaven. [2]

Many years later Bucke produced the book in which he explored the awakening of cosmic consciousness in Buddha, Jesus, St.
Paul, Plotinus, Mohammed, Dante, Bartolome las Casas, John
Yepes, Francis Bacon, Jacob Hehmen, William Blake, Honore de
Balzac, Walt Whitman and Edward Carpenter. He suggested a
possible awakening in numerous other major poets and philosophers
including Socrates, Swedenborg, Wordsworth, Emerson, Tennyson,
and Thoreau. Bucke's descriptions of illumination correlate with
literature describing what would be identified as Kundalini experiences
in the East, and echo descriptions of cosmic truths reported by great
sages in every tradition. They do not, however, describe a full range
of what can be identified as Kundalini.
    Great Western poets such as Walt Whitman and T. S. Elliot
allude in mysterious couplets to the power of spiritual consciousness
(as have Sufi and Indian poets), but it was Indian gurus and other
spiritual teachers who first specified the details of this personal
encounter with this numinous energy. Such biographical and
autobiographical material is invaluable for the study of this process.
Some of the stories from India available now for Westerners include
those of Anandamayi Ma, Caitanya, Sri Aurobindo, Yogananda,
Muktananda, Krishnamurti, Milarepa, Ramakrishna, Gopi Krishna ,
and B.S. Goel.
    Several Westerners who have followed Eastern spiritual
paths and teachers have also written of the Kundalini experience.
These include Da Free John, a self-styled spiritual teacher from New
Jersey who had experiences of light from early infancy and later
studied with Muktananda and others; Motoyama, a Japanese
parapsychologist and yogi; The Mother, a French woman who
followed Aurobindo and later headed his organization; Kennett Roshi,
a German woman who became a Buddhist monk, and founded an
Abbey in California; Swami Radha, a German woman who became a
yogi, and founded ashrams in California and Canada ; and Irina
Tweedie, a European who studied in India with a yogi who
incorporated aspects of the Sufi path in his teachings.
    Others have written of awakenings that occurred with little
or no structured practices but that led them to explore Eastern
mysticism, including Chilean Miguel Serrano, once an Ambassador
to India; American physicians Brugh Joy, Gabriel Cousens, and
Richard Moss; and technical writer Thomas Wolfe. A spiritual healer
and psychic from new Mexico, Chris Griscom, has written of her

profound spiritual and psychic experiences since early childhood, and
Serrano as well mentions "feeling a strange chilling sensation that
traveled along my spine and reached up to my brain" which occurred
often at night when he was a child.[3] All of these writers provide us
with insight into both spontaneous and disciplined approaches to
awakening and moderating Kundalini and bring clarity and understanding to the possibilities and difficulties of this process. I found
many of their experiences echoed in the cases of the Westerners I
interviewed for this book.

Most teachers describe Kundalini awakening as essential to
the spiritual process. However for some it is not defined as the ultimate experience but only a step in the right direction, usually the
fifth step in a seven-step process. Aurobindo viewed Kundalini as
the awakening of an "ascending current" of energy and said a
"descending current" occurs when one is fully open to higher consciousness, which may eventually enable the consciousness of God to
transform the condition of human life on this planet.

The following stories were selected from the writings and
contributions of those saints, teachers and spiritual voyagers who
have provided the most in-depth and detailed descriptions of personal
or observed experiences with Kundalini awakening. I recommend you
return to their sources and read in more detail of the lives of these
teachers and mystics for a deeper understanding of this process.

Part 1:
Self-Reports and Case Histories
of Eastern Spiritual Teachers

Caitanya

A biography of Caitanya provides the earliest story I have
found in the literature of Kundalini experiences endured by a yogic
spiritual teacher.[4] Born in 1486, Caitanya was the founder of the last
great Vaisnava sect in India, and his life and work coincided with the
development of middle Bengali literature. His adult life was spent
surrounded by writers and according to Mujumdar, who used many of
these men as original sources to put together a biography of his life,
58 of his companions became more or less famous poets of this era.

Caitanya's mother had eight daughters who died before his
brother was born, and he was born eight or ten years later. His father
reported 13 months before his birth feeling a divine light enter his

head and passing it on to his wife, who then had a vision of many gods worshipping her. After his birth he was found to have marks of a banner, thunder, conch shell, discus and fish on his feet. His grandfather, a famous astrologer, calculated from his horoscope and from his body that he had the 32 physical signs of a great man. It is said if he cried the only sound that would quiet him was the recitation of the name Hari (which means remover of sin, a name of Krishna).

There are many tales about his charm, cleverness and misbehavior. He was restless and precocious and easily able to get what he wanted, but at times he fell into a rage, once hitting his mother so hard she fainted. His demands included wanting to hold flying birds, the stars, and the moon and when he couldn't have them he had a tantrum. His unruliness grew when he started school and engaged with friends in fights and pranks all over the city, mocked other boys, threw and spat water at bathers in the Ganges or pulled their legs under water, poured water over the heads of meditators, took items of worship and food offerings from people who were bathing, and substituted the clothes of men and women bathers. He was often in trouble with the townspeople for these pranks, but they found it difficult to stay angry at him.

When his older brother became a monk and left the family, Caitanya calmed down and became extremely studious, telling his parents he would take over the duties of the oldest son. His father feared that he would eventually leave to become a monk the way his brother had done and so he was taken out of school. He became uncontrollable until his father relented and reenrolled him. His father died when he was eleven.

Throughout his youth he continued to have tantrums, and one time he broke everything in the house. The next day he gave his mother two gold pieces, the source of which was never accounted for. After this event he turned his full attention to studies and became an outstanding scholar. At age 16 he graduated and became a teacher in the home of a man who hired him to teach grammar to his son and other young students.   He was charming and extremely handsome, and would frequently be followed by contingents of students with whom he engaged in dialectic and philosophical arguments. During this period he once fell into a trance in which he "uttered unintelligible words, rolled on the ground, broke things, shouted very loudly, jumped and threatened to beat people, then became absolutely stiff..."   When friends brought him oils which they thought would calm him he shouted at them "My name is Visvambhar, because I uphold the world, I am He, but who recognizes me?" then rushed at people near him.[5]   Some thought he was possessed. After awhile he recovered.

He married a beautiful young woman but early in the marriage, while he was away giving a lecture in another state, she was bitten by a snake and died. He grieved intensely for her but eventually remarried to another beautiful woman of a well-to-do family.

In 1508, Caitanya went to Gaya to perform prescribed rites at his father's grave and he met Isvar Puri, a spiritual teacher who initiated him and gave him a ten-syllable mantra. He began meditating on the mantra and after a short time fell into an ecstatic state, lamenting loudly for Krishna. As he became more obsessed with the saint he decided to travel to Mathura to seek him. On his way there he heard a divine voice say "The time for going to Mathura is not yet . . . . you are the Lord of Vaikuntha descended to redeem man. You will dispense preman (love) and bhakti (devotion) all over the world. We are your slave. You are the Master, Lord of all, your will cannot be gainsaid, but please go home now and come to Mathura later." [6]

He returned home greatly changed. As he told a few friends what had happened he broke down and began to lament, repeating the name of Krishna over and over. The flow of spiritual love coming from him seemed overpowering to them. After this he frequently fell into ecstasies, begging for Krishna, at times falling or rolling on the ground.   Bhakti, or devotional worship, was not yet a common practice in India, but a group of worshipers had been patiently waiting for a savior. They came to see Caitanya and proclaimed him as the answer to their prayers.

His ecstatic trances interfered with his teaching of grammar, where he would fall into lengthy discourses on the greatness of Krishna and the excellence of devotion to him, most of which the students did not understand. At times he fell to the ground, rolling, shaking and crying, and then did not recall it afterwards. Eventually he had to quit teaching because of the complaints.

He became meek, bowing and falling at the feet of the Vaisnanvas, a devout sect of worshippers he had previously mocked. He would wash their clothes and carry home items of worship they had brought. He advised them to perform kirtan (devotional singing and dance) so that Krishna himself would eventually come to them. He became furious and threatened to kill people who insulted the Vaisnanvas. He exclaimed at times "I am he! I am he". Sometimes he would climb a tree in his fervor and then suddenly jump down and fall on the ground with closed eyes. He ground his teeth with a horrible noise, somersaulted, and rolled on the ground. Many people thought he was mad. However a highly-regarded holy man, Scrivas, saw him and said he wasn't mad but suffered from "maha-bhakti-yoga" (great devotional union).[7]

A leading Vaisnanva had dreams and visions seeing Caitanya as his Lord and master and during initiation ceremonies so did Scrivas. Soon afterwards he began to gather large group of devotees, who saw him as an incarnation of Krishna. It appeared he could read people's minds, giving them what they wanted before they had voiced the desire. He was 24 years old, and many followers were much older, highly educated and trained scholars, yet they never wavered from their faith in him. Frequently he would appear to people in the form of Visnu, holding a conch, discus, club and lotus in four arms. They would swoon, then fall at his feet in worship. Once he fell into a strange depression, feeling he did not possess love for god, and jumped into the Ganges to commit suicide. Two followers dragged him out.

After several months of instigating Krishna worship and devotions he had an encounter with some students which left them angry and wanting revenge. He felt the only way to redress this from the karmic position was to become a monk, whom no one hates and everyone respects, so that they would eventually fall at his feet. He gave up his family and possessions and became a sannyasin (a monk who takes a vow of poverty), and thereafter was angry if anyone compared him to a deity. He traveled broadly, often meeting with scholars and leaders of spiritual groups and converting them to Krishna worship. He introduced the Hare Krisha chant for meditation, encouraged groups to sing it together, including families, and later the practice began of large groups singing it as they carried instruments and walked in the city.

The last 12 years of his life are said to have been spent in a mood of acute emotional distress. He followed a strict routine, waking before dark to go to the Jagganatha temple in Puri. Then he returned home and recited Krishna's name for several hours. He observed great austerity, lost all taste for food and ate little. He often spent the entire night in devotion or in trance. His health gradually broke down. At one point he cried that after union with Krishna he had lost him. "In his trance, he beamed with pleasure, but when he regained his normal senses, he felt as if he had lost his treasure, and sang and danced in fury." He was said to be possessed by ten forms of love-sickness day and night. One night he was found laying by the main temple gate, "his body stretched to about eight to nine feet in length, each arm and leg was about four feet in length of bare skin and bones; feet, neck and waist were hanging loose, held only by about six inches of taut skin. Not only was he unconscious, his breathing had stopped; foaming at the mouth, his eyes were fixed in a deadly stare." By shouting "Krishna" in his ear his friends brought him back to consciousness, and his body regained its normal state. He did not remember anything except that Krishna had appeared and vanished in lightning speed.[8]

Another time he ran toward a hill like lightning, "each pore of his skin swelled like a pimple, oozing blood, and his throat made a throttling sound". He was unable to pronounce a syllable and tears fell from his eyes. "Then a quivering burst over his frame like a tempest on the bosom of the sea and he fell on the ground." His companions brought him back by chanting and pouring cold water on him. He described being in a beautiful place with Krishna and cried because they had brought him back.[9]

He frequently fell into trance and a slight stimulus could make him exuberantly happy or terribly depressed. Once in an emotional fervor he rubbed his face so violently on the floor that blood began to flow.

Sources vary in their reports of his death but it was probably in 1533, at the age of 48, several days after contracting an infection caused when a toe on his left foot was pierced by a falling brick during a festival in Puri.

Commentary

Although this biography does not specifically cite Kundalini, Caitanya exhibited many of the manifestations commonly associated with it. He went through a major personality change after his initiation, becoming meek, prayerful and devoted until he was totally obsessed with thoughts of Krishna, love and worship, and at some point identified himself with Krishna, exhibiting great inflation.

He had increased compassion for others and great influence over them. He exhibited many physical symptoms such as shaking, falling down, rolling on the ground, running at rapid speeds, suspension of breath, falling into trance, unusual stretching and lengthening of the body, and difficulty or disinterest in eating. He also had dramatic mood swings, lack of interest in any worldly activities, and ecstatic visions. It is probably safe to comment that the outcome of his ecstatic experiences is not especially encouraging in terms of Western psychology, for he seems to have lost the capacity to care for himself or his life in his singular obsession with God-consciousness. He clearly became inflated and obsessed in the process. In India this kind of God-intoxication is accepted, and sometimes worshipped, for Caitanya is seen as one of India's greatest saints, an incarnation of Krishna himself. Lost in the experience of union with the One, he entered the world of the gods and became an archetypal symbol, holding a certain numinous quality and an inspiration for others, with no regard for issues of individuation or balance in the process. His emotional extremes became who he was, and it appears there was little developed sense of personal self to contain the great numinous aspects of his psyche in any integrated fashion.

Sri Anandamayi Ma

A more modern Indian mystic, Sri Anandamayi Ma, was born in the Indian village of Kheora on April 30, 1896. A biographer, Bhaiji, writes that both her parents led simple lives, devoted to God, and had kind and loving natures.[10] There were many learned pandits and devotees in the family. When she was a girl various "strange phenomena" (not specifically identified) became manifest in her body, much of which went unnoticed by others. Since she was so detached and unconcerned many people assumed she was retarded; often she couldn't say where she was nor what she had said a few minutes earlier. She talked to trees, plants and invisible beings, often relapsing in a mood of abstraction. She was married at age 12 to a brahmin of her village who was a man dedicated to the welfare of others, and she spent the next nine years in obscurity.[11]

From age 17 to 25 she fell into trances, her body stiff and numb, while chanting the names of gods and goddesses. At age 22, it is told that people could see images of gods and goddesses flash out of her body as she recited mantras. At other times she would spontaneously perform various yogic postures (she never studied yoga). During one 15-month period she was unable to talk, and after the ability to speak returned she voluntarily continued silence for another 21 months. When she visualized gods and goddesses she performed spontaneous acts of worship and rituals (although she claimed to have no conscious desire to do so) and these were said to be exactly correct, again with no training. In these she described herself as the worshipper, the worshipped and the act of worshipping. She later said "The personalities and forms of gods and goddesses are as real as your body and mine. They can be perceived with the inner vision opened up by purity, love and reverence." [12]

Bhaiji wrote that the dominant tone of her mind during this period was "the natural expression of mantric symbolism and yogic practices", and later her quiescence and silence continued, "until a phase of intense peace and tranquility became the all-pervading feature of her life."[13] Her appearance had a blissful glow. While living at Dacca at about age 27 her peacefulness began to attract devotees. "It is difficult to describe the ways by which their souls became steeped in tranquil bliss in her presence." [14]

She often went into trance during kirtan (singing and chanting of hymns). Once while placing vermillion on a lady's forehead she dropped the case, fell and rolled on the ground. Then she slowly rose and stood on her two big toes. Both hands were raised straight up, her head slightly tilted to one side and a little backwards, and her radiant eyes stared with a steady gaze towards the far end of the sky. She began moving and dancing as if filled with a heavenly presence until finally her body seemed to melt down on the floor and she rolled. Then soft musical strains come from her lips and tears flowed.

During kirtan she might bend her head backwards until it touched her back, twist her hands and feet in movements until she fell flat on the floor, roll on the floor, perform great stretching movements, appear to expand in size or to shrink, and her breath would seem to stop. Her body might seem to be without bones, bouncing like a rubber ball, but her movements were as quick as lightning. The roots of her hair would swell, causing it to stand on end. Whenever a thought wave passed her mind, a corresponding physical expression swept over her whole body.

> In concord with her breath, her body was thrown into rhythmic surges like waves, and with its limbs stretched out it rolled on the ground in time to the music. Just as the fallen leaves of a tree roll on lightly, blown by the wind, so light and delicate were her movements. No human being, in spite of his best efforts could have imitated them. Everybody present felt that mother was dancing under the impact of heavenly forces, which moved her whole being in wavelike thrills.[15]

In private she went through a stage of spontaneously performing yoga asanas and mudras. Often with her breath seeming completely suspended, her hands, feet and neck would bend "with such a stiff twist that there seemed no possibility of them regaining their normal positions; a brilliant light flashed from her body illumining the space around her, then spreading, enveloping the universe. At these times she would cover up her whole body with a piece of cloth and retire to her solitary corner of the house."[16] During this period people who glanced at her might experience bliss, or if they touched her feet they could fall unconscious. Places she would lie or sit would become intensely heated. She would sit in one posture for hours, or fall silent in the midst of conversation. If left alone for several days in these states she felt neither hunger not thirst, and might forget how to talk, walk or laugh.

Ordinarily she ate very little, sometimes going days without even water, once passing five months with only a handful of food at night, and again spending five to six months eating a small quantity of rice only twice a week. During these times her appearance was bright and cheerful, her body healthy and vigorous. Later her eating habits became more restrained, and in 1924 she stopped eating with her own hands, taking three grains of boiled rice in the morning or evening. After she gave up eating rice altogether it appeared that she ceased to recognize it. Despite these rations she occasionally ate enormous quantities at a sitting. On one occasion she ate enough food for eight or nine persons; on another she ate rice-pudding prepared from about 40 pounds of milk, and asked for more. She said later that at these times she did not know she was swallowing so much food and would have eaten whatever was put before her.

It is written that "during samadhi her face lost all freshness of life; the body appeared to be very frail and weak and in her general appearance there was no expression whatever of either joy or pain."[17] In one five-day phase of samadhi there was no indication that she was alive or could ever become alive, her body being as cold as ice. When she recovered consciousness and was asked how she felt she said "It is a state beyond all conscious and supra-conscious planes -- a state of complete immobilization of all thoughts, emotions and activities, both physical and mental -- a state that transcends all the phases of life here below." [18]

Through her life she is said to have touched many people in dreams and visions, perhaps giving them a mantra and leaving flowers on their pillow, and to have appeared spontaneously in many settings. Her biographer said that she appeared before him often at noon in his office or at midnight in his bedroom, and he described experiences of psychic connection with her, such as knowing when she needed something, or her granting his desires automatically. Once, while walking in a field with her, he saw some ladies coming to get her and he felt disappointed that she would be leaving so soon. The field covered suddenly with a thick fog and the ladies could not be

seen and were forced to leave without her. She is also credited with
acts of healing.

Bhaiji also describes a number of his own Kundalini experiences including mantric sounds welling from his heart, bliss and
joyous vibrations, laying awake all night filled with joy, spontaneously going into yogic postures, and composing songs of love and
praise. When he asked for advice about the ups and downs of his own
process she told him: "That which takes a long time to come into
being matures into an enduring beauty after an equally prolonged span
of development. Why do you worry over it so much? Hold fast to
the guiding hand like a trusting child."[19]

Commentary

Although four hundred years later than Caitanya,
Anandamayi Ma's ecstasies are very similar. She had a great impact
on those who watched her moving, stretching and dancing in ways
the body does not ordinarily move. She had long periods when she
could neither talk nor move nor eat, lost in trance and ecstatic
experiences. She performed many yoga movements spontaneously
and seemed to know the teaching of classical yoga without any
learning of it, as if it were simply given to her. She seemed to be
completely motivated by compassion and love, saturated in peace and
light, and the kinds of emotional turmoil sometimes associated with
Kundalini are not recorded here. In fact she once said that the path of
perfect love is identical with that of perfect knowledge, and that if one
attains the final goal "exuberance, excessive emotion and the like
cannot possibly occur. Emotional excitement and supreme Love are
in no wise to be compared; they are totally different from each
other."[20]

Evidently the ability to cope with every day survival needs
was never an issue for Anandamayi Ma, who was well cared for by
her husband and followers. Her nature seems always to have been
quiet and introspective, tending toward peacefulness and silence, while
Caitanya's was clearly more volatile from the beginning. She also
brought forth and lived out an archetype of god-realization, showing
no concern for personal interests, but her gentle nature allowed her to
live a long and peaceful life, in which she effectively touched many
others who sought spiritual direction in their lives.

Gopi Krishna

Gopi Krishna, a modern Indian who had great difficulty with
his own Kundalini awakening, which occurred after intense but
unsupervised meditation practice for many years, became a prolific

writer offering many detailed descriptions and discussions of the Kundalini process. In <u>Higher Consciousness</u> he wrote about the mystical experience.

> Whether the experience is of a visionary type or unattended by visions and appearances, the most amazing feature lies in the alteration experienced in one's own personality and channels of observation. The observer finds himself transformed. He is no longer the puny, fear-ridden individual, unsure about the nature of his being and destiny. He either realizes himself as a widely stretched, floating mass of consciousness, released from the bondage of flesh, or he finds himself face to face with a celestial being, resplendent and sublime. Or he may see himself surrounded by super-earthly scene of unequaled beauty and grandeur. In almost every case the vision is unlike anything experienced on earth in the ordinary course of life. This feature is so striking that it sharply divides mystical experience from anything seen in dreams or witnessed under drugs. . . . [21]

> In the genuine mystical experience there is no distortion in perception, no riot of lights and colors, no unrealistic stimulation of emotions, no unprovoked laughter and no unrelated sentiments, but an inexpressible transformation of personality. The precision of the intellect and the accuracy of sensual images are never lost, distorted or blurred. On the contrary, the acuity of perception is heightened, the hues and colors become more clear and brilliant, the sounds more harmonious, and touch more sensitive.[22]

Krishna's personal experience of Kundalini is detailed in his autobiography, <u>Kundalini, the Evolutionary Energy in Man</u>. He wrote that he had practiced yoga from the ages of 17 to 34, seeking God-realization and feeling despair that nothing had happened, although he could keep the mind in a state of fixity for a long time and maintain mental absorption for long periods. While meditating and fully engrossed in contemplating the lotus one day he felt a strange sensation at the base of the spine, which extended upwards and grew in intensity until like the roar of a waterfall he felt" a stream of liquid light enter the brain through the spinal cord".[23] The illumination grew brighter, the roaring louder, and he felt a rocking sensation and slipped out of his body, entirely enveloped in a halo of light. He felt a sense of himself growing wider and wider, surrounded by waves of light, and becoming all consciousness, with no sense of his physical body. He felt himself to be "a vast circle of consciousness in which the body was but a point, bathed in light, in a state of exaltation and happiness impossible to describe."[24]

He could barely walk after this experience, felt a loss of appetite, mental confusion, and detachment from people and it plunged him into a period of intense ups and downs, leading eventually to a nightmarish experience where he lost all taste for work and conversation and became gravely ill. Two nights after the initial experience while he was lying in bed "a tongue of flame sped across the spine into the interior of my head." [25]

It appeared as if the stream of living light continuously rushing through the spinal cord into the cranium gathered greater speed and volume at night and when he closed his eyes he saw luminous currents swirling in circles, moving rapidly from side to side. It was fascinating but it terrified him.

Sometimes it felt as if a "jet of molten copper, mounting up through the spine, dashed against my crown and fell in a scintillating shower of vast dimensions all around me . . . at times resembling a fireworks display."[26]

He began hearing roaring sounds. These phenomena increased in intensity as the days went by. He became acutely anxious and exhausted, lost all appetite, his tongue was coated white and his eyes red. His face became haggard and anxious, he had acute disturbances in digestive and excretory functions. As months passed he felt such things as energy leaping through the nerves of his body, front and back; cognition which seemed unstable and continually contracted or expanded; mood swings from elation into extreme depression, and bursting into tears unless he gagged his mouth; insomnia; lack of love for his family; and inability to eat. His food intake dropped to one or two glasses of milk and a few oranges each day. He felt burning inside and great restlessness and his health deteriorated. He feared the supernatural and thought he had made a grave mistake. An ascetic told him he must not be experiencing

Kundalini since that was always a blissful experience, and he had great doubts, thinking himself the victim of evil spirits.

His panic grew and an "unearthly radiance" flooded his head continuously, often taking horrible shapes and forms in the dark of night. Finally, after a particularly intense bout of pain and heat, he lay on his bed one night "burning in every fibre, lashed as it were by a fiery rain of red-hot needles piercing my skin. At this moment a fearful idea struck me. Could it be that I had aroused Kundalini through pingala , or the solar nerve which regulates the flow of heat in the body, and is located on the right side of sushumna?" [27] Lying in bed convinced he was dying, he decided to make a final effort and he put all his energy into forcing an imaginary cold current up the ida, the lunar nerve on the left side. He distinctly felt the nerve and strained to divert it's flow into the central channel. "There was a sound like a nerve thread snapping and a silvery streak passed zigzag through the spinal cord, exactly like the sinuous movement of a white serpent in rapid flight, pouring an effulgent, cascading shower of brilliant vital energy into my brain, filling my head with a blissful luster in place of the flame that had been tormenting me for the last three hours." [28] He fell asleep in bliss and woke up an hour later with the luster still there, the burning sensation and fear nearly vanished. He began to eat in small amounts, and gradually returned to health, although he continued to obsess about his abnormal condition and feel uncertain about his future.

In future months he stabilized, and continued feeling heightened awareness of the senses, having inner vision where he saw the flow of vital currents, and experiencing a cranial "glow" that frequently drew his attention when he lay down to sleep. His body would shake as a current sent upward streams of a lustrous fluid, and he might feel at night raging energy from the genitals, abdominal and thoracic areas and the brain, with a roaring noise in the ears and a shower in the brain that felt like a life and death struggle.

Eventually he turned toward meditation again, and became caught up in a "boundless ocean of unconditioned being", losing himself in an "amazing, immaterial universe". He became inflated with the thought he was a yogi. He became obsessive about this and unable to sleep. One night he felt his head reeling, his ears buzzing with a discordant noise and a wide column of fire mounting up and shooting out flames around his head. This initiated three months of torture along the lines of his initial experience, insomnia, and extreme physical weakness. He went through another stage of inability to eat, becoming very weak, until one night he had a dream about eating meat, and began a careful plan of moderating a diet he could tolerate, eating every three hours, until eventually he was well again. This time he threw himself into work, helping the community and becoming involved in meaningful social causes, avoiding the supernatural. He became stabilized for the next 12 years. At that time he began spontaneously writing poetry and had intense visions that he believed reframed and restructured his consciousness, flooding him with ecstasy and verse. This led to the redirection of his life toward work as a spiritual teacher.

Commentary

In providing this first-person account Krishna offered many specifics on the interior experiences of Kundalini awakening, describing lights, energy, sensations, sounds, dreams and emotions in great detail. The reader can clearly sense the physical discomfort, fear, visions and fantasies that may accompany this process, along with the life changes in instigates over a span of years. At first Krishna had great difficulty maintaining normal work and social functioning but later he became tireless in his contribution to the community and charitable efforts. He clearly described intense mood swings and self doubt, eating disorders, and symptoms of agonizing heat or pain in the body. The possibility of inner redemption, the voice from within or the dream with the right advice, is revealed in Krishna's story. It suggests one might benefit from paying close attention to such inner guidance.

His difficulties seemed to have been the result of having no spiritual teacher, being full of self-doubts and denial of the religious aspects of his experience, and a tendency to obsessive thinking. Two of the supportive factors in his life were a wife who cared for his physical needs although he evidently told her little about what was going on, and a brother with whom he shared his experiences. Each forward step of this process seemed to emerge from some deep intuition that appeared whenever he reached a stage of desperation. Like many people he passed through several stages of this process, endured a lengthy gestation period before the experience stabilized.

Swami Muktananda

Many people I have met who report experiences with Kundalini once had at least a minimal encounter with Muktananda, who introduced them to the experience of Kundalini through shaktipat. In a series of magazines published by his organization (Shree Gurudev Vani Annual, 1972--1980) many of his followers described unique conditions that appear to be Kundalini awakening and discuss subsequent changes in their personalities and lives. Devotees of Gurumayi Chidvilasananda, his successor, also report these kinds of experiences. Muktananda wrote several books that describe Kundalini awakening, and in Play of Consciousness (1978) told in considerable detail of his own process. In this autobiography he said he became a spiritual seeker when he left home at age 15 to become a wandering ascetic. He described his temperament as fiery, impatient, arrogant and demanding. After meeting his guru, Bhagavan Nityananda, he became totally devoted to him, and practiced deep meditations in which he was completely identified with him and experienced overwhelming bliss. He described the dramatic ups and downs associated with spiritual practices, ranging from rapturous bliss to flare-ups of anger and abusiveness. One night he spent the entire night doing a detailed meditation in which he spent hours identifying every part of his body with the guru's body, until concentrating on the heart he felt prana becoming steady there, and felt a stab of pain at the muladhara "like a bolt of divine lightning... A wave of prana ran throughout my body and throbbed in thousands of different nerves. I was lost in meditation."[29]

Shortly after this Muktananda was initiated through a deep eye contact with the guru, and given the gift of his guru's sandals. He was told to go to a hut some distance from the ashram and meditate. There he began a series of intense experiences, suffering great pain and anguish. He was very restless, and his whole body ached as if every pore was pierced by needles. The ecstasy was gone. He had nightmares and his peace of mind was destroyed.He was flooded with "hateful and sinful" thoughts. At one point his abdomen swelled with air after which he exhaled it with great force. Spontaneous yogic breaths or the stoppage of breath would occur.

One night he went out into the dark, his mind confused, certain he was going mad or dying. He wanted to dance, jump and shout. His limbs and body became very hot, and he ached all over. He saw the earth, sky and trees spinning. He would stand up and sit down repeatedly. He saw images of his guru appear and disappear beneath the mango trees, and then the fields appeared to be on fire, with hoards of people screaming as if it were the end of the world. Creatures six to fifty feet tall danced naked before him with their mouths gaping open, screeching horribly. His body went into the lotus position and felt locked permanently in it. If he tried to close his eyes they would immediately open. Images of fires, ghosts and demons persisted. Then a moonlike, radiant white ball about four feet in diameter appeared. It struck against his eyes and then passed inside of him. He called this a " real" experience, not a dream. A second later the bright light of the sphere penetrated his body, his tongue curled up against the palate and his eyes closed. There was a dazzling light in his forehead and his head was forced down and glued to the ground.

After a while he saw a soft red light shimmering and flickering slightly, sending sparks through the universe, then slowly he came to body consciousness. He sat to meditate and felt pain in the muladhara and saw a light in the heart space. He made the sounds of a camel and the roar of a tiger, so loudly that villagers the next day thought a tiger had been loose in the fields. In the days to follow he had numerous experiences of energy in his body, saw the red light often, heard crackling and popping sounds in his body, felt great heat, had many conflicting emotions flooding him in meditation, and had intense mood swings.

In time the experience deepened, and the light became a steady red aura of his own size and shape that enveloped him inside and outside. Millions of tiny rays flashed within it and as he watched he became completely absorbed in meditation. His body would shake and swing, go into yogic postures, jump and hop like a frog, twist and hiss like a snake. He visited other worlds, and felt tremendous ecstasy. Yoga mudras and asanas occurred spontaneously, along with loud cracking sounds in his head. His head would roll so vigorously that it would bend below his shoulders and he could see his back. Later he suffered from an intense sexual desire, although he had been celibate for years and had no interest in sex. Images of a naked woman pursued him. Ultimately these experiences subsided,and deeper levels of bliss along with positive integrative images emerged, especially that of a blue pearl holding a divine being within.

Muktananda wrote that when Kundalini is fully awakened one sees the world differently, rising above body consciousness and duality until he/she experiences witness consciousness and feels "I am the Absolute". The world is felt as one's own Self, as the joyful abode of God. The body will become pure, well-proportioned, clean and beautiful with luster and radiance.[30]

Muktananda later advised those dealing with Kundalini primarily to trust in and obey the guru, understand and witness the inner process and surrender to the awakened shakti. He said "recognize and trust that whatever is happening is for the good. . . . Do not be afraid-- let whatever is happening run its course."[31] In addition, a yogi should stay pure and chaste, talk little, have noble thoughts, love solitude, and seek the company of saints and good people. He also believed that "To realize God one must first love oneself, and not indulge thoughts of being wretched, sinful and worthless."[32] One should neither torture nor pamper the body, but see it as a temple of God, keeping it pure, clean, healthy. "Do not punish the mind by calling it impure, restless and unstable. If lovingly led to a proper place, to rest in the Self, it becomes tranquil." [33]

Commentary

Muktananda's story offers a clear picture of the inner turmoil and overwhelming energy sometimes accompanying Kundalini awakening, even under the guidance of a master teacher . He described experiences with lights, visions, movements, yogic postures, irrational mood swings, sounds, ecstatic bliss and sexual energy with an intensity rare in this literature. He gives details of some specific images that commonly appear in this process: animals, fire, the destruction of the earth, demons, and the blue pearl. His Kundalini experiences were contained within a few years, and led to his lifetime of work as a guru and spiritual teacher.

If we look at his "fiery, impatient, arrogant and demanding" nature we have the flavor of the kind of personality pattern he brought into the spiritual life, which may be a reason for the fiery and intensely expressive processes he encountered during his Kundalini process. He also appears to have engaged and moved through this awakening fairly rapidly, under the direction of his guru, on which he had an intense and all-consuming projection of the Self. This is the Siddha Yoga path, using the internalization of the enlightened guru to burn away identification with the personal self and experience the true nature of Divine Self.

Swami Yogananda and Kriya Yoga

A less dramatic encounter with spiritual emergence seems to occur in the practice of Kriya Yoga, brought to the West in the 1920's by Paramahansa Yogananda who taught it to thousands of people over a 30-year span, using a special set of exercises and breathing techniques that promote a gradual stimulation and progression of Kundalini energy. He called this the "holy science" or the "science of religion", and spoke extensively of achieving continual bliss.

> The scientific method teaches a process enabling us to draw to our central part --spine and brain-- the life current distributed throughout the organs and other parts of our body. The

process consists of magnetizing the spinal
column and the brain, which contain the seven
main centers, with the result that the
distributed life electricity is drawn back to the
original centers of discharge and is experienced
in the form of light. In this state the spiritual
Self can consciously free itself from its bodily
and mental distraction. [34]

Yogananda emphasized the power of attention as a great di-
rector and discharger of energy, and described a controlled upward
movement of prana through the chakras, accompanied by various
sensations, which eventually, after prolonged practice, brings about a
state of conscious bliss and peace. He defined this as the universal
aim and highest necessity of life, because in it we are really
conscious of God, or bliss, and feel the expansion of our real Selves.
The more frequently this is experienced, the more personality or
individuality falls away, and a state of universality is reached. He
speaks of this merging as the true purpose and state of religion.
Yogananda said kriya practice is accompanied from the beginning by
feelings of peace and soothing sensations along the spine. It slows
down the respiratory rate, ultimately stilling the breath completely,
which feeds the physical cells with "undecayable light" keeping them
in a spiritually magnetized condition. He states that this prolongs
life, frees the mind from preoccupation with the senses and enlarges
consciousness.[35]
     According to scriptures, wrote Yogananda, a person requires
a million normal diseaseless years of evolution to perfect his human
brain and experience cosmic consciousness. Kriya practice enables
one to evolve much more rapidly because 1000 kriyas in 8 1/2 hours
produces the equivalent of 1000 years of natural evolution, 365,000
years in one year. In three years a yogi can accomplish what nature
brings to pass in a million years. But he warns that these practices
can only be undertaken by well-developed yogis who have carefully
prepared their body and brain to withstand the power generated by
intensive practice; a beginner does the exercises only 14 to 24 times
twice daily.[36]
     Yogananda wrote the personable Autobiography of a Yogi
in 1945. In it he described childhood memories of previous in-
carnations and great frustrations at being an infant in an impotent
body. He said he had a strong emotional life that was mentally
expressed in words of many languages, and with some difficulty

became accustomed to hearing his native Bengali. Born on Jan. 5, 1893, he was the second son and fourth of eight children in a family that expressed mutual love, tranquility and dignity. His father was a mathematician. His mother was a strongly feeling woman, who gave so generously to the needy that one fortnight she distributed more than his father's monthly income. Both parents were followers of Lahira Mahasaya, and were initiated by him in Kriya Yoga. Although this guru died when Yogananda was an infant he was part of his early childhood, with his picture on the meditation altar at home. He developed an inner relationship with him, frequently prayed to him, and at age eight experienced a healing of Asiatic cholera when he was nearly dead by bowing internally to his picture. A blinding light enveloped his body and the entire room, and he was instantly well. Shortly afterward he had a spiritual vision, where he saw in an immense flash of light a group of Himalayan yogis sitting in meditation postures in caves. As the image faded the light expanded in ever-widening circles to infinity and told him "I am Iswara (a Sanscrit name for the Lord, in his aspect as cosmic ruler), I am Light."[37]

Throughout his youth Yogananda met many yogis, had visions and made unsuccessful attempts to get to the Himalayas. As a teenager he met his guru Sri Yukteswar, also a disciple of Lahiri Mahasaya, who initiated him in Kriya Yoga. In this exchange he felt "a great light break upon my being, like the glory of countless suns playing together. A flood of ineffable bliss overwhelmed my heart to an innermost core."[38] He described many experiences with lights and visions such as closing his eyes and seeing flashes of lightning --"the vast space within was a chamber of molten light."[39] When he opened them the dazzling radiance continued outside. He says he later learned to experience this light at will. He also had many visions of Divine Mother after his meeting with Yukteswar.

Once when Yukteswar lightly slapped his chest he plunged into a deep silence, and all the world in the streets around became silent. He saw scenes in all directions simultaneously, and fell into ecstasy. When slapped again he came out of it. A similar vision occurred at Dakshineswar Temple years later, when after five hours of meditating he stood in the temple grounds and saw the goddess Kali and the temple appear in magnificent size, and his vision enlarge so he could see clearly for several miles down the length of the river and into the town. The walls of buildings glimmered transparently. Everything was bathed in white, blue and rainbow hues.

Yogananda had many inner messages, such as precognitive information regarding the death of family members, and visions of coming to the U.S., seeing the centers he would establish later in life. He often experienced advantageous synchronistic events, which assisted him in such areas as passing exams to graduate from college, and having funds when needed for various reasons. In 1920 he arrived in Boston, and began a tour of hundreds of cities where he taught the largest yoga classes in the world (at that time). During 32 years he initiated 100,000 students, and established the Self-Realization Fellowship with centers in Los Angeles and Encinitas, California. He died following a lecture in Los Angeles on March 7, 1952, and was said to leave his body consciously, in the ancient yogic tradition.

Swami Sivananda (1969) , who has also written several volumes on spiritual awakening, described the outcome of Kundalini awakening in an American man he met with who was swept into "cosmic consciousness" while hearing a talk by Yogananda. He said he felt indescribable ecstasy, bliss, immortality, eternity, truth, and divine love which became the core of his being and the essence of his life.

> He was aware, during this period of illumi-
> nation and during the months which followed
> of a number of physiological changes within
> himself. The most striking was what seemed
> an arrangement of molecular structure in his
> brain or the opening of new cell-territory there.
> Ceaselessly, day and night, he was conscious
> of this work going on. It seemed as though a
> kind of electrical drill was boring out new
> cellular thought channels.
>
> Another important change was felt in
> his spinal column. The whole spine seemed
> turned into iron for several months so that,
> when he set to meditate on God, he felt an-
> chored forever, able to sit in one place eternally
> without motion or consciousness of any bodily
> function. At times an influx of superhuman
> strength invaded him and he felt that he was
> carrying the whole universe on his shoulders.
> The elixir of life, the nectar of immortality, he
> felt flowing in his veins as an actual, tangible
> force. It seemed like a quicksilver or a sort of
> electrical fluid light throughout his body.[40]

He also reported that during the months of his illumination he felt no need of food or sleep, he awakened to a joy past all words or power of description, he had previously suffered from heavy colds and been a constant smoker but now the body was purged of illness and the desire for cigarettes was gone, and he went about his daily work as usual but with a hitherto unknown efficiency and speed.[41]

Commentary

Yogananda's biography is flavored with the charm of an Indian folk-tale, full of miracles, healings and visions that are recounted as natural and every-day occurrences. He reports none of the negative experiences of Kundalini, and seems from early childhood to be gifted with faith, love and psychic gifts. His relationship with his guru is in the classic Indian tradition, receiving shaktipat, insight, yoga practices, personal assistance, and lessons about life. He never emphasized Kundalini in his writing, and awakening seems to be a more subtle movement of consciousness and vision than we find in most other yogic literature. Since Kriya Yoga is said to be revived from ancient times, this path may be a secret process used by the earliest teachers, long before concerns about the materialistic age and the body ushered in yoga and tantra practices, although kriya yogis often practice energization exercises similar to yoga asana, and the kriya practice is essentially one of moving pranic energy up and down the spine in order to awaken the chakras and Kundalini. Yogananda said that kriya practices bring about complete control of the electrical flow in the body, causing only an attractive sensation at the beginning, and ultimately bringing a state of conscious bliss which counteracts the exciting state of normal body consciousness, and eventually causing individuality to fall away and a direct communion with God to be attained.

A number of centers in the United States and India, several of them established by former initiates of Yogananda, continue to teach Kriya Yoga. A few people I have spoken with who practice it do not report the kinds of discomfort or disruptive energy releases common to other kinds of Kundalini awakening, although they do report experiences of bliss, inner tranquility, light, joy and orientation of their lives toward spiritual concerns.

Krishnamurti

Krishnamurti is unique among spiritual teachers both in his personal history and his role in both Eastern and Western cultures. The eighth son born to an orthodox Brahmin family in 1895, his early rearing included learning traditional Hindu scriptures. He was a child given to daydreaming, occasionally experiencing visions of the gods or psychic awareness, and not much interested in academics.

When he was ten years old he was seen on the beach by C.W. Leadbeater, who noticed an intense aura around him. Leadbeater and Annie Besant decided he would be the prophesied great world teacher, and took him into the Theosophical Society, a movement based on the tenets of a universal brotherhood of humanity, which studied ancient wisdom and explored spiritual mysteries, psychic phenomenon, and the nature of subtle body energies. His father was persuaded to allow Krishnamurti and his younger brother, Nityananda, to live with Leadbeater and other Theosophists, in order to be trained and initiated into sacred mysteries and to be educated in Western ways. Twenty years later, after awakening, Krishnamurti renounced the value of attachment to any organization and to the dismay of those who had hoped he would be their new leader, disbanded the organization's Order of the Star, of which he was president, at a public gathering.

Krishnamurti taught and wrote as an independent teacher, never calling himself a guru. He didn't promote yoga techniques, although he practiced pranayama, hatha yoga and meditation, nor did he write much of Kundalini. But two biographies of his life provide a thorough description of his own intense awakening, occurring primarily in 1922 while living in Ojai, California, as witnessed by his brother Nitya and Rosalind Williams, a young American theosophist, who were both with him at the time.[42] The most painful and dramatic experiences lasted from August 1922 through 1924, and his spiritual process was deeply impacted by the death of his brother in 1925. By 1927 he seemed complete in this awakening, although deeper levels of it continued through his life, and he later stated it was not complete until 1948. In 1927 he wrote to Leadbeater: "I know my destiny and my work. I know with certainty that I am blending into the consciousness of the one Teacher and that he will completely fill me. I feel and I know also that my cup is nearly full to the brim and that it will overflow soon. Till then I must abide quietly and with eager patience."[43]

Some of the phenomenon reported in Jayakar's biography (1986) related to his Kundalini awakening include:

-- Acute pain at the nape of the neck, increasing for two days until he could not think, was unable to do anything, and was forced to bed. There he became almost unconscious, although aware of what was happening around him. During this time he saw a vision of a man mending the road, who was himself, holding a pickaxe which was also himself, breaking the stone which was himself. He felt himself identified with every element of the scene, including grass, trees, and a car driving by, being in everything, or "rather everything was in me, inanimate and animate, the mountain, the worm and all breathing things. All day long I remained in this happy condition. I could not eat anything, and again at around six I began to lose my physical body. . ."[44]

-- The following day he could not tolerate the vibrations of other people in the room, felt much worse, and was weak and tired, weeping from exhaustion and lack of physical control. His head felt as though many needles were being driven in. He imagined his bed was filthy beyond imagination, and he begged to go to the woods in India. Later, at the urging of his companions, he went outside and meditated under a pepper tree, felt himself go out of his body and saw himself meditating. Over his body was a star, and he felt the vibration of the Lord Buddha and beheld Lord Maitreya and Master K.H. (two Theosophical Society spiritual guides). He felt happy, calm and at peace, and that nothing could disturb the calmness of his soul. "Love in all its glory has intoxicated my heart; my heart can never be closed. I have drunk at the fountain of joy and eternal Beauty. I am God-intoxicated."[45]

-- For the next ten days all was calm, and then sensation in his spine and periods of acute pain began. Incidents started every evening around 6 p.m. lasting usually for two or three hours. The sequence of events began following meditation, after which he would lie down on a couch in a semiconscious state, start to moan and complain of a great heat, shudder a little and collapse. When he regained full consciousness he did not remember what had occurred although he felt a vague general discomfort.

-- He would experience extreme sensitivity and could not bear light, sounds and touch; he would appear conscious but then stumble and fall down. Sometimes he would sit up on the bed and murmur something, then fall backward or forward with a crash. He would groan and toss about murmuring incoherently and complaining of pain in his spine.

-- He would call for his mother who was deceased, talk with her, and relive early childhood experiences. Between spasms of pain he would converse with an unseen presence, who appeared to be a friend and a teacher.

-- His pain became more intense, as if his body was an open wound. It seemed to move to a new part of the body unaccustomed to the terrible heat. He would speak, sob, shriek with pain and beg for a moment's respite. His caretakers noticed two voices, one they called the Physical Elemental, the body, and the other Krishnamurti's natural voice. The time for the process seemed measured, as if a certain quantity of work had to be performed every evening. When he returned to consciousness the pain would be immediately wiped out.

-- One night the pain was much worse, and Krishnamurti began running at full speed, until his caretakers held him back, afraid he would be hurt. He tried several times to run from the pain. His body would contort in dangerous and awkward positions. On one occasion, sobbing and weeping, he put his head over his knees on the floor and turned over, nearly breaking his neck.

-- On one occasion he felt someone was lurking around the house, and went to a low-surrounding wall and told them loudly to go away. Then he lay down and started calling out "Please come back Krishna."[46]

-- For several days the pain shifted to his face and eyes, and he felt his eyes were gone, and sobbed and moaned. He felt his guides cleansing his eyes so that he might be allowed to see "Him" and he said it felt "Like being tied down in the desert, one's face to the blazing sun, with one's eyelids cut off". [47]

-- He saw visions of great beings, and his companions also felt the presence of energy and unknown guides and masters in the room. It was as if these beings were conducting or supervising the process.

-- One night he was heard to fall, and then to state he was sorry, that he knew he must not fall, he was to make no movement , so he clasped his fingers tightly and lay with them under his back, while the pain continued. It was so terrible that it was difficult to breathe, and he choked repeatedly and fainted three times. The process appeared as if he were enduring a very difficult initiation, and later he seemed to be aware of a roomful of visitors rejoicing at his success in completing it. He said "Mother, everything will be different now, life will never be the same for any of us after this." and again "I've seen Him, Mother, and nothing matters now."[48]

-- His pain continued, shifting constantly. Over several days he felt his scalp being opened, and he would faint repeatedly. This was accompanied by relieving significant early events of his childhood , including his mother birthing a child, he and his brother ill with malaria, and the death of his mother.

Gradually the intensity of these episodes decreased and he regained his physical strength. He frequently left his body, or had visions of masters and saints. One night he had an experience that was recorded by his brother as "the current starting as usual at the base of his spine and reaching the base of his neck, then one went on the left side, the other on the right side of his head and they eventually met at the centre of the forehead; when they met a flame

played out of his forehead". Nitya felt this could relate to the opening of the third eye.[49]
In later years Krishnamurti wrote in letters of an ecstasy that never left him, "I am full of something tremendous. I can't tell you in words what is like a bubbling joy, a living silence, an intense awareness like a living flame,"[50] and he reported capacities for clairvoyance and healing. He did healing infrequently, not wanting to be known as a healer, and he felt an antipathy to clairvoyance, calling it an intrusion of privacy.

Commentary
Krishnamurti did not put much focus on these experiences during his later years of teaching. His emphasis was on awareness, conscious living, mastery of thought and responsibility for the planet. Although the Kundalini process represented a pivotal point in his own awakening it does not seem that he regarded this as a process that ought to be encouraged, or for which one could train; nor did he have any inclination to pass along shakti to others, although he did occasionally do healing. His experiences provide us with another example of the intensity of this process, and of the need to recognize that there are powers at work here that appear to operate with a schedule and plan, over which the therapist/ doctor/ friends/ companions can have little influence other than to offer emotional support, physical care and protection. He was always adamant that two people stay with him while he was in these processes, even if they couldn't communicate with him. Ultimately the individual is faced with enduring the encounter alone, and ultimately the experience seems to lead to bliss, joy and a sense of universal compassion.

B. S. Goel
The biographical account of a much lesser known Indian, B.S. Goel, offers detailed descriptions of a Kundalini awakening which occurred from 1975 to 1985, disrupting and gradually re-shaping the mind and lifestyle of an Indian intellectual who had studied Freudian psychology.[51] Goel describes himself as a member of a deeply religious family but with no sign of religious interests as a young child. He was introduced to hatha yoga as a teenager, and in a few days could perform all the asanas automatically. He practiced yoga and pranayama through college, also studied Marxism and Freudian psychology, all to overcome what he labels a deeply rooted inferiority complex.
At age 29, during his Ph.D. studies, he was discussing Marx with a friend one day when a great force rushed up his spine to the

crown of his head and he was plunged into ecstasy. Soon afterward he began spontaneously writing poetry in English, something he had never dreamed of doing before. He had never even enjoyed poetry. This initial experience was followed by severe depression, and Goel saw a psychiatrist who said he had paranoid trends and religious delusions. In time he met a swami who taught him to meditate, and he entered Freudian psychoanalysis. The meditation produced beneficial waves of joy and peace, and taught him to observe himself and his mental behavior. He felt a compulsion to meditate frequently. Although the analyst was against all meditation and considered it a compulsion formation in him, he continued both processes and felt they were helpful, eventually writing a book on psychological analysis and meditation. The Indian guru Sai Baba appeared to Goel in dreams, and later during meditations and in visions, providing guidance for his process, although Goel had never met him.

After ten years of meditation, at age 39, Goel underwent what appears to be a major Kundalini opening. This was possibly triggered by the suicide of a friend. Staying the night at the friend's flat he felt depressed, and clearly with inner vision "saw that the two nerves laying just under the point where Hindus keep a lock of hair had slipped from their place making a fine downward movement."[52] He felt a nervous breakdown was taking place and that he was doomed forever. He became desperately depressed and tried to use psychoanalysis to pull himself together. He prayed intensely to Sai Baba and increased his daily meditation. Eight days later, while he was sleeping, someone pulled off his blanket. He opened his eyes and saw the form of Sai Baba. He tried to touch him and when he could not he decided it was an hallucination and turned over to go back to sleep. The blanket was again pulled off and Sai Baba made him sit up and asked him to meditate, focusing on the mid-point between the eyebrows. He sat in meditations from 1:30 to 4 a.m.

The next day, while doing the same meditation, he saw a thick, vertical red line appear at the mid-point between the eye-brows. He became very calm and the depression left him. Two days later as he concentrated the red line reappeared and became an exact eye. Sai Baba stood in the middle of it with a shiva-linga (an oval or phallic-like symbol) caught between his thumb and fingers of the right hand. Two days later the third eye opened and Sai Baba and he were both in it. He felt he received the full protection of Sai Baba and "experienced death". Soon afterwards he felt Kundalini rise in his backbone and move upward in the form of a cobra. A few days later he saw in the third eye Lord Krishna, Jesus Christ, and a five-headed cobra projecting some illuminating substance.

Goel says it is through the third eye that the grace of the guru descends, and this automatically breaks the center of ego, plunging one into such difficult stages he feels he will either go mad or die. Years of emotional and physical upheaval followed this opening for Goel, highlighted by numerous visions, particularly of the inner movement of Kundalini through the body. He wrote that in this process dark periods of depression were substituted abruptly with periods of great relaxation, which is why he did not break down completely.

Some of the symptoms he describes are uncontrollable weeping; seeing inner colors and visions; automatically repeating Om; his attention being riveted on the third eye from which streamed a powerful beam of crimson light; the loss of ability to engage in interpersonal relationships and all motivating force for work; and at one point an irrational infatuation with the daughter of a friend, on which he projected the goddess Kundalini. Psychological problems which he believes might have been diagnosed included confusion and bewilderment; anxiety neurosis with reactive depression; paranoia with religious delusions; God complex; auditory and visual hallucination; manic-depression; drowsy states; insomnia, extreme restlessness and delirium. He sees no hope in any kind of treatment for these problems during this process. He attempted the use of medication, suggestive therapy and catharsis with his brother, and self-analysis, none of which he felt had the slightest impact.

Five years into this process he had what he thought was a severe heart attack two nights in a row. He felt surrendered to the possibility of dying, and continued meditating and concentrating on the third eye. His attention slipped to the heart center, and he saw a vision of Lord Krishna there, which immediately put him into a state of happiness and confidence. Later he concluded that the various chakras are pierced by the guru through this process, and the journey is often marked by great happiness emerging in between two bouts of suffering. Piercing of the chakras tends to suspend conscious touch with the world, and may resemble the death experience. But after each attack of suffering one feels better than before, and consciousness is lifted further along. During each period of attack the feeling of estrangement and alienation from the world appears to increase. Goel believes the suffering of Kundalini is in direct proportion to the thickness of the walls of ideas, images and desires the soul carries.

Commentary

Goel, who established an ashram in India in 1982, has meticulously documented his progressive experiences in this book, which shows his change in consciousness over the years. Now the direction of his life is set, but there is a strong sense in his work of the ever-expanding development of spiritual awareness, so that images, dreams, energy and bliss may continue to bring him to deeper levels of evolution. I have recorded his experiences at some length because they reflect some unique aspects which mirror the experiences of some of my subjects. Some of these include inner vision, emotional upheavals, symptoms similar to those of a heart attack, egoic problems, bliss, spontaneous writing of poetry, and the appearance of a guru, Sai Baba, with whom he had no previous relationship. He offers interesting insight into the kinds of psychological problems that one experiencing Kundalini may be confronted with.

Goel's situation is also of note because he had what appears to be a spontaneous awakening, rarely described in the literature, following only short-term hatha yoga practices, at a time in life when his interests were not spiritual but more inclined toward Freudian psychology and Marxism. Yogic tradition would assert that his instant mastery of asana and spiritual awakening were the consequences of his spiritual efforts in previous lives. His path is similar to others, however, in the long-term progression, bringing a variety of experiences and insights over many years.

Part 2: Self-Reports of Westerners Who Followed Eastern Spiritual Traditions

Irina Tweedie

A remarkable biographical account of spiritual awakening under the tutelage of a yogic master, Bhai Sahib, has been written by Irina Tweedie (Daughter of Fire, 1986), a European woman born in Russia and educated in Vienna and Paris. This is an expanded version of an earlier biography, Chasm of Fire (1979). Following World War 2 Tweedie married an English naval officer, whose death in 1954 led her toward a spiritual quest. When she went to India, at the age of 52, she knew little of yogic practices, although she had been a Theosophist for seven years.

Her teacher defined his method (which he called a Sufi approach although it bears little resemblance to the Islamic Sufi tradition) as representing complete freedom. The disciple is never forced, but once surrendered to the guru, the guru initiates many processes. There are two ways open --" the path of Dhyana, the slow, and easier way; or the path of Tyaga (complete renunciation), the Road of Fire, the burning away of all the dross, and it is the Guide who has to decide which way is the best suited in each individual case."[53] The former path is for the many, and the latter for only a few. Once the disciple is committed there is no free will for awhile.

Tweedie's guru describes awakening Kundalini while on this path as much less troubling than in hatha yoga, since the opening is gentle and is initiated at the heart chakra. He acknowledges he is not much help with someone who has awakened Kundalini through hatha practices -- it is in the hands of God. "When awakened by hatha yoga it becomes a great problem. It is a difficult way. One has to know how to take it up and take it down again through all the chakras, and it is troublesome. But with us we begin to notice it only when it reaches the heart chakra; it means peace, bliss, states of expanded consciousness. We awaken the king, the heart chakra, and leave it to the king to activate all the other chakras."[54]

Tweedie is told no effort must be made other than to sit with the guru, who does not make conditions, and cares for and loves the disciple like a loving mother. In this system it is possible to achieve the goal of finding the Truth in one lifetime.

> In our yoga system the ultimate result is achieved in one life by Dhyana. Only one chakra is awakened: the heart chakra, It is the only yoga school, in existence, in which love is created by the spiritual teacher. It is done with yogic power. The result is, that the whole work of the awakening, or quickening, is done by one chakra, which gradually opens up all the others. This chakra is the leader, and the leader is doing everything. . .
>
> I told you once that we belong to raja yoga. But when you try to study raja yoga from books you will be told: do this, do that, concentrate, meditate, sit in this posture. Today it is obsolete. Times have changed. The world is progressing; those methods have been outgrown. They are dead. But our system is alive; it has preserved its dynamism for it is changing with the times.[55]

This emphasis on the lack of practices, and on the heart chakra, offers insight into some of the variations of Kundalini opening, and suggests one possible reason why some people seem to have an easier process than others, possibly because their heart chakra is opened initially, or has been active and open before the advent of Kundalini. Although in this tradition, it is the presence and action of the guru that initiates all of the activity. It is also helpful to remember that even a guru may not feel capable of healing or straightening out the Kundalini of someone whose process has been opened spontaneously.

Although Tweedie is told her process will not be so difficult, she does endure some remarkably difficult episodes during her months with this teacher. She provides one of the more dramatic descriptions in the literature of sexual energy as it can erupt with Kundalini awakening. It began as she lay comfortably in bed, and felt a vibration, and a sound she had never before heard like a soft hiss in the lower part of her abdomen. Suddenly she was flooded with powerful sexual desire, with no object in particular, an uncontrollable, wild, cosmic force that felt like madness.

> The whole body was SEX ONLY, every cell, every particle was shouting for it, even the skin, the hands, the nails, every atom. I felt my hair standing up as if filled with electricity, waves of wild goose-flesh ran over my whole body, making all hair on the body stand stiff... and the sensation was painful.
>
> But the inexplicable thing was that even the idea of any kind of intercourse was repulsive and did not even occur to me. The body was shaking. . . I was biting my pillow not to howl like a wild animal. . . I was beside myself -- the craziest, the maddest thing one could imagine, so out of the blue, so sudden, so violent!
>
> The body seemed to break under this force. All I could do was hold it stiff, still, and completely stretched out. I felt the overstretched muscles full of pain, as in a kind of cramp; I was rigid, could not move. The mind was absolutely void, emptied of its content; there was no imagery, only an uncontrollable fear -- primitive animal fear. And it went for hours. I was shaking like a leaf. . . a mute, helpless, trembling jelly, carried away by

forces completely beyond any human control.
A fire was burning inside my bowels. The
sensation of heat increased and decreased in
waves.[56]

In the morning she was shaky and weak, but the energy had
passed. However the following night it was worse, as along with the
desire and energy she saw strange hideous shapes and beings, leering
and obscene, having sexual orgies, and doing horrible sexual things
she had never before heard of or imagined. She was terrified of the
hallucinations and felt she was losing her mind. In the morning she
was again shaky and weak, and full of shame. This continued the
following night. Her guru advised her to control what was happening,
which she did somewhat by lying completely stiff, pulling in the
muscles of her lower body, trying to control the mind not to run
away with imaginings. In this position she experienced:

burning currents of fire inside, cold shivers
running outside, wave after wave, over legs,
arms, abdomen, and the back, along the spine,
making all the hair rise over the body. It is as
if the whole frame is full of electricity.
Gradually, all the muscles of the thighs and the
tummy begin to ache with tension. But this
pain, gradually increasing my prolonged effort,
somehow helps to relieve the desire. The
ghastly shapes are here, sometimes clearly
visible, sometimes indistinct. Strangely, I am
getting used to them. [57]

The struggle between the opposites is also documented in
Tweedie's book. She is told this friction is necessary to cause the
suffering that will defeat the mind. "The greatest obstacle on the
spiritual path is to make people understand that they have to give up
everything." This is why every order of the guru must be obeyed,
even should the guru ask one to deliver to him his wife or his child --
if not, the aspirant cannot survive. Whatever is dearest must go.
"This is the Law. One cannot serve two Masters. Either the world
or the Guru. Everything has to be given up, absolutely; nothing
should remain, nothing at all. Even the self-respect has to go. Only
then, and then only, can I take them into my heart." [58]
Tweedie's path is also unique in the interest the guru has in
her dreams, and her book offers many dreams and interpretations.

Bhai Sahib taught that much of a follower's karma is acted out and released through dreams, once Kundalini is awakened, and experiences felt and suffered in dreams are thereby avoided on the earth plane, thus speeding up the karmic process.

This work is a powerful exposition of the daily rigors of the spiritual life, even when focused on love, and under the guidance of a master. It demonstrates the nature of guru-disciple relationship, the intensity of sexual energy as it sometimes emerges in this process, and the austerities one embraces when seeking spiritual transformation.

Commentary

Tweedie's biography indicates the rapid path of spiritual awakening available even to Westerners once a commitment is made, and details the kinds of energetic phenomenon, visions, and ego-issues that are sometimes aroused in the company of a spiritual teacher. She courageously shares the trauma of her sexual energy and imagery. After less than a year with her teacher she was sent to London, with no money, to begin a new life on her own. She has since become a spiritual guide for many, inspired by her books and her teachings about love and enlightenment.

Kennett Roshi:
A Zen Buddhist Perspective

An interesting series of autobiographical books has been written by Kennett Roshi, a Westerner who experienced kensho (enlightenment or God-realization) in a Buddhist monastery and later founded Shasta Abbey, in California. Two of her books are of special interest to the study of Kundalini, one an autobiographical account of a deep healing and spiritual transformation that she underwent over several months, following medical advice that she was going to die shortly of heart failure; the other an in-depth description of ancient methods useful in helping people balance their energy. In her biography How To Grow a Lotus Blossom (1977) she described experiences and visions similar to the yogic tradition, sharing in a style radically different from traditional Zen teachers who keep such stories secret.

Kennett sees enlightenment as an on-going flow, rather than occurring in stages, beginning with a first kensho (enlightenment experience) which Zen Buddhists call the "great flash of deep understanding" or "Penetration of Heaven". [59] "It is the one in which one knows one's unity with the immaculacy of nothingness and which grows even deeper if one keeps up one's meditation and training."[60]

On-going growth following this experience is more subtle and tends not to be experienced as a particular event although there are small moments of kensho that "make one dance" and are signs of development. In many ways she feels the most difficult time for aspirants is between the first and third kensho because temptations are far greater and more subtle. One finds that in order to progress one must not only keep passions rooted out but clean up traces of them remaining from both this and previous lives. Kennett describes the third kensho as containing all the elements of the first, but the first occurs in a flash, like a lightning bolt, and the third is experienced much more slowly and deliberately with time to comprehend each step of the way. For example "the opposites are each looked at slowly and dispassionately and then deliberately discarded; the first kensho is a swift comprehension of grace; the third kensho starts as a deliberate act of will."[61]

Kennett advises that it is not good to do deep meditation and training alone, or to be in a place where one can be disturbed. She wrote "When advanced spiritual development is reached the world seems to treble and quadruple its efforts to distract and dishearten. . . and it is then that faith in the memory of the first kensho is absolutely vital; one second of doubt, even the possibility of thinking of the possibility of doubting, can cause the spirit to despair and death is the result. True meditation is not for cowards; it is hazardous, perilous and magnificent. For this reason a place of absolute peace and quiet is necessary. You will also need a friend or a disciple who is perfectly willing to go to any lengths to keep the world from bothering you." [62]

She believes all people can have these experiences, and the stages are always the same, but that each person sees and experiences kensho somewhat differently. She warns that no one should pursue these studies only for the sake of having such experiences. In her personal story she identifies 43 stages in movement toward her third kensho, the process beginning when she was extremely ill and close to death, and began 12 days of meditation. The experiences of the following months are expressed in vivid images depicting her difficulties, decisions, options, opposites and expanded awareness.

In the first stage she saw two roads, representing options in the world, and chose not to take either but to forge ahead, seeing nothing but a great mountain range with a face as sheer as glass before her. With determination, by refusing to consider any inadequacy, limitation, distraction or fear she moved straight up to the top. From this vantage point she saw the hopelessness and despair in the lives of those who stay on ordinary paths, but she was faced with a vast unknown, and soon a vast darkness. Her continually moved on, reminding herself that "nothing matters" and remembering her first kensho experience. She realized she had to put right every wrong act she ever committed. [63]

In subsequent experiences, framed by the images of a great abyss of darkness, or the seductive brilliance of lights which she must also pass by, she continued on in the process to question her purpose for living, to root out the deepest meanings of each of the Buddhist Precepts, and to view many past lives and resolve karma remaining from them through conversations with those aspects of herself. At this point her physical illness passed and she began to recover.

Commentary

Kennett's story depicts in detail her inner visions and awareness, and suggests how the expansion of consciousness may be accomplished with visions. Her descriptions echo yogic descriptions of light and energy and scriptural descriptions of samadhi.

In addition to describing the kinds of visual imagery that may accompany spiritual growth, she outlines specific tasks in the process such as reconciling past wrongs, reviewing past lives, letting go of attachments and temptations, holding to the goal by remembering past experiences, and penetrating deeply into the experience and meaning of image and scripture. Such experiences are rarely, if ever, recorded in Zen literature, which generally views visions and body sensations as "makyo" or distracting delusions. Her vivid images demonstrate the deepest experience of the intuitive and visual function in this experience. It is also notable that she entered this process on the verge of dying and experienced remarkable healing in the midst of it, and that a key part of this process was that a trusted monk be with her at all times during the ordeal.

Motoyama:
Japanese Parapsychologist and Yogi

Motoyama, author of <u>Theories of the Chakras: Bridge to Higher Consciousness</u> (1981) was introduced to spiritual practice at an early age, taken to Japanese temples and shrines, and taught to chant Buddhist Sutras and Shinto prayers at the age of four. He would chant with his mother and foster mother for hours at a time. He writes that he was told about and experienced the existence of non-human entities who reside in higher dimensions (he does not describe these).   At age 25 he began doing yoga daily, beginning with asanas at 3 a.m. and sitting for three or four hours, doing pranayama and concentration on specific chakras. His body and mind soon began to fill with an extraordinary amount of energy, and his physical and psychological states gradually changed. Within six months problems he had previously had with his stomach and ears disappeared, and nervousness ceased. Later he felt some new sensations:

> I had an itchy feeling at the coccyx, a tingling feeling on the forehead and at the top of the head, and a feverish sensation in the lower abdomen. I could hear a sound something like the buzzing of bees around the coccyx. In ordinary daily life my sense of smell became so sensitive that I could not endure offensive odors.[64]

These conditions continued for two or three months. Then while doing pranayama one day he had felt around the svadhisthana chakra a "feverish" feeling like a mixture of ice and fire accompanied by a vision of white steam. A month or two later he saw a round, crimson fireball in his abdomen.   At this time he began to have prophetic dreams and ESP experiences and to realize the spontaneous fulfillment of wishes.   He became overly sensitive, physically and mentally, so that the smallest noise in meditation startled him. His emotions became unstable and he was easily excited. He states that this chakra is thought to control the genito-urinary system and the adrenal glands, and is connected to the kidney, urinary, bladder and triple heater meridians of acupressure. He believes abnormalities in these meridians may indicate increased activity of the svadhisthana chakra. When tested he had a distinct abnormality in the kidney and urinary bladder meridians, although no malfunction was present.

A few months later, when he was meditating before the altar as usual, he felt particularly feverish in the lower abdomen and "saw there a round blackish-red light like a ball of fire about to explode in the midst of a white vapor. Suddenly, an incredible power rushed through my spine to the top of the head and, though it lasted only a second or two, my body levitated off the floor a few centimeters. I was terrified. My whole body was burning, and a severe headache prevented me from doing anything all day. The feverish state continued for two or three days. I felt as if my head would explode with energy. Hitting myself around the 'Brahman Gate' at the top of the head was the only thing that brought relief."[65]

As he continued his yoga practice, long-term problems with indigestion and gastroenteritis improved, and a new series of abdominal sensations began. He often saw "reddish light center on the naval that would become intensely white, seemingly much brighter than the sun. I grew dizzy and could see nothing for about ten minutes. I began to see a purple light shining between my eyebrows or in my abdomen."[66] He saw ghosts and spirits, some of whom he helped with prayers, some who made him feel peaceful and others who influenced him negatively and made him emotionally unstable. He would become ill or get angry for no rcason, and once stayed in bed with a fever for a week. He experienced enhanced ESP abilities such as clairvoyance, telepathy, and spiritual insight.

During this period, while playing a game similar to the use of the Ouija Board with an old man, he fell into a semi-trance. His body felt like it was on fire and began to sweat profusely, his right hand began moving violently. Then he plunged into the extrasensory vision of a man in ancient times who was a tribal leader, and wanted to guide him through a place where he had lived in a former life. The following day while bicycling he discovered the place the guide had shown him in the trance.

Two years into this process, Motoyama began to notice a pain between the nipples of the chest crossing the midsternal line, and he felt as if his heart was functioning abnormally. One early morning while practicing water asceticism (pouring ice water over his naked body) he saw heat rising from the coccyx to his heart through the spine. His chest felt hot and his heart was a brilliant gold. The energy moved upward from the heart to the top of the head, becoming shining white. It left the body through the top of his head and rose into a higher dimension. He was aware of his physical body standing in the cold while his consciousness was in the heights worshipping the divine. His mother, who was watching, said she had seen a golden light shining at the top of his head and at his heart. He believes this was the opening of the anahata chakra. After this he began doing psychic healing, he developed an attitude of non-attachment to worldly things, and he felt a constant optimism about everything, being internally peaceful and free.

Opening of the visuddhi chakra occurred four or five years later, after he began concentrating on it during pranayama exercises. Soon an irritation developed in the throat and breathing became difficult. After several months, he saw a dark purple light spread around his head. Consciousness of his body vanished, he became quiet and calm, and experienced a state of nothingness. Later he experienced a terrifying void, and felt such fear he wanted to give up yoga, and for awhile he saw a horrible devil-like being. In time he overcame the fear and he could enjoy the total silence and peace, work freely in the world with no attachment to results, and see the past, present and future in the same dimension. He became able to see the past, present and future lives of others. His hearing improved although he had had tympanitis in both ears since a child, and one eardrum and the bones of the left ear had been surgically removed.

The initial awakening of the ajna chakra began while focusing on it, concentrating on Om. After doing this one hour a day for several months he felt the Kundalini energy rise. His lower abdomen became as hard as iron, and his respiration became so slow that he was barely breathing. It felt as if the upper half of his body had disappeared. The ajna chakra vibrated and he was immersed in a dark purple light while a bright white light shone from between his eyebrows. He heard a voice call as if it were echoing in a valley. He was filled with ecstasy and a divine symbol of power was revealed to him. The outcome of this experience was deep calm and experiencing a state of widened and deepened consciousness, seeing past, present and future simultaneously.

The crown chakra , the sahasrara, awakened after only a year of yoga, according to Motoyama, while doing a Taoist practice called Shoshuten, the circulation of energy in the upper body. He had inner sight of the sahasrara and two or three other chakras shining, and began to see a golden light enter and leave his body through the top of his head, which seemed to extend ten to twenty centimeters upward. He saw a vision of the head of Buddha, shining blue and purple, resting on his own head. A golden-white light flowed in and out through the Buddha's crown. He heard a powerful but tender voice, and realized his mission, his previous lives, his own spiritual state and many other things.

Commentary

This biography echoes many of the conditions of previous stories including awareness of energy, light, inner vision of the body, visions of the Buddha and other entities, psychic abilities, fears about the practices, out-of-body experience, awareness of a past life, and feelings of ecstasy. It is unique in its careful exploration of experiences related to each of the chakras. Many of these experiences are found elsewhere in the literature but not with such specific correlations. Motoyama does not mention working with a spiritual teacher, other than his mother, who he says had experienced some similar openings, and who sometimes was with him during these experiences. However he followed strict disciplines and austerities, and meditated very consistently for long hours prior to and during this time of his awakening

Da Free John: A Western Teacher

Born Franklin Albert Jones (Nov.3, 1939) in Jamaica, New York, Da Free John, is a unique phenomenon in the West, an American who has encountered extensive spontaneous spiritual experiences since early childhood, who attended Western universities, and developed teachings that resemble Eastern philosophy which he presents through many books, classes and videotapes in an unusual personal style. He does not seem to teach yoga in any traditional form, but rather has developed his own approach to spiritual awakening, which he teaches at centers in several countries. He provides a fairly thorough history of his spiritual development and mystical experiences in his autobiography, The Knee of Listening.[67]

Free John claims that from his earliest memories he always enjoyed an experience of the "bright", an incredible sense of himself as radiant , with joy, light and freedom in the middle of his head. He felt "in touch with consciousness itself", aware he was the same as everyone and everything.[68] He writes that during his first twenty years this sense of consciousness and light was gradually undermined by the ordinary and traditional patterns of life. Several times, during serious illness, he felt a sense of a mass of gigantic thumbs coming down from above and pressing into some form of himself that was much larger than his physical body.

In 1957 he began studying philosophy at Colombia University and began what he terms "an experimental life along the same lines which controlled the mood of our civilization. I decided I would unreservedly exploit every possibility for experience. I would avail myself of every possible human experience, so that nothing possible to mankind, high or low, would be unknown to me." [69]

One night as he sat at his desk contemplating the exhaustion of this exploring and feeling deep conflict, he experienced a total revolution of energy and awareness. A rising force caused him to stand and he felt it draw him out of his depths and expand, filling his whole body and every level of consciousness with wave upon wave of beautiful and joyous energy. He felt mad, but joyful with an ecstasy in every cell that was almost intolerable in its pressure, light and force. He ran outside, hoping to find someone to communicate it to.

His head began to ache with it as it saturated his brain and he returned to his room.

In 1961 he finished Columbia and began graduate work at Stanford, continuing to experiment but seeing through this what he calls an end of contradiction. For six weeks he was part of a drug experiment at the VA Hospital, using mescaline, LSD and psilocibin at four different sessions. In one of these he felt profound emotion rising at the base of the spine and generating intense overwhelming love as it appeared in the heart. As it moved up through the head, the back of the neck and the crown he wept uncontrollably, as if all parts of his being had been simultaneously aroused, becoming conscious and alive. He had the thought "getting to cry is shaped like a seahorse."[70] In this process he believes he became conscious of the chakra body and Kundalini shakti which had opened in itself, and the internal form of consciousness (vital and ethereal attachments) became known to him. This "form" of the spiritual body was what he had known as the "bright" when he was a child. At this time he also felt the "thumbs" experience of his childhood, which also reoccurred later during meditations.

He lived with a woman who later became his wife, and became more secluded after this experience. He spent his time writing, although it was unproductive, and practicing intensive focusing on the mind itself, a training that ultimately made inner concentration and monitoring or witnessing of experience habitual. He came to understand what he calls the truth of Narcissus as the controlling force of the adventure of human life, that which keeps one from discovery of conscious being by covering it with the mechanics of living, seeking, dying and mortality. He struggled for several years with deep introspection, claiming he was close to madness at times. Then he pursued extensive studies of psychic and mystical literature. He found in Eastern literature keys to many of his own experiences and saw that his path and the meaning of all life was in the shiva-shakti process.

In New York he discovered a store front about which he had had a vision, and met a man called Rudi, who had been a student of Gurdjieff, Muktananda and Subud. He taught Kundalini Yoga and Free John asked to be accepted as his student. He was told to get a job and work six months first.   After leaving the store he felt a current of strong energy rising up his arm from his right hand: it passed into his body with a "profound and thrilling fullness" and his heart felt vibrant joy. His head felt swollen as if it contained an aura that extended around his skull several inches. He began to run, feeling on fire with joy and incredible energy.

Classes with Rudi involved receiving shaktipat, after which he felt energy move from the eyes down the heart and chest to the genitals, then travel upwards through the back of the spine to the head. Students focused on the "so-hum" (more classically identified as "ham-sah") mantra, and felt themselves going out into space, beyond all the universe. During his time with Rudi, Free John says he learned discipline, saw images of light, felt energy charges and kriyas in his body, began twitching facial muscles and making animal sounds in meditation, felt great peace and went into samadhi.

In 1966 he moved to Philadelphia and studied at a Lutheran seminary. A few months later he had an experience he believes was akin to a mental breakdown. It began with a cold and he noticed his flesh becoming massy and unpliable and his body, gray, disturbed and deathlike. He was overcome by anxiety and fear of death, and felt that all his physical and mental processes were dying. He lay in bed with a fever, his heart seeming to slow down, beat irregularly and stop. He was taken to a hospital and told he was having an anxiety attack. It continued for three days. One day he laid down on the floor and allowed the rising fear and sense of death to overwhelm him, experiencing the death of his body and mind, witnessing it and allowing it to happen. He went through it and came to a place of infinite bliss, oneness with the universe and pure consciousness. He felt wonderful, and aware that the motivation and error of his whole previous life had been avoidance of relationship -- creating separation.

In 1968 he went to India and studied with Muktananda. During the year he spent there he had many energetic and physical phenomena, transports to other worlds, and visions of the blue pearl or blue light within which he saw the supra causal or cosmic body. But he felt this was not the point and felt resistance to the ritual of Indian spiritual life and returned to the U.S. in 1969. In seclusion and constant meditation he probed deeply the meaning of spiritual life, and began to teach meditation and have discussions with students about spiritual life, practice and experiences. At night he reports having fully conscious meetings with saints, yogis and miracle workers and seeing miraculous demonstrations of yogic powers; he felt Muktananda's or Nityananda's presences as if they looked over his body. Later he returned to India but the ashram environment had changed dramatically, and was much less personal. He was given work to do and expected to follow the formal routine, which seemed empty to him. While working in the garden one afternoon, he had a powerful vision of Mary. She advised him to go on a trip to the Christian pilgrimage sites, and soon afterwards he left India.

After returning to the U.S., Free John became a spiritual teacher, gradually developing a following of several thousand. He lives in Fiji, heads spiritual centers in several countries, and has written numerous books on spiritual awakening and related topics.

Commentary

This biography includes many experiences reported by those who awaken Kundalini in the West including early childhood psychic experiences, drug experimentation, exposure to Kundalini Yoga practices, movements of energy in the body, light and visions of spiritual teachers, heart problems and overwhelming fears of death, and samadhi. His struggle to understand life and spirituality is outlined more fully than most teachers, and he provides an opportunity to see what it is like to attend Western colleges and seek spirituality within the context of Western culture. The assistance of a teacher seemed critical at certain junctures, but he also had lengthy periods without a guide. The financial support of his wife appeared to alleviate any conflict about making a living during most of his explorations, and his interest in spiritual matters appears to be a life-long obsession, factors not uncommon in the literature.

Part 3: Reports of Kundalini Experiences Outside of Eastern Traditions

Brugh Joy

Brugh Joy is an American physician who wrote an autobiography, Joy's Way(1979), in which he described what appears to be an awakening of Kundalini that occurred after a few months of meditation practice, which he learned from a spiritual teacher he identifies only as Eunice, who lived in Los Angeles.

> For me, the quickening began within a few weeks after I first met Eunice.I was sure that the big California earthquake had struck. I jumped out of bed and was heading for safety when I realized that nothing in the room seemed disturbed -- in particular, a hanging light fixture in my room wasn't swinging. The same thing happened several nights in succession, and each time it startled me. My

whole bed seemed to shake. I always checked
my pulse to see whether I was having heart
palpitations, and my heartbeat was always
regular. Finally I had to conclude that my
body was shaking or going into strange
repetitive muscular contractions. . . Now the
sensation is like a very fine motor or fast vibration centered at different times in different
areas of my body, primarily in the chest, neck
and forehead areas.[71]

Later he began to experience what he called "superbrilliant
light space. . . more intense than looking at the sun or any other
brilliantly lighted object I had ever seen " Then, one night, lying in
bed the motor feeling came on "like a diesel truck." He wrote:

It's vibration shook not only me but also the
kingsize bed. It was first centered in my chest
area, then moved into the lower abdomen, then
up toward my head. On came the superbrilliant
light. It was not just a flash, and it did not
stop. For a moment, I was terrified. Then I
heard a voice say, "What do you think you
have been preparing for?" I accepted it and
relaxed into the experience. It lasted for about
six hours: intense, intense, intense white light
and the quaking of my whole body. The next
morning, I felt unusually rested and nothing
appeared grossly different to my awareness, but
over the next few months I recognized that my
work was maturing and my ability to see
energy fields was beginning to increase.
Something subtle, yet profound, had happened
to me that night.[72]

After this the phenomena rarely occurred, although at the
time of writing his book he had noticed the beginning of the original
flashing pattern recurring.

Joy's experience led him to an exploration of psychic
phenomena and healing practices. He learned to read the energy field
of chakras with his hands, using this method for diagnosis and
healing, and he developed theories about the location of chakras,
much of it given to him by an inner teacher. He spontaneously

developed processes and exercises that awaken and transform energy, and he later discovered that some of the concepts he had been practicing and teaching were contained in the work of Theosophist Alice Bailey, Esoteric Healing(1953).

Commentary

Joy's experiences have many of the indicators of Kundalini awakening -- energy activity, lights and images, growing intensity of interest in spiritual matters, pursuit of healing and study of esoteric literature, changing his life as a physician to focus on work with chakras, healing and teaching processes to help others awaken their energy. He doesn't report emotional turmoil in the same style as other writers, but the awakening caused him to walk away from a successful medical practice, to spend months traveling on only 25 cents a day though India, and to undergo a personally directed initiation ordeal in the Great Pyramid in Egypt. He has reported psychic experiences such as sudden insight into esoteric truths, and has also been deeply influenced by his dreams, at times undergoing major personality shifts because of their insights. In one instance he reports, like Caitanya, hearing a voice that gave him a simple comment or message when in the midst of kriyas. I have interviewed several people who experienced spiritual openings while participating in the intensive two-week seminars he teaches, which emphasize the awakening of heart energy, using energy for healing, recognition of the dark side of the psyche, and psychic development.

W. Thomas Wolfe

An unlikely Westerner to write a book on Kundalini is W. Thomas Wolfe, an IBM technical writer who reports an awakening in 1975, following meditation and lengthy exercises using biofeedback. His autobiography, And the Sun is Up: Kundalini Rises in the West, (1978) is useful in providing a perspective on how Westerners who are not prepared may experience this phenomenon, and because some of his experience correlates with yogic tradition and with that of subjects I have interviewed. Wolfe's work also shows how technologies used in modern therapy can be used in ways that produce Kundalini responses.

The biographical information presented by Wolfe indicates a tendency toward psychic experience as a child, the experience of lucid and telepathic dreams as a young adult, and a period of reading and studying all aspects of psychic phenomena, dream interpretation, and various esoteric and exoteric religions. During a period of financial stress, and anxiety about his dying father, he had what he felt was a nervous collapse. One day when his legs had gone to sleep from sitting he stood up and was swept by a feeling of panic as the tingling in his legs spread into his upper body. His entire body began vibrating furiously, and he ran outside, throwing himself face-down on the grass where he lay without moving, his arms spread to grab as much ground as they could. He felt as if his whole inner foundation had been wiped away and he had completely lost control.

Wolfe put aside psychic interests after this, and during the next twelve years he married, had two children and became involved in his career in New York. He describes himself as a hard worker and very competitive, somewhat nervous, a heavy smoker, who eventually drank half a fifth of whisky and a six-pack of beer daily. Work intensity caused him to yell at co-workers and he developed chronic heartburn. Sometimes his heart would palpitate loudly and forcefully. At age 35 a challenge by a colleague forced him to see himself clearly, and he reevaluated his life, began to meditate, stopped drinking and smoking, and became friends with a couple of men who shared an interest in meditation and the psychic. After four months of meditation following a self-styled adaptation of TM he felt some relief of his chronic anxiety, and began recording dreams, and experiencing psychic events again.

Wolfe purchased a biofeedback machine and began practicing 30 minutes a day, trying various mental gymnastics to boost the amplitude of alpha waves and make them come and go at will. Within a month he had logged 54 hours of biofeedback time. Although he had mixed responses to the exercises he found that when he practiced them for any length of time he would be left with a feeling of residual bliss. He learned he could generate the most alpha when he let go and allowed inner volition to run the process. He noticed other strange effects such as heat building up under the electrodes on his head, coincident with periods of high alpha and theta wave generation. One night, after falling asleep, he felt a low-pitched humming current in his head.

Wolfe interprets a number of his dreams, which he feels are related to the Kundalini experience, and describes a number of experiences that followed prolonged biofeedback sessions. These include lying in bed and feeling a strong force in his head pulling him upward and to the right; feeling himself to be in a completely silent world; falling into an extreme ecstasy centered in the middle of his head; and having precognitive visions.

He believes his Kundalini awakening occurred one night when he was trying to sleep, and noticed a light pulsating in his mind's eye. It pulsed brightly, intensifying until it overpowered him and he heard strong, loud, discordant sounds. Then he felt a strong current run between the center of his head and his forehead, terminating just above the right eyebrow. His heart rate accelerated. The lights changed into a fixed, holographic pattern of large, luminous balls, which seemed to form a corridor he was either part of or traveling through. Wolfe calls this development a transmutation of consciousness, in which his body-sense changed into a sensation of being luminous spheres. An inner voice asked "Who is thinking now, Fred?" The thought seemed to give additional impetus to his travel down the corridor, and he became panicked. He tried to cut back on the intensity by recalling himself on his bed, and when he couldn't do so he felt trapped. Then he began to flicker between awareness of his childhood and his current homes. Finally the corridor vanished, the vibrations ended and he was able to realize where he was.

For seven months following this event his energy, experiences and psychic awareness intensified, and his body felt lighter. For two years more the experience abated and recurred periodically. His inclinations toward sex and negative emotions seemed deadened but the emotions of love, compassion and goodwill were magnified. In a series of dreams he felt beings trying to possess him, whom he believes were probably various personality components. Later on, during meditation, he had a vision of an immense burning sun breaking into his waking life, and he had experiences of a blue dot appearing, especially while reading.

He wrote: "There were many nights in this period that I spent sobbing quietly in the darkness before sleep to think that I would be losing my self and all my attachments, perhaps including my attachments to my loved ones. Becoming big was hard for me because I knew now that I had to cease being small. And it felt unstoppable."[73] He began meditations in which he pictured merging with Christ, and had dreams of merger, following which he seemed to feel more integrated.

Wolfe changed his work and moved and he began to spend time at a Muktananda meditation center learning yoga. During this period he had symptoms that put him in a coronary care unit for three days, thinking he had a heart-attack, but it could not be diagnosed. He began to have digestive problems and had to eat lighter and more frequent meals so as to digest food properly, and cut down on the amount of formal meditation and biofeedback sessions. After a few months his problems waned.

Wolfe's experience with Kundalini caused him to conclude that "One must pause at the heart of one's activities and know one's self. Life must be lived free of attachments, free of encumbrances of the senses. A man must accept what will come. He must let his Godhead live through him. He must be fully aware in all aspects of life. He must abandon all labels, including the label of self. . . The small self must dissolve -- go away. And this is not something one can force or do. It is what remains when one just gives up and surrenders oneself to what will be."[74]

He advises that the preparation for Kundalini is to become sensitive to small internal stimuli, to discriminate between desirable and undesirable stimuli, to become more receptive to possibilities and open the mind. He advocates recording ones dreams and experiences, and sharing them with others, and holding to the expectation that this awakening can occur.

Commentary

Wolfe's history contains many of the elements reported and commonly misdiagnosed in Western subjects following Kundalini awakening, and demonstrates that this experience can happen to someone who has not led a particularly disciplined or spiritual life before the awakening. Changes in Wolfe's energy impacted his life in nearly every area -- sleeping, eating habits, emotions, psychic and physical. He reports great emotional upheavals, losing attachments, temporarily deadened sexual energies and negative emotions, experiencing awareness of a blue dot (similar to the blue pearl of Muktananda), conditions similar to a heart attack and numerous other experiences. He was reoriented in this process to Eastern spiritual practices, seeking out a guru, and feeling increased love and compassion. Some of the factors that may have assisted him through this process were his work with dreams and a journal, talking with friends who gave him emotional support, having a context of spiritual opening for his experience and seeking out a guru and a spiritual community.

Jung's Client With Kundalini Symptoms

In an appendix to <u>Collected Works Vol. 16: The Practice of Psychotherapy</u> (1954/1966), Jung describes a case in which a 25-year-old woman had physical problems and corresponding dreams that clearly indicate Kundalini activity. At the time he was working with her he found her "neurotic" symptoms undecipherable. He had no knowledge of Eastern religion and he felt at such a loss in understanding her process that he repeatedly considered transferring her to another therapist. When the analysis felt stuck Jung had a dream in which she was sitting at the topmost pinnacle of a castle tower, high on a mountain top, golden in the light of the evening sun.

When he told her the dream her symptoms emerged rapidly, beginning with "an undefinable excitation in the perineal region, and she dreamt that a white elephant was coming out of her genitals."[75] (A white elephant is a symbol associated with muladhara chakra, representing the carrier of the universe.)
Soon afterwards symptoms of uterine ulcers appeared. Her physician found an inflamed swelling of mucous membrane, about the size of a pea, which refused to heal for months and merely shifted from place to place, and then suddenly disappeared. Then she developed extreme hyperaesthenia of the bladder, although no local infections could be found. At Jung's urging to express herself, she began to draw vivid flowers in symbolic patterns. The bladder problem ceased and intestinal spasms developed, causing gurgling noises and sounds of splashing that could even be heard outside the room. She developed problems with the colon, ileum and small intestine, which abated after several weeks. Then she had the feeling "that the top of her skull was growing soft, that the fontanelle was opening up, and that a bird with a long, sharp beak was coming down to pierce through the fontanelle as far as the diaphragm."[76]

Although Jung felt he could not understand two-thirds of her dreams or give her any help, she felt the work was going "splendidly. . .I always have the craziest symptoms, but something is happening all the time."[77]

Synchronistically, after many months of analysis, someone gave him one of the first books published in English on tantric yoga, Avalon's The Serpent Power, and Jung could see that her dreams and experiences correlated with the symbolism of the chakras. He attributed this possibility to the fact that her psyche may have been influenced by living in Java for a while as a very young child, a rare lapse from his usual recognition of the universal symbolism of the collective unconscious. Jung wrote:

> When the Kundalini serpent had reached the manipura chakra . . . it was met by the bird of thought descending from above, which with its sharp beak pierced through the fontanelle (sahasrara chakra) to the diaphragm (anahata) {sic}. Therefore a wild storm of affect broke out, because the bird had implanted in her a thought which she would not and could not accept. She gave up the treatment and I saw her only occasionally, but noticed she was hiding something. A year later came the

confession. She was beset by the thought that
she wanted a child.[78]

With the experience at the crown chakra the patient became
obsessed with the idea of having a child, which seemed a great let-
down to her. But by understanding a "little bit of Tantric
philosophy" he helped the patient to make an "ordinary human life
for herself as a wife and mother -- and to do so without losing touch
with the inner psychic figures which had been called awake." He
defined her symptoms as "neurosis caused by the forgotten early
childhood influences which estranged her from her European
consciousness" and he saw the cure as helping her have "a lasting
spiritual possession instead of nebulous spiritual fantasies, as she led
an ordinary life with husband, children and household duties." He
cites this as an unusual case but not an exception. He writes of it as
a "saga of blunders, hesitations and doubts" due to his ignorance of
Oriental psychology. He adds "No psychotherapist should lack that
natural reserve which prevents people from riding rough-shod over
mysteries they do not understand and trampling them flat." And he
adds, "the ultimate cause of a neurosis is something positive that
needs to be preserved for the patient ."[79]

Commentary

Unfortunately Jung neglected to report whether his client
had any unusual spiritual, energetic or emotional conditions that
might be correlated with Kundalini awakening. However, this case
presents an opportunity to view how symptoms can be illusory and
poorly diagnosed using a medical model or traditional psychoanalytic
approach, and demonstrates how Kundalini imagery and conditions
may arise in psychotherapy. He diagnosed her condition as a neurosis
and used the therapy to help her adjust to an appropriate role in her
society instead of addressing the spiritual implications of her
obsession with having a child. It is possible that the dreams and
physical symptoms may be only coincidentally related to Kundalini,
and more appropriately symbolic of a developmental stage in her
consciousness having to do with taking on the feminine/mother
aspects of her psyche, bringing her own creative forces into life.
Jung does not define the nature of the "spiritual possession" she
received from this analysis, and it would be necessary to have more
information about her later psychological/spiritual evolution to
accurately identify this case as a Kundalini experience.

References: Chapter 5

1   Bucke, R. (1969) Cosmic Consciousness, p. 3.

2   Op. cit., Foreward, unnumbered pages, p.4.

3   Serrano, Miquel (1974) The Serpent of Paradise. London:
     Routledge & Kegan Paul.

4   Mujamdar, S. (1969) Caitanya: His Life and Doctrine.
     (-- Caitanya is pronounced as if spelled Chaitanya. The Sanscrit
     word means Pure Consciousness, with an absolute freedom of
     will, knowledge and action.
     -- Stories of Jesus, St. Paul, St, Catherine of Genoa, Hildegarde
     of Bergin and other Christian mystics predate the Caitanya
     story.
     -- Stories of Jesus,Buddha and Mohammed are so overlaid with
     myth and dogma they are not appropriate for comparison with
     "ordinary" people.)

5   Op. cit., p. 126. (Visvambhar is another name of Vishnu, the god
     who sustains the universe.)

6   Op. cit., p. 134.

7   Op. cit., p. 185. (Maha-Bhakti-yoga is devotion to supreme yoga or
     union with the divine)

8   Op. cit., p. 241.

9   Op. cit., p. 242.

10 Bhaiji (trans, by G. Gupta) (1962) Mother as Revealed to
     Me.Varanasi: Shree Shree Anandamayee Sangha.

11 Op. cit., p. 34.

12 Op. cit., p. 46.

13 Op. cit., p. 12.

14 Op. cit., p. 13.

15 Op. cit., p. 50-51.

16 Op. cit., p. 67.

17 Op. cit., p. 92.

18 Op. cit.

19 Op. cit., p. 32.

20 Atmananda (1971) Words of Sri Anandmayi Ma, Varanasi: Shree
     Shree Anandamayee Sangha.

21 Krishna, G. (1974) Higher Consciousness: The evolutionary thrust of
     Kundalini. New York: Julian, p. 28.

22 Op. cit., p. 37.

23 Krishna, G. (1970 rev.) Kundalini: The Evolutionary Energy in
     Man., Boulder: Shambhala, p. 13.
24 Op. cit., p. 49.
25 Op. cit.
26 Op. cit., p. 51.
27 Op. cit., p. 66.
28 Op. cit., pp. 65-66.
29 Muktananda, S. (1978) Play of Consciousness, Ganeshpuri, India:
     Gurudev Siddha Peeth, p. 61.
30 Op. cit., p. 32.
31 Op. cit., p. xix.
32 Op. cit., p. xxiv.
33 Op. cit., p. xviv.
34 Yogananda, P. (1967) Science of Religion, pp. 79-80.
35 Yogananda, P. (1945) Autobiography of a Yogi, p. 181.
36 Op. cit., p. 279.
37 Op. cit., p. 12.
38 Op. cit., p. 125.
39 Op. cit., p. 166.
40 Sivananda, S.(1969) Spiritual Experiences (Amrita Anubhava), p. 45.
41 Op. cit. p. 46.
42 Jayakar, P. (1986) Krishnamurti: A biography, San Francisco: Harper
     & Row; Lutyens, M. (1975). Krishnamurti, the Years of
     Awakening, New York: Farrar, Straus and Giroux.
43 Jayakar, Op. cit., p. 73.
44 Op. cit., p. 47.
45 Op. cit., p. 48.
46 Op. cit., p. 52.
47 Op. cit., p. 53.
48 Op. cit., p. 54.
49 Op. cit., p. 57.
50 Lutyens, Op. cit., p. 282.
51 Goel, B. S. (1985) Third Eye and Kundalini, India: Third Eye Fd.
52 Op. cit., p. 10.
53 Tweedie, I. (1986) Daughter of Fire, Grass Valley, CA.: Blue
     Dolphin, p. 21.
54 Op. cit., p. 36.
55 Op. cit., p. 55.

56 Op. cit., p. 109.

57 Op. cit., p. 116.

58 Op. cit., p. 87.

59 Kennett, J. and MacPhillamy, D. (1977) How to Grow a Lotus Blossom, Mr. Shasta, CA.: Shasta Abbey, p. 1.

60 Op. cit., p. 2.

61 Op. cit., p. 3.

62 Op. cit., p. 6.

63 Op. cit., p. 26.

64 Motoyama, H. (1981) Theories of the Chakras: Bridge to Higher Consciousness, Wheaton, Ill.: Theosophical Pub. House, p.240.

65 Op. cit. p. 241.

66 Op. cit. p. 243.

67 Jones, F. (1972) The Knee of Listening, Los Angeles: The Dawn Horse Press.

68 Op. cit., p. 10.

69 Op. cit., p. 11.

70 Op. cit., p. 18.

71 Joy, B. (1979) Joy's Way: A map for the transformational journey, Los Angeles: J. P. Tarcher, p. 197.

72 Op. cit., p. 198.

73 Wolfe, T. (1978) And the Sun is Up: Kundalini Awakens in the West.   Red Hook, N. Y.: Academy Hill, p. 123.

74 Op. cit., p. 127.

75 Jung, C. G. (1954/1966)   Collected Works Vol. 16: The Practice of Psychotherapy , (R. F. C. Hull, trans.) Princeton: Princeton University Press, p. 333.

76 Op. cit.

77 Op, cit., p. 334.

78 Op. cit., p. 336.

79 Op. cit., p. 337.

CHAPTER SIX

KUNDALINI AWAKENING IN THE WEST

When Westerners pass along their personal stories of awakening spiritual energy, having visions of the divine, or being thrust into the maelstrom of psychic upheaval generated by Kundalini it is usually with a sense of puzzlement, wonderment and anxiety. Nothing in western science or religion provides any rational foundation with which to understand and integrate this experience. People sometimes wonder if they are deluding themselves, if they are crazy, if they have a disease or if some great joke is being played -- for certainly they are not "holy" enough to "deserve" a genuine mystical encounter. To the extent that fear, doubt and self-deprecation persist the path will be more difficult, for these negative emotions cloud the capacity to focus one's attention on spiritual development, and can lead to compulsive fixations on emotional or physical symptoms.

Spiritual openings in the West occur in many patterns, following the diverse exploratory processes which engage Western psyches and sometimes occur with no apparent cause or trigger. These cases, collected through many hours of interviews, are less complete than those in the previously recorded literature because the subjects are for the most part still actively engaged in their spiritual journey, still in process. They are not gurus, spiritual leaders or saints, and never expect to be. They have experienced openings, insights, visions, energy phenomena, change -- and they have a new sense of certainty and awareness about who they are -- a connection with Self in it's most profound sense. But they live ordinary lives, struggling in ordinary ways with the demands of professions, relationships, families, schooling, and self-development. For some the events of Kundalini are ten to twenty years past, yet the experience is still having an impact on their lives.

The uniqueness of each experience is a reflection of the individuation of each life, showing a multitude of paths, all of which ultimately converge into the knowledge of the same transcendent Self. We can see many of the conditions associated with Kundalini in each history, yet can never be entirely certain this is a "classical" Kundalini awakening. What we can see clearly is that each individual is engaged in discovering that which is greater than ego, which brings the numinous forward in consciousness and creates the possibility of knowing a range of experience beyond the ordinary life.

Sarah

Sarah was born in 1918 to a widowed mother who was a Christian Scientist and a Theosophist. As a child she developed psychic and spiritual interests, especially feeling a connection with her deceased father, and was encouraged to explore these interests and to take responsibility in helping others less fortunate than herself. In her twenties she married a young law student, who later became a successful attorney, and she gave her energy to family and community service. For years she led a full life involved with community, church, and the rearing of six children and 30 foster children. She taught Sunday school and bible class, was a board member of many charitable groups, and was concerned with addressing social problems and doing meaningful volunteer work.

In her forties Sarah became disillusioned with this work. She found herself moved by the retarded children to whom she taught religion,struck by the simple way they approached God. She began to study meditation, at first following practices one hour a day such as concentration on a candle, a match, or the breath. Over the next ten years she learned Transcendental Meditation (TM) and practiced meditations, yoga mantras, movement, concentration and/or problem-solving techniques up to two hours a day. In her fifties she became interested in parapsychology and Jungian psychology and returned to college to earned both a BA and MA in psychology. During this time she was also involved in a women's therapy group, producing much art with symbolic content. Then she attended a seminar with Brugh Joy at which her awakening occurred.

During the sessions with Joy she spent one hour daily meditating, and two sessions daily that began with listening to high intensity sound. She experienced inner sight (seeing with the mind's eye inside the body) so she could see the chakras. Brugh recommended that she visualize triangles joining at her solar plexus.

Normally this visualization joined seventh, sixth, fifth, and fourth chakras but in one meditation she saw it going down all the way to the base chakra. As it hit this point it exploded all the way upward through her body, like a tremendous whole body orgasm, sending tears down her face. She felt "unhinged" for two days afterwards. She felt rather diffuse, unfocused, and quieter than usual. Her energy stayed very intense and she was awake all night with it. She felt rushes of joy, laughter or tears. She felt almost no boundaries and whenever she went into meditation the experience returned.

Since this event she sees this image and feels intense energy when meditating, sometimes several times a week, sometimes with months passing between experiences. Listening to music sometimes triggers the energy. Visions may come either spontaneously or in response to requests for information. An inner spiritual guide named Michael came and offered her guidance. She did many spontaneous works of art using symbols such as crosses, the AUM symbol triangles, circles, fires and snakes. She reports no kriya activity (shaking or jerks of the body), dreams, or physical difficulties that seem related to Kundalini. She recalls several fearful visions, one in which she felt herself cut up piece by piece, and another in which swords were being taken out of her. She states that she learned to detach from negative visions, and "get the ego out of the way", and they stopped. One night she was awakened three times by a man's voice saying "Call to commitment". She feels this marked a deepening of her spiritual experience.

Sarah continued her work with Joy, and while doing meditation practices at his workshops that involve listening to high intensity sound she sometimes sees visions, or experiences intuitive knowing about the future. She has written three books, most of which came to her involuntarily as she listened to music. "Each day I would have a piece of an overall vision and in two weeks I would have a complete story which would tell me what was happening in the psyche. These were very easy to see and understand." Sometimes she sees guides and entities associated with clients who assist her in healing them, and she has had many psychic experiences. She once smelled a Havana cigar in meditation and saw a big, craggy Englishman. He dictated information for his wife, who was her house guest at the time.

Since the awakening, Sarah has acquired a Ph.D. in psychology. She continues to practice psychotherapy and teach, primarily doing small group work using imagery, music, dreams, art, dance, movement and meditation practices. When she teaches a group the format for the meeting is always channeled to her, although sometimes only at the last minute. She can see blocked chakras in others and help to release them. She often sees lights, and sees many colors in all of the chakras.

Sarah believes that "Kundalini energy feels like a tremendous invasion to some people and they are just resisting the invasion when they have many kriyas". Trust is the most important aspect in dealing with it. "I can take people to the level where they can see what they need and bring it back. We must trust the healer in them." When she works with others with Kundalini experiences she mainly listens and does a therapeutic process called voice dialogue, talking with the Kundalini energy. She feels it calms them down just to talk with her since they know she experiences it, and they feel less fearful of being crazy. She also helps them get in touch with blocked energy, by going fully into the experience of it and asking what the body needs. She works with dreams, art, dance or movement to express and release blocks. At this point she believes Kundalini "is no big deal. I used to think it was but never thought it would happen to me. I know it signifies a level of consciousness. It may be my focus is just different now. I used to focus on things that were unjust in the world -- now I see it all going on inside of me."

Sarah does not report radical life changes related to this opening, but sees a deepening of her spiritual awareness which she regards as part of a growing process in which she was already engaged. Her concept of God changed to a more impersonal view, seeing god as part of everyone and everything, and letting go of concerns about the past and future in favor of living for the "now". Where once she was an activist she is not anymore, but sometimes she "feels so much compassion it hurts". She comments "The more I am in it the less I know. I used to think I knew a lot but I'm not sure now. I'm moving into not-knowing, which is like Ken Wilber's concept of 'no-boundaries', and is not a very comfortable place."

Commentary on Diagnosing this Experience:

Sarah's experience is the least intense and frightening of any in this collection, and yet her subsequent productivity, psychic capacity and creativity is the most extensive of any of the subjects I interviewed. She has reported the least amount of physical difficulty or illness and is probably the most energetic and yet she is the oldest, 68 at the time of the interview.

I recall Swami Tirtha's comment that Kundalini can arise through selfless work, because this has been the tenor of her entire life. She has done the equivalent of karma yoga, caring for numerous children and supporting many social causes. She has also experienced psychic tendencies throughout her life, a pattern that corresponds with at least half of the biographies and cases I have studied. These became significantly more pronounced and integrated after the awakening. She has clearly been devout spiritually and was seeking an experience of deeper awareness of God in her ten years of meditation practice. As a mature, spiritually-committed and stable person she may have had few of the doubts, personality conflicts, and insecurities that seem to trigger panic in others. Her life does not seem to contain the ambivalence, experimentation, introversion and drug use of some who seek spiritual awakening; instead she was self-disciplined, led a well-ordered life and was content to be of service.

Sarah also had a context (Joy's work) and support system (a husband who was also involved in this work) to help her integrate and contain the experience. She had studied psychology deeply and had considerable therapy, as well as relationships with other people who had been in similar processes. Awakening presented no major conflicts about what to do with her life, but instead offered her a deeper spiritual dimension and greater intuitive power.

There may be many people like Sarah, seriously committed to God in the nature of their own religious traditions, who are unable to break through the barriers into direct experience because in their own tradition it is not considered a possibility, and there are no techniques for finding it. Belief systems, even in many religious orders and theological institutions, may prevent one from learning the practices that release the psyche into direct awareness of the divine.

Jayne

Born in 1943, Jayne was the only girl in a family of five children. She was raised in the Congregational church and describes herself as always spiritually searching, and having psychic experiences as a small child. She would frequently leave her body, and fly down the stairs at night, and wrote a poem about this when she was eight. She felt a strong psychic bond with her mother, who also had out-of-body experiences, and who went through a spiritual opening during a near-death experience in childbirth. Her brother, father, and husband were all alcoholics who died in recent years.

Jayne practiced hatha yoga, kriya yoga, pranayama and meditation exercises regularly for 20 years before her Kundalini experiences. She was widowed at the age of 31 when her husband died in an accident. She feels the death of the men in her life led to significant inner growth. Her energy and personality changes after her husband died and she began playing the piano and dancing, changed her style of dress and felt intense personal power. She had a sense of putting her house in order. She was in therapy for three years and began a spiritual study group. Then she went on an Evolution of Consciousness cruise around the Mediterranean with Patricia Sun, Robert Monroe, Jack Schwarz and many healers. They went to a number of power spots in Europe and the Middle East. In the Great Pyramid she had a strong sense of having been there before. As she lay in the king's chamber a spontaneous sound of Aum emerged from her. She had out-of-body experiences during this trip, following which she remembered many past lives of being in Egypt and doing initiation ceremonies there. After this she visited a yogi at a healing center periodically, and she felt an inner connection with Sai Baba.

The first time Jayne felt Sai Baba's presence she was with a psychic in New York who saw East Indians around her and told her that Sai Baba wanted her to see him right away. She felt his presence and chills went through her body. Several times after this she felt he was present with her, and sometimes she saw his form and talked with him. During this time, from 1978 until 1984, she practiced pranayama and hatha yoga almost daily, meditated three to five hours a day, and was celibate.

For five years she experienced many physical symptoms such as energy in her head, starting often with a bursting feeling in the throat that felt like an enormous goiter, heavy and pulsating; she had shooting pains to the right of the third eye, and through the middle and back of the head; and she saw white and yellow lights. This occurred often when a psychic healer did chakra healing on her, when meditating and when working with clients as a masseuse. She often (daily) felt tingling, itching, tickling sensations, kriyas, spasms or orgasmic blissful feelings in her entire body. She sometimes had shooting pains from her chest down her arm. The first of these occurred at a yoga retreat in 1975, when the chest pains were so intense she thought she was having a heart attack.

In the winter of 1984 she was mugged and her foot was broken by an attacker. Feeling very upset by the incident she visited a Tibetan Lama to find out why it happened and he told her there was a karmic reason for it. In April she visited a friend in the country and felt intense chills. A friend recommended a therapist who works with Kundalini and when she met him she recognized him from a dream she had had and felt an immediate bonding and intense infatuation. He had very intense energy or " shakti."

In June she began to experience extreme symptoms. For three months on an almost daily basis she lay in bed having sponta- neous rebirthing experiences (Rebirthing is an intense breathing process which resembles hyperventilation, and produces birth memories and other images and experiences.) She saw visions of herself living in an apartment across the street (where she later moved), and became obsessed with the idea that she lived in the wrong chamber and needed a place to do healing. One night she "moved a table to the center of the room and lay on it all knives, tools, straight edges, scissors, razors -- everything you separate with. I knew I was getting at the bottom of things, seeking clarity. I knew I needed more clarity because of the merging I was doing in meditation." She smelled perfume and felt it indicated the presence of Sai Baba. She lined up plants in terms of male and female, and thought of her desire for the alchemical marriage, blending of male and female within. She decided where each plant needed to be. She bought a sack of salt and sat in it. She felt frightened to be doing these things without her therapist there. Later she walked outside and "saw the world turning into many colors, and people seeming to be so nice to each other. I couldn't understand who was putting on this show." She went through a week of wearing white, feeling very pure and light, and seeing joy and kindness in everyone, dazzled by the brilliant intense colors of the world.

In another incident she put all of her furniture on the sidewalk outside, and locked herself indoors to do a rebirthing process. A friend came over and called the police when Jayne did not answer the door. When they arrived she convinced them she was okay and just wanted to be alone.

On another occasion she wrote an entire book of poetry in one sitting, and felt she was beginning a birth process. "I took off all my clothes, got in bed and said this is the day of my birth." But shortly afterward she fell into an intense depression, and went to a medical center for help. She was labeled manic-depressive, and felt even more desperate about herself, afraid she was going crazy. It happened shortly afterwards that she met a male friend and brought him home, where they made love. During the experience she felt intense Kundalini energy, starting in her legs and going up through her body. Her depression lifted completely and did not return.

She followed a number of practices to become more grounded, including eating meat, having bodywork with people who understood her symptoms, and having a daily massage, especially having her head and feet massaged. Other practices that seemed to her helpful were reflexology (foot massage), ginger soaks, relaxing in mud baths or tranquility tanks (where one floats in body-temperature water), bringing routine and structure into her life, eating regularly, walking, using color healing, and balancing the endocrine system with minerals such as potassium, broth or mineral soups. She found she was more comfortable wearing a turban or tie around her head when she felt energy pulsating there.

In retrospect she feels this opening was the biggest event of her life. "Colors were so beautiful and music sounded so beautiful. I had an awesome appreciation of it all. For a week everything was just heavenly, and I couldn't understand why everything had gotten that way." Since this time she is "over all more certain of my world view -- it would be hard for anyone to convince me I was wrong. I am positive of past lives and precognitive dreams."

Jayne says she is content with her life now, follows yoga practices, but limits pranayama and meditation. She does healing and massage for a living, and is clear-headed and open in talking of her experiences. She continues to experience periodic rushes of energy and bliss, along with visions of light .

Commentary on Diagnosing this Experience:

The key to evaluating whether or not Jayne had a Kundalini experience lies for me in her extensive prior spiritual practices. She had followed these with intensity and devotion and experienced symptoms of heightened pranic activity and/or Kundalini for many years. Although the erratic behavior and depressive aspects of her response are more intense than many would suffer, this is clearly described in the biographical histories of Goel and Krishna She also had a number of personal traumas in her life -- an alcoholic father, brother and husband, the death of all these men in recent years, and the mugging and injury.

As a child who was psychic one would suspect Jayne to be sensitive and more open to the impact of psychic phenomena. Her sensitivity may have intensified her reactions to the trauma of being mugged (which under many circumstances can cause breakdowns in some people). Her profound projection on her therapist may have heightened her emotional intensity, along with the lengthy period of celibacy. Rebirthing is an extremely cathartic breathing process, in which the body hyperventilates and seems to slough off all the old stored pains and blockages. It may be that Jayne went into a temporary emotional overload, either as a response to Kundalini or creating a trigger for the Kundalini to erupt in her system, which had been preparing for it for many years. The spontaneous writing of poetry and its curative influence is also common to many experiencing Kundalini.

The initial irrational psychological states are past her now but the energetic and light manifestations continue, and further levels of awakening will probably continue for many years.

Nan

Nan describes herself as a child who was always spiritually oriented. She felt she could commune with trees, animals and stars, and felt a presence with her that she believed was God. She sometimes saw the image of a triangle, and heard mantras being sung. She felt "the order of the universe as her mother, and the divine presence as her father".

She was a college student in the Midwest in the '60's and involved in much drug experimentation, especially using LSD. She had intense mystical episodes on drugs at times, but during two of these trips she experienced an arching in her lower back and an uncontrollable panic and fear of isolation and annihilation. After this she stopped using all drugs. She felt despairing, and that on LSD she had "reached for everything she ever wanted, God, and had failed". She had continual feelings of being terrified for six to eight months. She saw a psychiatrist who gave her Mellaril and Ritalin, which she took for a few months. She began reading yogic books and saw some of her drug experiences in them.

When a yoga teacher came to the area where she lived Nan learned to meditate, and while doing so would hear street sounds blocks away and see the color purple. She felt the presence of a "being" with her. She would have the urge to move into different asanas, but her teacher discouraged her and told her this was her imagination. This frightened her and she gave up her practice.

A few months later she and her husband were evicted from the farm where they lived, but another farm on 1000 acres became available and they moved. The first thing she did there was set up a meditation room, and begin meditating again. Soon afterward she visited a small cult group that claimed a mystical Christian tradition and taught classes related to power and psychic phenomena. She and her husband felt in their presence that a psychic force was being applied that prevented them from leaving. She felt riveted to the couch. She was frightened and began internally chanting the mantra she had been taught by her yoga teacher. It brought up an image of her guru and immediately the group seemed to stop what they were doing.

She continued to meditate regularly for 30 to 45 minutes two times a day, but was plagued with fear and feelings of inadequacy. One night she had a dream of Hari Kan Baba (a deceased Indian spiritual teacher) in which he came and talked with her. She woke up in the cold night, her body burning up, and found her husband had just had the same experience, waking up with great heat in his body. She heard the voice of an inner guru or guide in her mind and suddenly realized she had been hearing it for at least two months in meditation but had been forgetting it when returning to normal consciousness. These memories came to her and she "felt the power of this inner guru's love and caring". She felt deeply in love with this being who was guiding her.

She began to feel overshadowed by a divine presence who was controlling her life and protecting her. Falling in love with him was very frightening. It was a powerfully beautiful experience but painful because she feared she was losing her mind. She spent hours wandering alone in the woods with this being, meditating and feeling unity and ecstasy. "I had a very personal experience of God as the beloved, which was very different than my LSD experiences, which were of God in an impersonal form. I would hear a phrase or comment and in one word there would be a power and intensity of absolute love and compassion beyond description and impossible to withstand without melting. "At times when she drifted out of the ecstasy she was fearful that she was going crazy. "All I wanted was to merge and have no separate identity, having a separate individuality was painful. I had a desperate longing for unity which wouldn't end."

Nan had been very dependent on her husband because of her fears. He went out of town for two weeks and she stayed alone. She was so unstable she could not take care of herself and the inner guru told her what to buy at the store and when to eat. She wouldn't have eaten otherwise. She was not in her body, and felt the physical was being taken care of by his instructions and she was protected so that nothing bad could happen. It was an experience of feeling guided. Her guide told her he was her "kulu guru". She had never heard Sanscrit before, and found in a dictionary that kulu meant sheepherder. Later, while in India, she learned that kulu referred to the coiled or dormant power of Kundalini, and the term kulu guru "was used to designate the guru of the kulu Kundalini opening".

She describes three main issues overwhelming her at the time -- the tension of longing, fear of her sanity, and obsession about the meaning of the experience. She was told by the guru she was not intellectually capable of understanding it since it was "outside of her present construct of reality", and also that "the experience is an expression of the universe's love for itself". He told her to write down her early childhood experiences and then to read them aloud. In this way she gradually relived her early childhood, birth and womb experiences during the two weeks she was alone in the house. During this period of isolation at times she felt there were monsters walking around, and heard footsteps. She believed the guru was creating these experiences to desensitize her and help her overcome her fears. When she was finished writing he told her to burn them.

At the culmination of this period she lay on the grass, feeling his presence strongly with her. She reports: "He told me that he had come to assist me, but that he would be leaving soon because he was angered by the way I had wasted my life thus far. He told me that I had gotten myself in such a mess that I needed this intervention to get out of it. I felt like surrendering, and yet I did not want him to leave and mentally asked him to stay with me. There was a silence in which I felt him assessing my being and I saw my past lives flash by like on a deck of cards. I then felt a surge of energy, love and expanded consciousness. As it rose the external world fell away entirely and I felt merged with him in total unity. I have never had such an intense experience. If this had been complete I would have died, and this world of form would be gone."

After this the fears and experiences gradually began to subside. However, when Nan meditated an excruciating pain would develop at the base of her spine and begin moving upward. After about 15 minutes it would become intolerable and she would have to stop meditating. It would then subside. This lasted for two weeks. Nan continued to feel her guide's presence with her.

She decided to go to India and moved to a large city in order to earn some money for the trip. At this time she would fall easily into a trance. She would "experience a word or a quality of God and feel a manifestation of it flood over me, such as the feeling of perfect justice or perfect compassion". She would meditate for hours, experiencing bliss and unity. She felt a passion for a level of unity she couldn't attain, was very ungrounded, and felt unable to express herself through her previous persona.

Eventually she went to an ashram in India, where she meditated up to eight hours a day and did not eat very much. She often went into samadhi during and after darshan (sitting with the teacher). She experienced ecstatic energy, coming in waves, and sometimes extreme sexual energy moving upward, with strong sensations around the heart chakra, "feelings of expansion, surrender and ecstasy". She would fall over backward when meditating. The ashram practiced tantric yoga, and Nan and others frequently experienced kriyas such as making sounds, humming, jerking their bodies, rolling around on the floor and falling over. She experienced "twisting-snaking energy that was blissful, moving from the lower back or base of the spine upward, that caused my body to writhe around, moaning and groaning, twisting, swaying, falling forward or backward and then having a sudden backward jerk of the head accompanied by the sound 'hum'. There was also an arching backward until falling over."

Sometimes she fell over and rolled on the ground or moved into asanas or mudras, and once she danced in a trance of ecstasy.

Nan practiced pranayama, asanas, lessons for cleaning and balancing chakras, developing the seed qualities of chakras, mantra meditations and visual meditations. None of these calmed her emotions, "only serving to intensify my passion for spiritual unity and relationship to the inner guru". She felt her spiritual experiences were respected in this environment -- she was a spiritual person and not a crazy person, which helped resolve her fears about her sanity. But after several months, she became ill with chronic amoebic dysentery and a kidney infection, and spent two weeks in the hospital. She became very thin. Her physician said she would die if she didn't go home, and suggested that her symptoms were related to her spiritual practices. So she returned reluctantly to the United States.

She has completed college, raised a family and engaged in charitable work in the years since this awakening. She continues to meditate and experiences blissful feelings of unity, waves of energy, kriyas, and the presence of spiritual guides. At times in meditation she has out-of-body experiences, experiences shaking, vibrations, ecstasy, and spontaneous yogic breathing patterns (rapid breathing or stopping of the breath). Sometimes she feels a "downward-blessing type of energy from the crown, often accompanied by a visual picture of a white lotus with petals dripping down amrit (nectar)". She often sees white or purple light or a thousand-petaled lotus while meditating. At the time of her father's death she saw a vision of her father and her guru (whom she had asked mentally to assist her father at death) walking into her room, and she reports other psychic experiences such as an ability to "read" people at times, or knowing a lot about a topic as if she has "hooked into information from a collective body of information". Sometimes she does healing.

Nan feels the major impact of her spiritual experiences is the "precious gift of love". She feels grateful and that she was given something that no matter what she did she could never repay. "Many people never have that kind of love in their life. Relationships with people are like reflections of the divine. The experience with the guru is more like direct light. It is a tremendous gift. My whole value structure is based on the experience, so that my whole emotional structure is based on it . . . the important thing is to live for the welfare of all sentient beings and try to complete this journey and be one with the divine."

Commentary on Diagnosing This Experience:

The pattern of Nan's life clearly suggests this was a Kundalini awakening although at the time it could easily have been diagnosed as reactive to her heavy LSD use, and in a hospital setting encounters with a luminous guide would be interpreted as hallucination. But this kind of psychic guru experience is common in the literature. It is quite similar to that described by Krishnamurti who saw two guides in times of crisis, and both B.S. Goel and Dr. Gabriel Cousens have reported seeing appearances of Sai Baba, as has the previous subject, Jayne. Gurus such as Sai Baba, Nityananda, Sivananda, Muktananda, Babaji and others are frequently experienced by devotees, often giving specific information and advice, sometimes before they have even heard of them. The literature also refers to receiving shaktipat through a guru who is no longer in the body. Kennett Roshi describes encounters with an entire group of sages. It seems possible, if one accepts eastern cosmology, that the etheric or astral plane contains many highly conscious beings who influence events in our lives, either with or without our awareness. This experience of Nan's appears far deeper than any hallucination for she is given very specific and useful direction which seems entirely beyond her ordinary consciousness at that time.

Nan was feeling desperate, frightened and depressed as she entered this crisis. She reports herself as following spiritual interests from early childhood, and the intensity of her spiritual aspiration may have brought her to some profound openings under the influence of LSD, for which she was totally unprepared. It is difficult to say how or when her Kundalini energy awakened, but she demonstrates many of the characteristics -- heat, energetic phenomena or kriyas, involuntary asanas, seeing light, psychic contacts, wandering disoriented in states of ecstatic bliss, seeing monsters in ways described by Irina Tweedie, Muktananda and others, seeing past lives, and having a passionate desire to meditate. Since the time of this occurrence over 18 years ago she has continued to experience the bliss, light, and occasional kriyas while leading a productive and stable life.

Nan's physical problems are similar to those Gopi Krishna endured but could also be related to the illness in India or a generally weak constitution. It is likely the intensity of Kundalini energy will cause more difficulties for someone who is not constitutionally strong, and that preoccupation with spiritual experiences that take one out of body consciousness may cause damage over time to the energy system in the physical body. Perhaps yoga, said to be given to the more materialistic people of the Kali Yuga, was also developed to build a body-consciousness and control that would keep the yogi more healthy despite his/her out-of-body consciousness.

Margaret

Margaret was raised on the east coast, the only child of an upper-class intellectual father and vivacious French mother. The family was Catholic, but neither parent attended church, and they were surprised to find their daughter very interested in catechism classes, mass and God. She had a sincere and loving interest in religion but twice experienced humiliating incidents at church, once with a bishop who did not like the confirmation name she had chosen (her grandmother's name) and loudly commented on it when she made her Confirmation; and another time when a 13-year old friend came and waited for her outside the church and the pastor called her a hussy for wearing shorts. She lost interest in formal religion after this.

Margaret was ill frequently as a child, with many allergies and every known childhood disease. Her vision was poor. She had her tonsils removed three times. Twice, at age 8 and 11, she had near-death experiences when she had extremely high fevers and rashes, lasting one or two weeks, and she would be out of her body. These could not be diagnosed nor treated by doctors, who advised her parents to pray. As a teenager she had constant lower back pain, generally labeled growing pains by doctors. Finally at age 18 she went to a specialist who thought she had a tumor. They did surgery and discovered two crushed disks near the base of the spine. These were removed and a two-inch space was left just above the first chakra, wired up but never filled with a metal plate. Immediately after the surgery she was totally paralyzed, only her eyes moved, although she was aware of everything going on in the room. Doctors did not know what was wrong, nor what to do. After a few hours she came out of the coma, slowly feeling the paralysis dissolve, beginning in her toes and fingers and spreading through her body. The doctors did not know if she would ever walk again, but she was determined to attend college in the fall, and insisted on getting out of bed, and within a week and a half began walking, building her capability up over the next three months and entering college.

In her twenties Margaret began religious seeking, attending many churches and reading about religion. During the 1960's she tried growth and encounter groups, some sexual experimentation, and alternative lifestyles such as living two years in a commune, and occasionally used marijuana and psychedelics (always under strict guidance). She read the Seth books which made her see a new way of looking at God, without judgement and sin. She studied psychology, especially Jung. She began meditating regularly, and taught others to meditate, initially using TM. She became interested in Robert Monroe's book on out-of-body experiences and tried to learn to leave her body at will and to do astral projection, with no success. During morning meditations she experienced some phenomena of light and energy, and sometimes saw golden lights emanating from things or the molecular breakdown of furniture or objects so that she could see through them. She had spontaneous out-of-body experiences, and saw auras. She began to hear messages as if from an inner guide.

One day she began a meditation ritual of holding herself in white light and love, making a few notes on questions she wanted to bring up, then sitting in a meditative or trance-like state and doing a visualization of walking down a tunnel and seeing one or more figures in white forms. As she listened to a guide or guides who spoke to her, she would speak into a tape recorder their responses. She is not sure if they were outside herself or sub-personalities in the deep unconscious, but their information was supportive, and led her into self-awareness. A voice would talk with her very much as a therapist might, focusing on growth, reflection and self-examination. There seemed to be several entities, and they told her they were a conglomerate energy, and called themselves Pi. Later she discovered that "in Chinese symbolism the Pi symbol is a disk with a central hole signifying heaven or the doorway from temporal to non-temporal existence".

During these dialogues her body would vibrate as if electrical currents were running up and down her legs and out her fingers, and she would feel extreme pressure or denseness of her head and neck. She might get very cold, and need to wrap in blankets. She would sit without any movement for an hour or more and be very stiff when she stood up. In the beginning weeks lights in the house would blink at times, and electrical problems occurred while she meditated. She sometimes heard music on the tapes later that she knew had not been in the background.

A friend sat with her during sessions, and Margaret recorded them and wrote everything she learned. She was taken into very deep issues around her childhood, and given a new perspective about these. She ended up writing a complete autobiography. Sometimes scenes would be presented and the guide would make comments or ask her about it. At times she would witness and experience past lives, and the guides told her the point was to make them relevant to issues she was working on. She felt incredible compassion and nonjudgmental guidance. She was in Jungian analysis at the time and would take huge amounts of personal material to her therapist, who worked with her and supported her although he was somewhat apprehensive about the risks of channeling. Although she worried about her sanity she reassured herself that she must be sane since she functioned well at work and could take care of all her needs.

Margaret continued these processes for several years, doing them three times a week. At times the energy would come up in other settings and she always recognized it when she felt "slightly spacy" with heaviness in her head. She spoke with the guides one day and asked them not to bother her while she was driving or working, and the experience stopped happening at those times.

She began doing psychic reading for a few friends, but this raised many questions for her, as she did not want to "get into this level of messing around with the universe." She felt people wanted guidance and answers that they would be better off seeking for themselves, and she stopped this kind of activity.

During this time and since then she has had consistent back pain, throbbing and aching, but this has been true all her life, and she feels she has learned to live with it and barely notice it. The pain varies in intensity at different times, and she doesn't know why. Mainly it strikes the lower back and between the shoulder blades. In the morning she has to move slowly due to the pain on waking. Sometimes at night she feels one or a few waves of energy that begin at her feet and sweep through her body and the top of her head. She often wakes at 2 a.m. in the morning as if someone has shaken her or called her name, but she feels this could be a menopausal symptom, along with the sweating and heat flashes she often experiences. Twice she has done major healing on herself. At one time she had lifted heavy boxes and hurt her back so badly she was unable to move. Lying in bed she had a dialogue with her back in which she felt deeply in touch with that part of herself, listened to what it needed, and promised to take better care of it. She fell asleep and a half hour later woke up to answer the phone, realizing as she stood in the kitchen that the pain was gone. Another time she severely scalded her hand, and went through a similar process which healed it. At other times she has been unable to heal physical traumas, so this is not a consistent practice.

She had many vivid dreams at the height of this process, and in some lucid dreams the guides came to her and said "Come with me, there is something I want you to see" and would show her a place or a representation of something. In the most powerful of these she was shown a dark rectangle, and was told that it was a representation of a person's life. It was black except that for little twinkling lights. She saw many rectangles, some with a few lights scattered here and there, some with more lights clustered. She was told the twinkling lights were places where love was given and received in that lifetime -- nothing else in those lives matters, the only thing that matters are moments of love.

Sometimes she goes into a hypnogogic state, where she suddenly enters a third or fourth dimension, rather like wearing 3-D glasses where "dimensionality shifts somewhere i.e. to the astral plane". Then she sees beautiful nature scenes.

Margaret eventually felt that all the world was God, and learned "to see beyond the ordinary conditions of life". God became less personalized. "I am more and more aware of God being everything and we are all part of this. All we do or do not do is part of a learning pattern." She is deeply attuned to nature and experiences bliss, weeping at times before the beauty of the sky, ocean, and mountains, seeing God permeating everything. "This planet is incredibly beautiful." She feels great love flowing in her and her heart expanding before nature, or when listening to classical music. In recent years, although she rarely does the channeling, under the surface is a constant sense of the beauty and infinity of God. She feels she still needs to accept that the dark side of life is also God. She has an intense affinity with animals and feels that a growing edge is to improve relationships, since she has always been extremely introverted, and to create or experience more of the twinkling lights shown in her lucid dream.

Commentary on Diagnosing This Experience:

Margaret experienced a psychic opening of major dimensions, and it is probable the Kundalini has awakened in her system, although her symptoms are quite different from that of the other subjects. It is possible some of the back pain, heat flashes, insomnia and other symptoms that she attributes to ordinary physical problems are related to Kundalini. Without the back disorder and the fact that she is menopausal we would certainly have to consider these symptoms as originated by Kundalini, but it is possible they are not. Other aspects, such as the waves of energy sweeping through her, remembering past lives and the hypnogogic states are seen commonly in the literature. She had many preliminary manifestations in meditation, common to other subjects and in the literature.

Margaret's case interests me especially because I had questioned whether people with major back problems could awaken this energy, and the part of her spine missing is where the Kundalini energy is reportedly housed. This could explain why she would not experience the intense whole-body symptoms. Of course, if the physiology of Kundalini is related entirely to the subtle body rather than the material body this would not be a factor. Perhaps Kundalini energy has primarily activated only her upper chakras, particularly the heart and the third eye, sweeping her into consciousness through visualization and psychic awareness.

It is clear that many kinds of psychic experiences happen without Kundalini awakening, and it is important not to assume they are the same thing. But psychic openings such as Margaret's, especially those involving spiritual guides, are found in the literature related to Kundalini openings. Theoretically, psychic manifestations could provide education and psychological readiness for some people prior to awakening. Margaret has also moved into profound experiences of love and joy, as well as a new consciousness of God as being all of the universe, which correlates completely with scriptural references to Kundalini awakening.

Chris

Born in California in 1941, Chris was raised Catholic by a devout mother and non-Catholic father. She reports feeling a close connection with Jesus as a child, and took religion seriously, but she had difficulties with the philosophy of the church and left it in the early years of her marriage. She was the oldest of three children, and felt loved and secure in her family life until the death of her mother at age 14. Her father did not cope well with the loss, and she felt distant from him after this. He remarried when Chris was 16 to a woman she could not relate to and she left home at 17. She worked and attended college for two years before marrying.

As a young housewife with three children she had little interest in spiritual activities until her early thirties when she became involved in an organization that used group processes in psychology and meditation to promote personal change and growth. At their meetings she studied Jung, engaged in encounter groups and began meditating. She became close to the members, who formed an extended family with which her own family became very involved. After four years she left the organization because of its demands on her time, but she felt grieved, certain she would never experience such a place of belonging again. This brought back the earlier loss when her mother died and her family connections disintegrated, a loss she had never fully mourned, and she cried for days.

As she struggled to get through this period Chris began to practice meditating seriously, seeking a relationship with God, or at least an answer to life that would reassure her she was not so alone. She attended weekly meditation groups with followers of Muktananda and Yogananda, and meditated at home for several hours a day. She felt an inner connection with Yogananda, after reading his book

Autobiography of a Yogi (1945). She went to a Christmas program with Muktananda at his ashram in Oakland, but felt shy and distant from him and the intensity of the followers there. She experienced darshan, being tapped by him with a peacock feather after waiting in line with several hundred people, but didn't feel any reaction.

A few weeks later she went to a week-end program with Roy Eugene Davis, a spiritual teacher who had been a disciple of Yogananda's, and received kriya initiation. When she tried the kriya yoga practices she imagined energy moving up her spine and into the crown of her head, and it was slightly uncomfortable. Eventually she let the practice go. Sometimes she experienced intense energy when meditating, and it was hard to sit still. One day when she was practicing a zen breathing practice she felt a sense of letting go, of expansion into space, which made her feel wonderful.

Something about this opening worried her however. She thought later "I knew if I could be happy just being a 'housewife' and washing dishes I would never do anything else with my life. I might lose my ambition and my dreams. I knew nothing of the philosophy of yoga, or the potential of this opening". She then enrolled in an MA program in psychology and became very busy, and meditation became infrequent with concentration difficult. Soon after "I lost all the facility I once had in reaching peaceful, joyful places."

During the next ten years she attended college and taught handicapped young adults, worked in rehabilitation, established a private therapy practice, engaged in Jungian analysis, took numerous courses and seminars, raised her children, and maintained a home and marriage. She traveled to Switzerland and Egypt, and found both trips influenced her sense of independence, making her feel that limitations in life are primarily self-imposed. Eventually she felt "There were many things I could do, but they were all just passing time. I wanted to reestablish a relationship with God."

Chris became interested in working with the body as an adjunct to therapy, and took courses in Jin Shin Do Acupressure and neo-Reichian bodywork. She attended a training with Gay and Kathlyn Hendricks in which for the first time she saw clearly a relationship between spirituality and energy. She began doing individual therapy with Gay and told him her intention was to release any barriers she had to having a complete relationship with God. In the first session they worked with her body, breath and energy, doing deep rapid breathing, kicking, and flowing into an altered state of consciousness. About two hours later, sitting in a rather dull class, her body suddenly began to feel gentle charges, or tremors, filling her with bliss. "It was as if I were on a drug, becoming more and more high, waves of orgasmic-like pleasure flowing through me." This continued for about two days.

The following week-end she attended a Vipassana meditation retreat, and fell into deep and peaceful meditation. Following these two experiences she felt compulsively drawn to meditate, and began to practice one or two hours a day, taking short breaks during the day to go back into meditative states. "I began to experience a great variety of energy releases, sometimes waking in the middle of the night shaking, or feeling streams of gentle blissful energy pouring through me from my feet through the crown of my head. Once, while reaching to pick up a book of Yogananda's I felt pressure as if a hand were on my shoulder, which gently pushed me down to the floor, and for several hours I laid in an altered state full of ecstatic energy, light, and joy."

During the following months she went through several intense emotional experiences, at one point feeling so needy for love and caring she wanted to die from it. "It was as if all the neediness of the world was passing through my body. I learned that if I was willing to completely feel whatever the universe was laying on me at that moment, if it was God's will or part of my karma, that in the act of surrender the entire complex could lift spontaneously and I would reel with a sense of freedom and new energy."

A friend introduced her to yoga, and she began to explore books that discussed Kundalini energy. As she read she recognized her own experiences and her body seemed to respond to some of the scriptures, sending so much energy through her that she would frequently have to put the books aside and fall into meditation.

Deep in her studies of Kundalini, she would feel occasional doubt that what she experienced was really Kundalini, since it was more pleasant and less intense than that of many of the people she read about, and one night after wondering this she was awakened about 2 a.m.: "I felt as if I had been tossed into a galaxy of energy and light, my body stretched out and quivering while rushes of blissful energy rolled through me. I heard a voice deep inside say 'Of course this is the real thing, we're just taking it very easy on you.'" This energy flow lasted several hours, until she decided she needed to go back to sleep. At one point she distinctly heard a sound, that she had never heard before and has been unable to recall, except that it seemed to come from some distant echo chamber.

In the several years these experiences have continued they have come in many forms. Sometimes she feels afraid of being so entangled in a process that is clearly not common, and she feels great emotional swings and depression; at other times she feels she receives a gift of pure wisdom, as if someone is teaching her something she needs to know. She often falls asleep in a meditative state, and it is the first practice she is drawn to when she awoke in the morning. At times life seems more joyous and at other times she feels very uninvolved in life and frightened that she may have destroyed her life by taking the meaning from activities she used to enjoy. She frequently experiences bliss.

During a yoga retreat while meditating in the sun she felt "intense awareness of a column of brilliant light running through me, which was my Self or higher consciousness, completely free, and the activities of personality or 'prakriti' swirling around this column to get my attention and keep me earth-bound. It seemed as if I could identify with either one and each would direct where my energy would go." This was a profoundly centering and moving event. She recalls the image when she wants to feel centered and calm.

Chris's body shakes, vibrates or jerks often while meditating, when resting in bed, or following sex. She felt no pain until about two years into the process, when she reported great stiffness on getting up in the morning, especially in her ankles and legs. Sometimes her waist was numb and she could not turn over when she first woke up for several minutes. At other times she felt aches and pains or flashes of heat and cold, and several times a month she has difficulty falling asleep because of feeling so highly charged energetically.

She reports a period of intense depression and despair, accompanied by her body feeling as if it were dying internally, dull, aching, and sluggish. These symptoms seemed to abate during meditation. She began having Jin Shin Do Acupressure treatments weekly with someone who understood and supported the energy, and would go into intense kriyas during the sessions, shaking, jerking, doing asanas, and feeling a loss of conscious awareness. "It felt as if my energy body was sucking all the energy the bodyworker could give me and flooding the entire system with it, becoming very charged and enlivened." Over several months most of the aches and sluggishness of her body disappeared. During one experience, she felt an intense powerful upward surge of power "like an electrical charge from the muladhara through the crown chakra, with uncontrollable vibrations for several minutes, feeling wonderful and shocking, which left me whimpering. The energy seemed to stay in my head, making me feel strong. It was as if a lot of the questions and problems that bothered me became insignificant, as if I were identified with a wiser and stronger part of my inner Self."

She reports seeing light only rarely, usually in meditation or during bodywork, and she has had no spontaneous visions. She does not feel she has psychic abilities or other yogic "powers", although she is strongly intuitive in her work, and is exploring methods of using energy for healing. Her eyesight is significantly less sharp than when this process began. She has rushes of blissful energy at unexpected moments, such as when walking down the street, and feels lots of energy in the crown of her head, tingling like electrical charges. This happens especially when she is around someone else who has awakened Kundalini. There is a consistent steady hum or vibration in her entire body, and she easily goes into deep states of meditation. She has had experiences in which she felt her awareness was outside time and space, and in which she was plunged into unitive consciousness.   Chris has felt some support in having someone else to talk to, but relies on a strong sense that she needs to turn inward, through meditation, for any answers she needs. She believes that several past-life regressions, in which she relived spiritual lives, were immensely helpful in integrating the spiritual part of her psyche. She became involved in yoga, and frequently attends meditation programs and retreats. She says she can easily assimilate spiritual texts that she would never have understood before.

She believes that two factors that may have supported her process are her study of Jungian psychology, which taught her to witness and wait when she experienced splits between opposing desires or difficult truths about herself; and her 25-year marriage. In addition, having friends and therapists who she could talk to about it was extremely helpful, along with learning about yoga and reading the scriptures. She finds also that "over and over I must resort to trust in the inner Self and in the positive intentions of the infinite or divine force of the universe to sustain me. It seems it is fear, anger, mistrust and emotional attachments that consistently block the positive energy and bliss." She cites breathwork as a major practice that helps her to release blocks. She believes Kundalini awakening is a process along the way to a spiritual life, and not that spiritual life itself, calling it a cleaning-up process, although the energy itself is blissful when it is not hitting barriers in the physical or subtle body.

Commentary on Diagnosis of This Experience:

Chris demonstrates many symptoms of Kundalini awakening -- bliss, physical sensations, kriyas, emotional upheavals, and samadhi experiences.. It is possible this happened because of shaktipat experienced years before with Muktananda, or because she was intensely seeking it and meditating, before the time that bodywork opened her system more fully. Her case shows how spiritual opening can occur in stages, if we consider her earlier experience a precursor to the later opening.

She says "At some level in my being I gave up the desire for anything else -- I really deeply wanted to know God. And I feel the therapist who opened my energy up knew exactly how to assist me in this intention. I also feel Yogananda, although I've never seen him, has been with me in my spiritual search since the very beginning when a friend recommended his autobiography to me in a grocery store years earlier. I have continually turned to him and asked him to push me through into the next stage of awareness as far as I can go and I always feel a response."

Her maturity and years of analysis, her stable relationships, friends who support her in this process, understanding bodywork therapists, having a context for understanding spiritual awakening through both breathwork and yoga, her in-depth study of yogic literature, and her commitment " to allow God to do whatever is needed to help me become more free" may be some of the factors that make the process generally pleasurable and manageable for her.

This history shows the potential of body therapies in this process, both in the energy awakening that occurred in work with Hendricks and with the Jin Shin Do practitioner.

Beth

Beth, born in 1951, was the youngest of five children, raised in Arkansas in a family in which she "was not especially happy as a child." Her father was a car mechanic. Her mother was often depressed, but Beth recalls no traumas or major difficulties. She had a basic Christian upbringing and attended a Baptist church occasionally, but felt no affinity for it, even though she thought a lot about God and why she was here. She believes she may have had energy experiences around the ages of six or seven, and has a vague memory of intense energy in the perineal area as a child, and precognitive awareness. This went away after puberty.

Beth became interested in Eastern books at age 15, mostly Zen Buddhism, and at age 18 she began practicing meditations she learned from these books for a few minutes a day. "Mostly I would sit and think about things a lot" she says, " and I became more and more preoccupied with thoughts of God and the meaning of life, sometimes thinking all day long on these questions". She began working as a hospital aide and when people died it would trigger deeper questions. She attended junior college and enrolled in a four-year school to study nursing.

When she was 21 Beth was awakened one night unable to breathe. "I felt as if I was being electrocuted. My body was paralyzed. I could not even move a finger or call out for help. I was wide awake but terrified. Two giant hands were squeezing my chest, preventing me from breathing. I felt certain I was the victim of a freak accident involving lightning or wiring. For no apparent reason the current suddenly withdrew from my upper body to my spinal cord. Then it moved simultaneously down my neck and up from the plantar region of my feet and concentrated at the base of my spine. It then more or less subsided altogether." Although the experience lasted only about ten minutes it seemed like an eternity. Afterwards she spent hours looking for an electrical problem in the house.

A day or two later as she slept in the afternoon the episode repeated itself, and thereafter the phenomenon increased steadily in frequency, soon occurring in waking as well as sleeping hours. She was fearful she was developing a disease of the nervous system. Soon she was having mental and visual experiences. She saw at times "radiant halos and weird luminous colored lights". A round blue light seemed to be a permanent part of her peripheral vision, following her around. She heard sounds such as the buzzing of thousands of bees, felt a snake-like movement up her spine or a flash like a lightning bolt at her side, while sensations of heat or cold went through her head. "It would be like being bathed in radiant energy and I was completely at the mercy of it. I felt like it was a higher intelligence. Sometimes I was paralyzed and I went out of my body."

Beth found the out-of-body experience nice at times, but worried she wouldn't come out of it and might die. While walking she might feel hot energy sweep up through her body, see lovely beautiful lights, feel bliss, feel free of time and space, and sense her consciousness being attached to her body by only a thin thread.

For about six weeks she was struck with an energy experience several times a day while in class, or driving, working, or walking. Her whole body changed, her pulse raced and her heart pounded and she felt hungry all the time. She could barely eat enough and in one week she lost seven pounds. She would meet people and could know about them psychically, becoming confused between what they told her and what she already knew. Colors were more bright and intense and she saw lights, and heard what seemed to be celestial singing, bells, and chimes.

If she focused attention on her head, energy would go there and the results were unpredictable -- sometimes energy shot up powerfully, sometimes it was hot or cold, usually it was neutral. There was no pain. At times she felt a tearing sensation at the base of the spine but again there was no pain. She appeared to faint at times, and her skin would be clammy. At times her body shook and rocked as if a train was going by, and often it felt full of buzzing and electricity. If she relaxed or she talked about or thought about the energy it intensified. For several months she would sit in a chair each night at the same time and be flooded by the energy pouring upward and making her hair stand on end; she would be filled with bliss and waves of light, and feel an "irresistible smile". One night she felt the energy rise to her neck, and closing her eyes and looking inwards she saw "golden energy swirling incessantly around my organs". It seemed to move with determination and intelligence as if familiar with her anatomy, bathing her in a glistening sheen.

Anxiety and fear made her unable to concentrate and she flunked out of college, becoming reclusive and barely able to function or sleep. She was nauseated all the time, often had the taste of copper in her mouth and her lips tingled. She had constant vertigo, even falling down once or twice. She had vibrating sensations on the top of her head and between her eyebrows and couldn't sleep much. There was often a sucking sensation around her cervix, as if vaginal fluid was needed by the energy. She often felt sexual arousal from the energy and at times the sensation of having a spontaneous orgasm lasting 10 or 15 minutes. Occasionally this was a mild sensation which lasted several hours. Eventually she left her job at a nursing home, and her ego strength faded. "I felt I was not in control -- I was a servant at the mercy of this energy." Her moods would sweep from euphoria to depression.

The energy continued for two years, the most intense phases being the first few months. During the early months she also had a long series of dreams, many about nuclear war. Some foretold her meeting her future husband. Every night she received "a different gift of a vision of the future - extremely life-like, sort of symbolic and seeming to be in a whole different world". Two dreams included a unicorn, which brought happy feelings.

Beth did not seek professional help at this time, but a friend gave her Gopi Krishna's biography, which filled her with relief, and hope that she had no serious illness. She wrote to him and he responded, and she eventually went to meet him in Europe. He told her the experience was genuine, and gave her basic advice about sleeping and eating right and being a good person. "It was helpful to have it confirmed." She says that although she felt isolated and lonely during the worst of the process, she felt she knew best about her body. It was important to figure it out for herself and come up with her own answers. "Even at the time I could look at it as if it were God but also as if it were an evolutionary process, or a higher knowledge or intelligence." She feels the awakening opened up a whole new world, adding a new dimension to her world view, and giving her life meaning.

Beth still has occasional experiences with the energy (14 years later) although they are mild, and when she was pregnant in later years the energy seemed to go away, except during the delivery when she shook all over. After years she now is able to relax and says she has "a little more faith, that it will take care itself and take care of me." She lives a quiet life with her husband and children.

Commentary on Diagnosing This Experience:

Although Beth had done some meditating and contemplating about spiritual life she followed no specific practices that could be said to lead to this dramatic spontaneous awakening, and relates no traumas that might account for the difficulty of it. She has many of the symptoms reported in the biographies in the literature, ranging from violent energy charges, hearing yogic sounds, precognitive and psychic abilities, emotional swings, visions of light and of the inner body, spontaneous sexual energy, and out-of-body and blissful samadhi-like experiences. It is impossible to judge why she would go through such an intense awakening, and it is easiest to surmise it must be related to samskaras or karmic destiny. She sees it as possibly related to a genetic readiness for this stage of evolution, and speculates that there is a biological source for the experience related to nucleic acid and DNA. She is one of the few subjects who has not followed a yogic path, or aligned herself with any teachers or traditions to continue the process, but was able to get the context and understanding she needed from Gopi Krishna. The most significant assistance she received was in reading his book, over and over, and realizing "that my experience was not unique and aberrant but belonged to a process recorded also by others." In the ensuing years as the process has abated she has put her focus on leading a balanced and integrated life, and finding service-oriented work.

Karen

Karen is a slim and graceful college professor in her early 40's, raised in the Midwest by intellectual parents, who were active in the Methodist church. She was sensitive as a child, always feeling herself to be different than other children. She reports that "As early as age three I was troubled by the suffering of others, and always had big questions, thinking deeply, much to the dismay of my parents." She worried about pollution, war and the needs of orphans. She also reports psychic experiences in childhood. Once she dreamed that the stables behind her house burned down, killing the horses, an event that soon occurred, leaving her anxious that she might somehow have been responsible. Years later she had a precognitive vision of the John Kennedy assassination the night before it occurred.

One summer in a high school camp worship service she had an "incredible sensation of someone's energy hands on my shoulder, communicating that I needed to come with him. I was overwhelmed and wept. I went out into nature. Later the counselors were upset and wanted to interpret the experience but I couldn't hear them." A year later she had a similar experience, "as if a large energy body was touching me." Around this time she also had an out-of-body experience, seeing her body on the bed as if she had a dual-consciousness. "I remember feeling it was God holding my energy body up above my physical body, and I marveled at it. I felt I began to understand what some of the spiritual experiences were that people talked about." At age 9 Karen suffered with glandular fever for three months. By age 14 she began having migraine headaches once or twice a year. These were preceded by an aura. As an adult she learned to deal with these by going to bed, playing "passage music into another realm and just going into a deep state of rest. What I learned was not to fight the energies, and to go with them. I let myself float with them into a more expanded environment."

In her late teens she became very interested in Buddhism after a stay in Japan, where she was very attracted to the Buddhist temples and Shinto shrines. Then the book The Religions of Man by Huston Smith brought Christianity alive for her. In a later university course she wrote out the eight-fold noble path and tried to live it and meditate on it, but she felt she went too deep too quickly and she eventually limited her meditation.

After college graduation Karen married and moved to the West coast. She met a a woman who was a follower of Yogananda and practiced Kriya Yoga, and began studying the Self-Realization Fellowship courses and practicing visualizations, which she found exceptionally easy. She eventually gave up this interest because her husband was not interested, and she feared it would jeopardize her relationship. During this time she had several psychic experiences.

During the early years of marriage Karen had three children. She began Jungian analysis, did group therapy processes, had some acupuncture treatments and began lucid dreaming. While doing a process in a workshop one night she began spontaneous rapid breathing, felt she was about to jump into an abyss, and saw an image of a door opening and something beckoning her through. "I knew I couldn't go through or I would die." During the workshop her energy changed, and each day it felt as if something new changed in her body. A white eagle appeared in a vision as a guide, and she felt something running across her body. She had a sense of coming out of the experience carrying a globe of light, and as she walked barefoot with the globe, a snake slithered across her toes and she felt she was crossing a threshold of fear.

"As I walked into the woods alone I could feel the texture and energy of each living thing. I heard something calling to me. I looked ahead and saw it was a huge boulder. Rationally, I thought that could not be, but the sense was unmistakable. I laid down on it prone, arms outstretched, for a long time. Then I knew I had to hug a tree. After this I felt I could return to the people at the workshop. This was a very big opening, a complete confrontation with fear."

When she returned to the workshop she could barely speak. When asked by the leaders what was going on she simply said "I was called upon by that very big boulder." They told her the Dalai Lama had been there a few months earlier and identified that boulder as the center point of a vortex of energy for the entire Northwest -- a power spot, and an ancient Indian ceremonial spot.

A few years later a major physical problem triggered another deep psychic experience. She suffered from an intensely painful illness in her right eye, when the cornea eroded and raw nerves were exposed. She never knew if she would be able to see when she awoke in the morning. She went into a depression, believing everything was being taken from her. Her eyes were taped shut for two weeks as even the slightest movement caused excruciating pain. This seemed to trigger profound inner visions, and holographic dreams with multiple perspectives. Once she woke up to see everything in the room very clearly, forgetting her eyes were taped shut.

Some time later she met a man with whom she felt an instant affinity and energy connection and began a long term relationship with him. Her first intense experiences of energy awakening occurred with him. The initial experience happened following a long day of love-making, feeling the rising of energy moving through them as in tantric practices, which she did not know at the time. During these hours they shared intense energy and saw visions, one of which was a clear blue single eye.

That night they were sleeping in a vacation home on a small island when he awakened with a dream of small entities who were outside the house wanting to come in. He dreamed that he told them to leave but they came into the room anyway, and that he ran to the bedroom door and slammed it. As he did so the actual door in the bedroom slammed shut and woke both of them. As he told Karen this dream she felt a wave of fear and she recalled the same vision she had seen years earlier at the workshop of the door opening and someone beckoning through. The knob on the bedroom door turned and the door opened and light poured through. "Suddenly all of my energy was thrown down to the base of my spine and then built upward. As the energy rose, my body arched back. Deep breathing patterns took over, came all the way up and over my head and through my mouth and I screamed an incredibly loud high-pitched sound. When the sound stopped the door slammed shut. During this experience my lover saw light energy forms spinning around in a whirl, and then saw an enormous eagle sweep up and over our heads as the sound was made. After the door shut the space was clear and very still. We began to repeat a mantra -- a rune in which you invoke the power of light -- which we knew vaguely, until light came through the skylight above us in the morning."

After this whenever the two were together Karen experienced strange body phenomena. "It felt like the original experience was a preparing of my body to tolerate energy, to learn to tolerate pleasure and bliss. As the energy continued it felt as if my body was getting remade, every cell being restructured. The feeling was often like a vibratory frequency working through every part of my body." She began having kinesthetic dreams, where an image would be given to her and she would hold on to the image while her body would have physical sensations and unfold in movements as in a dream. With this unfolding "whole chunks of awareness and knowledge would be there -- cosmic glimpses of relationship to the cosmic plan." After the original opening the couple, who lived in separate countries, met every two months, always experiencing tremendous body energy and synchronistic experiences, and simultaneously remembering what seemed to be past lives. They experienced visions and dreams in common, even when sleeping a continent apart.

During this period she often became ill with flu-like symptoms of nausea and malaise following time with her lover and returning to her habitual life, but gradually she learned how not to get sick. "I set some intentionality. My body was so open and beginning to reject some of the energy patterns in my day-to-day life that were not okay for me. I asked that I not have to suffer that particular illness, that I find a way to hold it and integrate the experience in my body. After a year I didn't get sick."

One day while alone in a hotel room in Europe she fell down on the bed and felt she was leaving her body. "My head felt like the vessels in it were going to burst and my breath changed. It came on so unexpectedly I thought I was dying. I was aware my body didn't want to die since it was gripping life with such tenacity. A female guide came to me and told me that the leaving is not the dying and that I needed to learn to love without attachment. I went into a deep hypnogogic state, and she introduced me to knowledge which she said I had once given to her. She offered me deep affirmation for the inner work I was doing and told me lovingly that I needed to distinguish between earth plane affections and attachments and my larger purpose here as a being from another dimension. I had to learn to sustain the light and to not distract myself by recording everything that happened to me. I became profoundly aware that the description is not the experience. She told me that when the whole body energy moves to a point of light above my head my consciousness is connected to another plane. She also said I was being taught something very important in dreams every night."

In 1987, also in a hotel room, she experienced vibrations and tremors through her legs, spine, and face and performed yoga asanas spontaneously for three hours. Energy rushed first up the right side of her body, and then moved up the left side. Then her entire body was shaken by energy streaming upward and vibrations. She went into a prayer position with her head down, pulling at her hair and saying "I used to be bald". It felt as if the energy wanted to do things with her body that she was unable to do, and her body felt like clay. "I pulled at my face as if my body was not light enough. It felt strange to have this 'funny' body. I felt I was almost taken 'home' several times, and experienced deep grief over being here (on this planet). I was aware of having had a previous body, a light form. I knew this other body could move easily and do anything. I was pulled into extreme postures, -- underneath, backward and curled forward, and then began rocking. Then I fell entirely backward and upside down, my fingers rigid, and I went into a head stand against the wall, my head between my knees. Then I stood up with a full body vibration and went forward to the ground. I was surprised to see little red lights flashing as well as a soft yellow peripheral glow. I felt extreme heat, and heard crying which turned to laughter. Then I realized it was my own voice but I didn't know if I was laughing or crying. I heard the words 'siddha yoga', and my head jerked from side to side. I distinctly felt I needed to keep my spine open. My stomach was upset. I coughed often, and then felt cold. Then I had a sense of a butterfly body living within me as if my body was it's cocoon. It seemed to break out as a new body through my back with still wet wings beginning to unfold. I found myself making loud, high, sustained sounds." After this event she felt very vulnerable for a few days, and her whole body seemed to be slow, delicate and vibratory.

A year later she had great pain in her left big toe, which hurt all afternoon and became increasingly worse, swelling until she could barely walk. She began laughing and crying at the same time. She tried to work with the energy and "felt it kick off in my body. I kept cradling the toe, saying 'my baby, poor baby'. Heat came up through my body and an unusual breathing pattern took over. Then I had phlegm in my throat and began growling and pawing at the floor. I found myself saying 'I am a leopard; I'm a South-American leopard'. I felt I was hanging onto life by by toenails and fingernails."

She felt completely embodied as this animal, growling and moving to clear her energy. Her body went into postures, some of which choked her, and she felt like vomiting but held it back. It seemed to her that she must clear her body of all impediments for the light and energy to go through. She became aware of the need to take spiritual practices seriously, and made tones which cleared the higher chakras, causing energy to move upward. She began meditating, and spontaneously saw beautiful crystals, growing like corals, standing before them groups of frail, bald beings of light -- "my people." She had a realization that inner dialogue distracts from experiences, and "wherever you put attention is where energy is." Then her energy felt more like silk -- warm, and rising, and she went into ecstasy.

During another period she felt heat coursing through her body and her hands and feet tingled with electrical charges and burned for five days. Afterwards it seemed as if "a healer was working through my body. The energy would rise when I was around anyone who had a problem, I would feel the energy move through my palms and fingertips and if I allowed it to it would intensify and find a way to work with the energy of the person I was with. I would always say a prayer that the energy would be used for the highest good." During this time she caused a surgical scar to fade, warts to fall off of someone's foot, and stopped a nose bleed instantly. This experience continued for about six weeks, and then receded into the background after she stopped responding to it.

Karen continued to feel a cellular changing and restructuring of her body, as if cells were unfolding much in the way a flower opens. Sometimes at night a radiation-like energy pours through her, waking up both her and her husband. At times she feels she leaves her body at night and goes out into the stars. One night, in such an experience, she felt drawn to leave and not return and was awakened by a phone call from her lover who said "I felt you were going away." At another time she had a major dream in which "I dreamed of myself as a vertical shaft of light, surrounded by layers of different colored lights and energy wraps unfolding in a spiral and coming off."

In August of 1987 she had what she calls a "star-body" experience, after awakening at night in her bedroom at home, and not knowing where she was or who she was with. She could see outlines in the room but didn't recognize anything. She saw her husband but couldn't think of who he was, and she felt out of her body. She knew who she was in her larger self and had no fear, but felt a sense of having forgotten her particular identity in this time and space. "I knew that I couldn't just radiate this genuine loving energy to people, that they wouldn't understand or be able to receive this unconditional love as love. It was as if the human form seemed to elicit a need for a particular personalized form of love -- that until an individual totally recognized who he/she was, his or her ego still needed to be acknowledged an an individual. I had to work hard to remember the seemingly insignificant differences between people so that they would believe they were seen for themselves; it seemed such a limited condition of receptivity for love. At the same time I felt tenderness for the human condition of embodiment and witnessed my own body struggling up to the body next to me for a kind of human animal comfort and warmth. Gradually I was able to recall the particulars of this life and my husband next to me, without losing the exquisite consciousness of the other dimension."

Karen has experienced many other movements of energy and awareness. She feels energy rocket up from the first chakra at times, causing her whole body to vibrate and shake. Sometimes she arches backward and her head goes almost upside down beneath her, or her shoulder blades are pulled together as if they want to touch. The body will lock into such postures for a period of time and then release. Waves of energy and heat and unusual breathing patterns occur. She sometimes feels the energy stuck at the top of her head unless she is free to make sounds. "Something about sound is for me utterly central to moving energy." Sometimes fist-size balls of energy roll upward through the spine, pushing through the center of her head or slightly to the left. She falls into raptures and ecstatic states, and has spontaneously performed what she later learned to be mudras. The first mudra she performed was that of equanimity, where the hands are held out palms upward. She has had a variety of aches and pains, and at one time was diagnosed with adrenal exhaustion.

Karen sometimes follows a macrobiotic diet, but at other times wants to eat meat. She has had several years of Jungian analysis and participates in other psychological and spiritual programs. But she does not engage in regular meditation practice since she can go into such deep states and the experiences demand attention that she feels she must allocate to her family.

When asked how this process has impacted her life she stated "I think I've changed dramatically from believing in the connectedness of all beings to knowing it. The presence of 'God' is no longer a question for me, and God isn't anthropomorphic anymore. God is here in every cell of every creation. At a deep level I feel more secure in life because I've reached a source of truth -- a quality of truth about the nature of our beingness. . .I don't feel that there is anything I absolutely 'have to do' in this life -- I used to fret and worry about that. My compassion has grown -- expanded in depth and breadth. Much of what I feel is not so personal anymore. I am not so concerned about 'personal little me'. It's like being a cell of a larger organism, a small part of a vast mind. I feel more committed to a spiritual life, it's the most important dimension of consciousness; living this spark of Spirit in the gift of incarnation. I no longer seem to engage in searching and longing for so much; every cell is informed with the divine."

Commentary on Diagnosing this Experience:

Although these experiences sound extreme and dramatic, Karen carries a presence that is very gentle, centered and loving, and she is extremely capable in her roles as a mother and teacher. She is passionate and intense and often exhausted by the emotional demands of her life, but is much more stable than a review of this history might suggest. She has a strong capacity to witness and accept the volatile energy, and the visions and dreams that come to her, along with the conflict of her life circumstances.

Karen's history demonstrates the correlation between certain kinds of intense emotional and sexual involvement and the awakening of the latent energies, which can take a couple mutually into transpersonal realms of experience. There is clearly a powerful link between Karen and her lover and both of them have most likely awakened this energy and used it to expand their range of energy and psychic awareness. It appears from their experiences that they may have powerful past life and karmic links.

She demonstrates every level of the Kundalini experience including samadhi states, pranic activity, physical problems, involuntary asanas, visions, extra-sensory perceptions and psychic and healing abilities. We can also see stages in this process similar to those of many cases, with early signs of sensitivity and psychic openness, preliminary experiences of energetic and psychic openings, followed by a more dramatic experience some years later. She is engaged in intense personal conflicts and pressures that may make the Kundalini experience more difficult than if she were living a quieter, ashram-style life, yet she has a great sense of acceptance and attunement to the path with which she is presently engaged.

Mark

Mark, born in the south in 1925 , had many traumatic early childhood losses. His biological mother died at his birth, and an aunt he was greatly bonded to and who was his caretaker died when he was seven. When he was 12 the uncle he lived with separated from his second wife, to whom Mark had become attached. At this time he went back to live with his biological father, who had led a transient life. He had nine older brothers and sisters and never fit well into the family. He left home as a teenager, went into the Air Corps in World War l, worked and eventually made his way through college, then became a teacher. During his youth he had two automobile accidents, and once fell out of the box car of a train, all causing damage to the right side of his body. He was later told by a chiropractor that his back was "zig-zagged curved".

Mark married late in life and when the marriage broke up a few years later he was deeply wounded and depressed. He experimented with Gestalt therapy, bodywork, and group therapy, and attended an intensive group process for several weeks that promoted deep introspection. He became even more depressed at this time, withdrew from therapy and worked alone with his dreams. He used marijuana frequently, feeling it "helped to interiorize my experience and relate to parts of myself that had been repressed".

About this time Mark practiced meditation for about two months by sitting and following his thoughts daily. Then he heard about Muktananda and went to Oakland to meet him. In the darshan line he was introduced to him, and they spent about 15 seconds talking. As he left he took a poster of Muktananda with him. He had an altar at home where he placed it, and used it to focus on in meditation. Beside it were two candles, and beads from the bark of a Tulsa tree. He would smoke marijuana to deepen his meditation on the poster, and see 20 or 30 faces in it, especially seeing the images of three women in Muktananda's face -- a young girl, a young woman and an older mother. He would practice this after doing exercises in the morning. One morning he felt a tug at the end of his right finger as he did the Salute to the Sun asana, and then as he bent over one leg the muscle contracted under his right knee. He leaned over his left leg to get more leverage. Suddenly his right hand grasped the leg and yanked it. It was so painful his mouth flew open to scream, and out of his mouth came a soft sound "ta". (He was later told this is an ancient mantra.)

Mark was terribly frightened by this experience, although at the same time he felt the soft sound and ritual movement was in some sense trying to help him. He began to experience more ritualized uncontrollable spasms and movements, usually on the right side of his body, and to perform asanas involuntarily.He became paranoid about these episodes, feeling he was possessed. He sought help from past-lives therapists and mediums, believing something was trying to take him over, and felt very negative, fearful and uncertain. He submitted to the strange movements because he feared that if he didn't something awful would happen.

A month after this experience Mark felt the energy force move him to throw away the marijuana in the kitchen, give away the liquor in the liquor cabinet, and take the necklace he had used as part of his ritual and flush it down the commode. He then knocked the candles down from the altar and demolished the whole thing. He felt panic about this and stopped meditating. He kept a daily journal and found it made him feel better, and he continued to seek out people who could tell him what was happening. A well-known psychic told him it was Kundalini, and was the first to suggest it was related to God and he should surrender to it. He felt a contradiction between the beneficent experience she described and the bizarre movements he had.

He felt desperate to change his life and didn't know how. He had already tried a number of group processes, Esalen and individual therapy and it seemed nothing had helped, Something was pushing him. He had became more and more dissatisfied and the marijuana had come from desperation. He felt prepared to do anything. He began meditating for three hours a day beginning at 4 a.m. One morning his attention was drawn to the phone number at the bottom of the Muktananda poster, and he called the center and heard a talk on Siddha meditation. When he heard that they recommended meditating 20 minutes a day, he put a huge clock on the table, feeling he had been in perversion of real meditation. He called a therapist who was a devotee of Muktananda. She told him he was experiencing Kundalini and it was out of control. This terrified him and he imagined a conspiracy between her and Muktananda. She told him to call the retreat center in New York and they could help, and reluctantly he did so. He talked to a secretary and when he called back for a message he was told "The Kundalini will take you there. Come to the Intensive." He feels this became the story of his subsequent travels.

Shortly after the decision to attend the intensive Mark began to have experiences of feeling frozen in movement, such as standing in the shower until the water became ice cold. He met a friend in a restaurant and when he tried to get up his right arm flew out but his body would not move. Finally with help he pitched over on his right side, and then could not get up. A doctor was called who came and ministered to him for an hour and a half, using imagery, guiding him with his hand at the base of the spine. Finally Mark got up, did some mudras, and blessed everyone in the restaurant.

At the intensive in New York he reports "I came in and sat down and keeled over. I was given sweets, and felt warmth, friendly faces and reassurance. Then I went upstairs and performed a ritual, pouring water over my head. I gravitated between terror and exultation. In the hall when Muktananda came to me I began shaking. Muktananda's peacock feather struck me on the right side and I crouched over like an animal." He loved the chanting and music of the program and felt as if he were in a magic hall at times, but when he left fears and anxiety would hit him. Although Muktananda was not to do darshan at this time except with children, Mark implored the coordinator to let him in, so she did. "I was struck with the thought 'Accept ye be as little children ye can not enter the kingdom of heaven' as I stood in line behind the children, and when I reached Muktananda I was no longer afraid. I knelt and raised my right arm above my head. Muktananda said to come closer and looked in his eyes for a few seconds. Then I returned to my place on the floor and began to feel internal snake-like movements. A smooth soft feeling moved up from my fingertips and my agitation ceased; I reached out to hold hands with the black and white men on either side of me, searching for family. The white man curled up in a fetal position to avoid me, and some helpers in the hall came over. But I said loudly that Muktananda wanted me to do this and they went away. Then my his hand stopped moving, and I cried, and said 'I tried, I could only save one of them'.

On the bus going home from the ashram Mark tried to touch everyone, and believes this came out of a desire to help them. He behaved similarly on the streets of New York, touching and blessing people. "I saw terrible faces in the clouds above the city. As the cab drove to the airport the hood flew up, and I freaked out, paid the driver with all of my money and walked the rest of the way. I was very confused at the airport and had the wrong ticket, and then I collapsed onto the floor at the counter. Finally a stewardess got a ticket for me and helped me into a first class seat on the plane."

As the plane took off he had the impression that he was being "zapped" by people who were controlled by evil spirits, whenever they pointed something at him i.e. an elbow, knee, or toe. He had a bible, and opened it to the chapter on three temptations. He drew pictures of Muktananda and of tabernacles from Jewish stories, which made him feel protected. To stop the evil spirits he leaned toward a girl with his hand like a cobra, and did the same to the man behind him and another with a newspaper. Then he leaned over and did a karate chop to a man's groin. When the stewardess came over he said "I was doing my meditation and they bugged me" in a child-like voice. An inner voice said he would be arrested for assault or incarcerated for a mental check. When nothing happened all his social expectations of how things should be fell apart, scaring him even more. "I didn't know how to deal with a world in which anything could happen."

After a friend picked him up at the airport he settled down. The support of this person was very important, as he assumed it was an emotional problem he was going through. For the next few weeks he slept only two hours a day and went through a number of psychotic-like episodes. One of these experiences occurred between 2 and 3 a.m. "I woke up and went through my house to separate the good guys from the bad guys, sorting through shoes, records and other items. By 10 a.m. the whole house was divided, and I zapped the bad guys. Another time he awoke and went out on the patio in his shorts. He was "assisting in the dying of Muktananda". He wrote the time in pencil on concrete. Anything that moved was experienced as an enemy. He performed rituals until 5 p.m. when he had a dinner engagement. At one point he heard his voice sounding like a boy saying "Come on and die man -- I have things to do."

IIis ex-wife called and advised him to go to a massage and healing center in the mountains. He went for several days, where he relaxed in a nature setting, using a pool and hot tubs. People recognized his need to be touched and did massage with him. One woman did Trager massage, which he feels opened his heart.

After this Mark realized increasingly that he wanted to work with his hands, and saw how unhappy he was as a teacher. He became aware of the desire to touch, as well as to be in nature with people, and work with the body. He still felt fear about his body but at another level felt more accepting. He began to release inhibitions and accept the aesthetic and sexual needs of his body, rather than judging them. He decided to study massage and Trager work. This proved difficult at first because his body, particularly the right side, would spontaneously go into movements he could not control. He stopped taking classes for several years, realizing he needed more grounding and to integrate his experiences. He visited psychics and therapists and felt none were very helpful, that he had to find the answers within himself.

Following these initial experienced Mark began to exhibit a wide range of physical symptoms and frequently underwent testing at Kaiser Hospital. He felt if he could prove something physical was the matter they could fix it. Neurologists observed his spontaneous movements but their tests were negative. One doctor called it myelonic movement (involuntary movements with a physical cause in the brain), and ordered a brain scan. At one point he was referred to an oncologist because an x-ray found a mass in his right lung. The surgeon who was to do a biopsy decided there was not enough evidence to justify it. He was told his problems were emotional, and given a prescription for Haldol. He took one of these and nothing happened, and he decided he would need a massive dose if there was to be an effect so he stopped them completely.

During one phase he had difficulties with his heart. He would wake up at night convinced he was not breathing and unable to detect a heart beat, He would stamp his feet and pound his chest, thinking he was dying. He had chest pains and tightness, felt constriction in his chest while jogging and went through cardiac testing, again with no diagnosis.

Other conditions he has experienced are :

-- Agitation and a burning sensation in his right toe with his foot turning out and pressing the ground; feeling as if lightning is flashing down his leg.

-- Constant internal pressure that causes pains and body spasms. Sometimes he shakes from head to toe.

-- Itching or feeling like ants are crawling over him.

-- His arms raising and his hands tracing movement of the energy as it circulates in a spiral in his body.

-- The lobes of his skull becoming very sore and soft as if he could poke his finger through them.

-- Getting stuck in a trance-like state until someone or something releases it. Occasionally while driving his eyes are fixed ahead and they "glaze over" for a few moments.

-- Numbness and extreme cold in his toes and fingers, especially on his right hand. His fingertips turn yellow or white and this might last for three hours until they turn purple and come back to normal. He was tested for diseases of the lymph system because of the extreme temperature difference between his left and right side. He also has felt burning sensations on his feet, especially his right toe, and at times extreme tolerance of heat. Once he burned his skin with a hot pad and did not feel it.

-- Sometimes he spins in circles with his hands held together as in prayer and he feels this is an attempt to find a new balance: for awhile this happened two or three times a week, at the time of the interview it happened about every two days.

-- Once the energy pushed him against a rock and adjusted his vertebrae and aligned his back. He believes when the energy wants him to take over it will cause pain. When he is uncertain what to do he starts the 23rd psalm and" all movement ceases if it wants me to take over".

-- He sings old songs or whistles involuntarily, and makes monosyllabic sounds such as "ta"; hearing the words "peace", "God" or "God be with you".

-- He feels easily susceptible to the energy of others when getting massage or bodywork, and often sees colors, especially orange and yellow in a swirling mass as if he is looking into a fire. He was unable to meditate for years, but more recently has experienced falling into meditation spontaneously.

Mark has not experienced many visual phenomena, but once, early in the process, he saw light within as if there were no outer skin covering the body. He saw with his eyes open channels of energy with a flash of silver running across.

During his struggle to integrate this process Mark retired from his job to spend time studying massage and other forms of bodywork. He is trying to shift from an intellectual orientation to a holistic view of life. He still has many symptoms but they rarely occur in public. He practices hatha yoga and some meditation. He finds that staying physically active, being in nature, and putting his focus on what he is doing in the moment are very useful practices in managing the energy. In addition to hatha yoga he feels the most helpful kinds of bodywork have been acupressure and Trager work, in the hands of a competent and sensitive person who understands the energy. He felt Rolfing and Polarity Therapy were not helpful. Massage is relaxing. But none of these can make the energy go away. When he feels relief from bodywork, which he says releases negativity, and the energy comes back afterwards, he knows the work "is something only the energy can do. . . .The bodywork will open a channel and the energy start moving as if a gate has opened."

He has had many significant dreams involving women, and his views of women have changed as he sees them helping him relate to the feminine part of himself. Other changes are in recognizing his need to accept people and "be with them in a more spacious and free environment". Also he says "I needed to become more responsible for my behavior and my anger. I believe much creative energy is channeled through anger and I want to transform that form so it can be used."

Commentary On Diagnosing This Experience:

Mark has had the most persistent and painful problems with Kundalini of anyone I have interviewed, although I have talked with several other people briefly who reported a similar ordeal. He is unique in that bliss seems elusive and snatches of light, peace and understanding are rare. He has all the physical manifestation of Kundalini awakening, and has been racked emotionally, primarily with fear, doubt and anxiety regarding the uncontrollable movements and pain in his body. His opening occurred without any systematic preparation and while using marijuana. The shaktipat experience combined with mental confusion and an already depressive and despairing frame of mind allowed the opening, but did not nurture it.

I theorize that the tremendous psychological losses of his early life, loneliness, significant injuries to his right back, lack of context for or understanding of eastern spirituality, leftover anxieties from southern Baptist religious beliefs, and the use of marijuana created a fog of fear and confusion that simply swamped him in the early stages of the process. He was a thinking and analytical person, not in touch with his body or emotions, and desperately seeking something he knew was missing. This experience plunged him into his shadow and he has struggled for years since to come to terms with his body, emotions and relationship needs. It is as if two sides of his psyche have been in hand-to-hand combat throughout this process giving him no opportunity for bliss, surrender, ecstasy, or the other potential boons it offers.

Mark is getting in touch with his feminine side, softening, searching for his wholeness. He believes now that he is in a spiritual process, but he understandably views it as closer to hell than to heaven. It has clearly brought immense change and growth in his philosophy and self-awareness. He cites both bodywork and nature as nurturing for him during this process.

Jay

Jay, a 34-year old self-employed consultant, is a personable, easy-going, educated man who has practiced Transcendental Meditation for 14 years, beginning when he was earning an MA in business. He is the son of Jewish parents, raised without much religious influence in the home other than attending a Sunday school he hated. He rejected religious practices. He is the youngest of three children. Although there were tensions in the family there were no significant childhood traumas that he recalls. He is bisexual, and has been in a long-term relationship with a woman but never married. He had a six-month period of intense drug use in 1971, using mostly marijuana and hallucinogens, which he says he probably took 50 or 60 times. The first twenty times he used mescaline or LSD the experience was gentle and pleasant, but it then became very frightening in terms of fear of death. He felt his heart would burst. He gave up drug use but for the following year and a half had recurring anxiety attacks.

He began meditating in college, and found meditation practice quiet and enjoyable the first few years. He learned a few asanas and one pranayama technique but seldom practiced them. Looking back on his experiences he believes it is possible that an event in 1976, following four years of meditation, may have been part of his Kundalini process. He was at a three-month TM retreat, and felt at a plateau in his practice. He had a light case of flu and took extra time to rest, having a massage to relieve the aches. Two meditation periods later he felt blocked and then "I felt suddenly as if I had broken through a layer of ice and could feel myself dangling above an ocean of bliss, feeling my toes touching it, experiencing intense thrills, warm, flowing from my toes up my body, flowing everywhere. I was plunged into this ocean of bliss, and then I lost awareness of what was happening; it was indescribable" His meditations continued to plunge him into bliss for several days afterward but outside of meditation he was gripped by anxiety -- a tremendous fear would overcome him about an hour after meditation, twice a day, whenever he had the bliss experience. He would lie down on the floor in his room to get his bearings before getting dressed to leave the room. At the time he assumed these symptoms were a release of the old drug experience from his body.

This continued for three days. He does not think he was sleeping at night, although he would wake up feeling refreshed. He kept asking people "Is this real -- am I really here talking to you?" He felt no tangible sense of reality. He had known of the spiritual experience of detachment conceptually, so he felt it was not to be worried about, yet he felt frightened at the lack of connection with people. After three days he was back to normal.

The next time he attended an extended retreat he heard on several occasions a loud noise that sounded as if it originated from somewhere in his spine and rose to his head. He felt a dramatic physical movement up the spine at the time. He had felt small jerky movements of his hands or legs occasionally before, but this was more intense, and yet he isn't sure the body moved or if it just seemed like it did. During the next years he sometimes heard a roaring ring beginning at a low intensity and rising to a high pitched ringing sound in his head, lasting five to ten seconds, and he would feel smaller body movements and a small internal thud occasionally.

In 1979, Jay attended a two-week retreat, where he learned the TM "flying technique", or levitation. He had observed others "going nuts" with these practices before, making noises, shaking, and bouncing around and he had felt there were getting carried away, and could have controlled it.

While doing these practices and in a deep state of meditation he felt disturbed by someone moaning. It was so loud that he felt pulled out of his blissful meditative state and he felt slightly annoyed. Suddenly he realized it was him moaning, and felt "this can't be happening, I should have control over myself." It was a very sexual sound, and he was flooded with rapturous, orgasmic sensations, and drooling on himself. It was the first time he had had such an experience and been conscious of it and stayed with it. It became more and more intense, very active in a subtle way. "The vibrations felt like a spring was getting compressed so that the spring was growing, as if potential energy in the body was getting more and more powerful so when it would let go it would really let go. I felt energy and warmth building in the solar plexus, building and building -- until it popped open. It felt like intense radiation moving out and up at the same time and I was flying -- bouncing and bouncing." He burst out laughing uncontrollably, his body felt very light. As energy moved into his head he felt light, like a glow, his whole body felt it was glowing. This lasted about an hour,

Following this event he felt continued intense energy, very blissful and good all the time. When he sat to meditate the process would continue, always beginning with the groaning, the building sensation, and breaking loose. It felt like a "cosmic orgasm". The rising occurred in meditation, or while sleeping, and soon happened in public as well.

At night he woke up with sensations going on, especially in his legs. He felt restless, with vibrational feelings in the legs and needing to kick them hard. Sometimes he felt warm and flushed. He began having drenching night sweats, so heavy he would have to change the bedding several times a night.

He dreamt of being in a store with a shopkeeper -- "someone I recognized and could not quite place. As I dreamed I started to wake up and the nausea was there. It moved up to the throat and I made a groaning noise; my head felt as if it were filled with a porous material like a sponge. The nausea moved up and penetrated all the pores. It felt like an uncomfortable warm fluid. My body became tense everywhere, as if preparing to burst, as if something were pushing through. I shook and groaned, and I couldn't control it, but could only wait for the experience to pass." After this, similar episodes occurred periodically about twice a week for a month or more. Today, seven years later, they occur every four to six months, usually lasting one or two minutes. Sometimes he feels only a preliminary "spaced-out" sensation and nausea but it subsides, although usually the whole process follows.

In 1983 he experienced severe headaches and extreme fatigue, and had a recurrence of extreme night sweats. The headaches began at the temples, radiating into the top of the head, and were extremely painful. He saw several doctors including a chiropractor, acupuncturist, holistic practitioner, Homeopath and Ayurvedic physician. He tried white flower oil on his head, and could not tell whether it helped or aggravated the headaches. Acupuncture made the headaches less severe but did not help the fatigue or night sweats. He used an Ayurvedic treatment of drinking a mixture of many herbs in fresh almond milk, eating asparagus root candy, making minor dietary changes, and getting Ayurvedic massages with sesame oil with garlic cooked in it. In about six weeks he felt better with the headaches diminished and the night sweats less frequent. From this point on he felt better and slowly regained strength. He still has occasional night sweats, but they are not so severe. Recently they increased again and he saw an acupuncturist for treatment, who needled two points in his body that released sweating. He hasn't had the problem since. He continues to see the acupuncturist because he understands the spiritual process and is helpful to talk to.

Jay is presently feeling an upswing, although with a tendency to fall asleep in meditation. He is alert and energetic during the day. Sometimes he awakes in the night with little flashing bolts of lights in his head, which feel expanded beyond his skull. They tend to be white; he rarely sees other colors. Sometimes he wakes up with a glow above him, penetrating down into his head. This may be a subtle white or slightly gold color. He sees these lights before his eyes, or off to the side, always inside his head. Twice, once in 1983 and again in 1986, he had a profound experience of being awakened from sleep about 2 a.m. feeling a sweet and tender glow from the top of his head, dripping down like honey, seeing visions and feeling great sweetness in the heart area. He describes this as a wonderful, delicate and delicious feeling beyond description.

Another condition he has noticed since the opening is that when he has sex he feels a warm trembling vibration at the muladhara and below the naval, and he will laugh uncontrollably. He feels sexual energy in his whole body and may shake or go into kriyas, or into an involuntary yoga posture.

Jay reports no major emotional upheavals related to this process, although he feels listless and fatigued periodically. It has not interfered with establishing a successful business. On the whole the experience influenced him primarily at the spiritual level. "It woke me up to the possibilities of what spiritual experience was like and made my drive to spirituality much stronger. It is my main goal now, and I try to make everything in life fit it. It opened me to look outside the system I was in (TM) which was a big change -- emotionally and conceptually -- I had to, because Maharishi hadn't talked of these things."

He has not experienced many visual or psychic phenomena. Once he saw a vision of a "being" in meditation and said "What is this?" It answered "a Being of Light". He has noticed in the past year, after a class in Neuro-Linguistic Programming, that he may have some capacity to visualize. He went to an aura reading workshop and learned that by looking at auras in the mind's eye (creating pictures in the mind) instead of seeing them actually around people, he could identify an aura and pick up impressions of people or things that seem accurate. Sometimes he gets images of someone's past life and can describe it in detail. He believes it is impossible to tell if someone is right or wrong about such things, and is not attached to this kind of experience. He does feel he has a strong sense of what to do in his life, and trusts that good things are coming.

Commentary on Diagnosing This Experience:

Jay may have experienced most closely what a yogic adept might be expected to experience with Kundalini -- being plunged into the process while practicing intense, sustained meditation, and doing advanced yogic practices. His physical difficulties -- primarily night sweats and headaches, the moaning, bouncing and energetic phenomena -- as well as the up and down mood swings, the two-stages of opening, and the continuity of his experience are typical of Kundalini patterns. He reports no occult powers or personality changes subsequent to this opening, and it is difficult to assess it's impact on his lifestyle because he was already engaged in the transitions of completing college and getting established in the world during these years.

He has not had emotional trauma or serious physical difficulties due to Kundalini, perhaps because he had a strong context and support system for the experience, even though the organization that initiated the process did not adequately educate him about it. This seems typical of much western yogic training. The TM tradition is one of integrating spiritual practices and everyday Western lifestyles, which is what he seems to be doing well.

Rob

Born in 1933, Rob was the eldest of two sons of upper-class Christian Scientists living in the Midwest, who practiced healing frequently in their family life. His feelings about church were indifferent, but he was taught to see spiritual values in a context that viewed the material plane and evil as non-existent, and that people were made in the image of God. At age 16 he was in a motorcycle accident and his leg was completely shattered, the bones splintered. It was put in a cast while doctors waited to decide what surgery to do, and Christian Science healers and his parents worked on it for a wee. When he returned to the doctors all of the bones were back in place.

In college Rob became disenchanted with religion, and became angry at God for not attuning him to the hard sciences. He plunged seriously into intellectual pursuits and resisted any spiritual teachings. He believes now that he often had energetic phenomena in his body at this time which he ignored and suppressed. He went into the military, then moved to the west coast and earned an MBA in business, and worked for major corporations until starting his own business years later.

In 1965 his interest in psychology, abandoned in college, reemerged and he began attending numerous workshops and programs. In 1968, when he was 35, Rob attended a lecture given by Bernie Gunther, who taught tantric energy exercises using breath, color and sound. As he listened to Gunther talk of energy he had an"Aha!" experience, recognizing that he had been in touch with this energy, and he began doing the practices recommended for expanding it. He next attended a program on eastern energy perceptions which led him to take the Self-Realization correspondence program through Yogananda's organization. He began doing energization exercises and meditating regularly. But he resisted the teachings, convinced they weren't right for him. In 1970 he attended a meditation program, and while sitting in the audience meditating his body felt like it was exploding. He felt on fire, his skin prickling all over.

In 1971 he began TM meditation, and began a regular practice that included some tantric exercises, stretching and energizing exercises, visualizing white light, doing chakra cleansing exercises, and activating the medulla and third eye centers. He meditated for 20 minutes two times a day. In 1973 he enrolled in the Course In Miracles, which helped him resolve some of the philosophical split he had had between material and non-material reality, giving him a new perception regarding a spiritual path. Before this time, he had sought scientific reasons for the energetic phenomena he felt. These phenomena increased as he meditated. He felt at times as if his skin was rolling back on his head, with intense energy gathered at various chakras, and sometimes having tingling sensations and pressure or contraction of the chakras. On some occasions he felt tremendous activity at the forehead and crown chakra, as if his head were opening, with prickly sensations at all points of his body.

He became interested in Carlos Castenada's books, a series of shamanic adventures in Mexico, and traveled to the Yucatan. While touring Mayan and Aztec ruins, visiting pyramids and sacred pools, he had many altered-state experiences, such as being charged with ecstatic energy while standing over the site of an ancient high altar (and not knowing until later it was there). Walking on the beach at night he saw a crow pass over the moon, flying rapidly downward at about 60 m.p.h. He wanted a photo of it and focused his mental energy on communicating with it. It came back and hovered with wings outstretched before the moon, leaving immediately after the picture was shot. He feels that Castenada came alive for him on this trip and he and his wife "terrorized" themselves with some of their experiences. His energy was almost unbearably intense at times.

During these years Rob used alcohol, marijuana and tobacco consistently, although never in conjunction with meditation. He used them to deaden himself from the rising energy, which he believes allowed him to be functional by depressing the central nervous system and helped him remain oriented to the material world and feel comfortable. He had insomnia and much restless energy at night, and a couple of puffs of marijuana helped him sleep. Later he recognized a dependency on these drugs and cut back on their use.

In 1980 Rob began conscious work with energy, after reading a book by Brugh Joy and attending a two-week intensive seminar with him to learn ways of heightening and using healing energy. While there he experienced a psychic opening, felt a unitive experience with the universe, and had a shamanic experience where he could perceive entities and move clouds. At times he would feel physically and emotionally contracted, or experience mood swings, but when he could move away from his personality he would feel unified with nature and God. While drawing a tree he felt merged with it. He experienced kriyas, or involuntary jerking and spasms, concentrated mainly in the second and third chakra areas; if he induced the energy by feeling himself open to it and visualizing, it became unstoppable. He also experienced passing tremendous amounts of energy in healing.

Two weeks later Rob attended a workshop with Richard Moss, using energy exercises to alter consciousness for healing. His energy became even more intense and when he looked into the sky he felt he would disappear unless he held onto a tree. Grounding exercises he tried were useless. He was terrified at times, and felt he " was absolutely on fire". He would smoke and drink "to keep from exploding", and exercise, walk, and run.

Coming home he felt completely out of control. " I felt schizophrenic -- I saw the world in a new way -- and it was warped and uncontrollable and I was unable to be rational." He also wondered if he were manic-depressive, with "mood swings from euphoria to total contraction, expansion to suicidal, and thinking the energy would probably kill me anyhow". His wife tried to use energy-balancing techniques with her hands to balance his energy but he only became worse. She called Moss who told her not to give him any more energy but to have sex with him and to have him run. At times following this experience he would feel wide open, and meditate in front of the full moon, feel himself go into the moon and feel out of his body, then come back and use the hot tub, swimming, walking, sex, drugs and work to try to dull the energies.

He continued to work at programs with both Joy and Moss, which always brought new levels of energy, and greater understanding of the process. He began working consistently with his contraction. He describes it like energy in a hose, which has intense pressure built up. It will pop out in the weak spot on the hose, bringing up physical problems or psychological issues. He came to recognize that over and over it would break out in the same spot, until he resolved the issue. He began what has become a lifelong pattern of self-introspection, using processes with his wife and children to gain greater awareness, and began to work with emotions as energy instead of emotion. If emotions came up he would move them as energy into the heart chakra. As his state of being became more clear his moods such as depression or anxiety could be relieved more quickly.

In 1982, at another conference with Joy, Rob's work required him to hold energy for a group in his heart chakra, and do many psychic exercises. During a three-day break, in which he had fasted and kept silent, he was sitting by a pool listening with a walkman to some highly dissonant and disruptive music of Phillip Glass, which made him feel open,"as if losing touch with the time-space dimension". It was 120 degrees outside and he stepped into a very cold pool, on the first step. As he did he felt intense energy move upward from his feet. As he stepped down each step the sensation increased, moving upward to each chakra. Leaving one chakra "it would expand the chakra above it, building intensity like a crescendo, and I felt very open, with no resistance, like flowing into the wind". It was a "totally incredible and intense experience that I followed until my nose was in the water."

The following day, while at a restaurant, he felt some pressure in his chest and couldn't eat much. He felt agitated and became irritated at a colleague. That night when he went to sleep he awoke around 2 or 3 a.m. His stomach ached and he was extremely cold. He felt as if his food had impacted and left a burning sensation in his stomach. All the events and learning of the conference felt packed into the psoas muscle. He was semi-conscious, and only half aware. He felt freezing and put on several sets of clothes, a down jacket and five or six blankets. His energy would contract and constrict in cycles, intensifying until his whole being felt condensed to the size of a pea at the base of the spine and the physical agony was incredible and unbearable. The following is an excerpt from his journal:

"Suddenly energy exploded upward from the root chakra to the high third chakra under the heart, where it exploded like a neutron bomb going off in my chest. I expanded spherically in tiny pieces, which were all that remained of me, like bits of energy traveling fast like warp speed to the ends of the universe. I felt I was passing through and interacting (like holographic interference) in thought forms and sources of collective knowledge like the Akashic Records and Dead Sea Scrolls and said to himself 'Hey -- I know all that stuff.' I became waves of energy passing on and on past the edges of the universe. Nothing was left. Then very slowly the bits of energy began to fall back. As they came near me they got feathery and essence like, shimmering inward very softly, nurturing me and feeling exquisite. I hang suspended in this feathery stuff and wonder what its about. A voice answers very loudly, clearly and firmly 'This is a state of grace.' I'm loving it. Soon I feel a little form tugging at the edge of the feather ball --'Let me in, let me in -- you left me!' I know it is my ego -- I know if I do it will get control of me. But I know I must accept it and love it."

When Rob woke up from this experience he found he could neither move nor speak, he had no energy and was completely immobilized. He watched his roommate move around and tried to speak but couldn't. He wondered if he had disappeared. Finally he made a "hymph" sound and the roommate came over and asked if something was wrong. When he was touched, Rob was able to mumble "Get the others -- I need help." Six of Joy's assistants came over and gave him hands-on energy treatment for 20 minutes and he could feel life slowly coming back into his body. Since this time Rob has continued his usual practices of meditation and exercises, sold his business and become more involved in community service programs, especially working with people who are dying. He says he has increased compassion, is much more service oriented, and works constantly to manifest his spiritual awareness in his life. He has moments of pure bliss and samadhi in meditation and spontaneously, sometimes several times a week, sometimes not for a month or so. He has difficulty tolerating alcohol. Sometimes his energy arises and he gets flashes of awareness and the answers to problems.

While traveling in Europe he had an intense psychic experience in a church called the Knights Temple, where he felt and saw with great details scenes of being a knight templar in the first Crusades. He knew nothing of the stories of these knights, who were a small band that took pilgrims to the Holy Land, nor did he know at the time he was at the scene where the Holy Grail was supposedly kept. Another time, in Carcassone, France, the center of epic battles of the Crusades, he had a similar experience involving being on a battle field and killing hundreds of men with grey and blue hats.

Rob had consistent lower back pain for many years that became worse until it ended six months before this interview. It focused in the area of the second chakra, and often he would lie in bed feeling his legs shaking and energy blocked in the lower back. He used yoga asanas and four kinds of bodywork to become more open: Hellerwork, which focused on his fascia and deep tissue; energy work as taught by Joy; Jin Shin Do which treated his organs and meridians; and Polarity which affects bone structure. He feels Hellerwork saved his life at one point, when there was so much pain he could not lie in bed more than a half hour at a time. In addition, there were internal components of self acceptance and letting go of control that had to occur to release the pain. He works with the pain in the body as holding psychological content, learning from it, being in it, and seeing what it is telling him.

Rob has had heart attack symptoms frequently, although mild enough that he does not think about them, saying they are just contractions of the heart chakra. Only once, when he was working in industry and under stress, did he feel it might be a real heart attack. Tests show he is in great health with no heart problems. He has no other physical problems he would attribute to Kundalini, but after his

228 ENERGIES OF TRANSFORMATION

last major opening the cartilage tore loose in his ribs, and he still
has a floating rib.

He often sees lights when meditating, in varying colors at
different time. When his state of being shifts he may see color
flashes, as if there is a dark sky with pinholes through which
luminescent blue and purple come through and grow a bit. At times
the world looks luminous or he sees auras.

Rob advises others dealing with this energy to expand into it,
rather than contract against it, and to breathe fully. He believes the
problems people have with it are due to resistance. He has found it
essential to keep his body loose in order to move the energy, and he
consistently does yoga exercises plus nautilus work, running, and
bodywork for this reason. When asked about the meaning of this
experience for him he said "It is my life".

Commentary on Diagnosing This Experience:

It appears Rob has had life-long experience with pranic energy which came into full awareness and focus after the lecture with
Bernie Gunther. I have met other people who felt similarly in touch
with this energy field since childhood and work as psychics and
healers. Rob is similar to many new-age people who are willing to
try many experiences and push themselves constantly in order to have
a breakthrough in consciousness. He continued vigorous pursuit of
energy experiences despite the difficulties they caused him, and
learned to work nearly constantly on his personal process. He
managed a successful career and marriage, raising two children while
involved in these experiences. Eventually he experienced the intense
openings associated with Kundalini, and felt a powerful shift in the
focus of his energies toward greater service in society. His description of the opening during the second seminar resonates with a
number of those in the literature and a developmental or progressive
pattern of this process seems clear in his story. His experiences with
kriyas, back pain, insomnia, heart pains, past life memories and
lights while meditating are all consistent with the literature, as is
bliss, psychic capacities and his growing spiritual orientation.

Rob is an example of someone who has learned to work
consistently with this energy, using it in a conscious process of
psychological as well as spiritual growth. He also used a variety of
bodywork modalities effectively to alleviate some of the difficulties,
along with other forms of physical release. His process seems
greatly enhanced by having spiritual teachers who not only assisted in
the expansion of the energy but taught him methods that have helped
him to integrate and understand it.

CHAPTER SEVEN

NURTURING SPIRIT
IN THE BODY

The case histories show us clearly that this act of transformation by its very nature is a catalyst triggering change in every
aspect of being -- physical , emotional, mental and spiritual.
Whether the transformation is recognized as a mystical event or
viewed as a biological process there is no way to avoid the impact of
its many physiological and psychological components. In order to
integrate this experience and tap into its inherent nature for the joy of
living, one must learn to sustain and channel freely very high levels
of energy. It is essential to come into acceptance and appreciation of
the energetic process, and to open to it and let it motivate new ways
of being. The egoic task is primarily to remove barriers and develop
a physical and psychic structure which can help us in this task of integrating spirit.

As I began to consider the problems that accompany this
process from a therapeutic perspective I concluded that there are five
major tasks necessary for a successful integration to occur. They are
described briefly as follows:

1. UNDERSTANDING:

Understanding and education regarding the essential spiritual
and transformative nature of this process, and the nature of the
conflict between ego and Self. It is then possible to recognize the
symptoms and endure them with a modicum of witness-con-
sciousness, so as not to add undue anxiety at such a stressful time of
life. Having friends who also understand greatly facilitates progress.
The therapist must provide a loving and supportive container that is
theoretically broad enough to hold this process.

2. LIFE STYLE ADJUSTMENTS:
Setting the intention to make essential life-style adjustments in order to reduce stress, live moderately, follow spiritual practices, and find one's personal rhythm through deeper contact with the inner being. Living closer to nature and bringing simple structures and supports into one's life can be nourishing and supportive, along with self-expressive creative activities, movement and dance.

3. EMPOWERING THE BODY:
Strengthening the body and opening energy blocks through body therapies, massage and oil treatments, practices such as hatha yoga or chanting, pranayama or breathwork, dietary changes, and grounding activities.

4. PSYCHOLOGICAL or KARMIC CLEAN-UP:
Finishing up old psychological business. All the old karmic debts have come due and one must come to terms with unfinished desires, unexpressed emotions, and self-destructive habits before the spiritual life can come to full fruition. This can be assisted by writing, drawing, dancing, talking things through, crying it out and various kinds of therapy. Above all one must learn patience, faith, love, self-acceptance and to trust the natural flow of life. This is a stage of letting-go.

5. OWNING THE INNER SELF:
Connecting with ones inner guidance through processes such as imagery, dialogue with various aspects of oneself, dreams, art, and most essential, meditation. Learning to witness external behaviors, and listen with the heart to inner voices.

This book addresses in its entirety the issue of education and understanding. The other tasks are considered in depth in this chapter on the body and the following chapter on psychological and emotional factors related to Kundalini. We will explore some of the specific problems, and provide insight and advice gathered from the perspectives of spiritual teachers, therapists and individuals who have experienced awakening. None of these suggestions are proven nor experimentally validated. There exists no precise method of treatment for this transition, other than the ancient admonition to be under the guidance of an enlightened teacher. But there are many possibilities to explore.

Am I Insane? Or dying?

I passed every minute of the time in a state of
acute anxiety and tension at a loss to know
what had happened to me and why my system
was functioning in such an entirely abnormal
manner. I felt exhausted and spent. The day
after the experience I suffered loss of appetite
and food tasted like ash in my mouth. My
tongue was coated white, and there was a
redness in my eyes never noticed before. My
face wore a haggard and anxious expression,
there were acute disturbances in the digestive
and excretory organs. I lost regularity and
found myself at the mercy of a newly released
force about which I knew nothing, creating a
tumultuous and agitated condition of the mind
as the sweep of a tempest creates an agitation
in the placid waters of a lake. Gopi Krishna[1]

The most distressing part of experiencing the many body
symptoms of Kundalini is the anxiety that erupts around the thought
"I must be crazy -- only crazy people hear voices and jerk around like
this", or "I must have some terrible disease -- maybe two or three of
them." Once the possibility of organic cause is eliminated, the most
important step in overcoming such doubts is to understand that one
is not alone in this condition, that it has been defined and described in
over 4000 years of written history, and is experienced by many who
follow the spiritual practices of mystics. Because higher levels of
energy rush through the physical system, there are many disruptions
of the normal biological and neurological processes, and random
stimulations of the brain will produce spontaneous reactions, most of
which pass without any treatment. On the other hand, if this experience is triggered by an accident, if there is any history of seizure
disorder, or if the disruptions are uncontrollable and lead to long
periods of trance and exhaustion, it is advisable to get the evaluation
of a neurologist in order to rule out complex motor disorders.

If there are frequent physical manifestations, not attributable
to any medical cause, there are several ways these might be
interpreted. According to the principles underlying most body
therapies blocks in the physical body are related to areas of stress or
holding due to a contraction that occurred during a past trauma.

Bodies contract in response to pain, both physical and psychological, and we develop rigidity and tension through holding contractions or repeatedly responding in particular ways to unpleasant stimulus. When people breathe, bend or are manipulated in new patterns during therapy release occurs, often along with shaking and vibrating movements. Such movements may also occur while doing breathwork or hatha yoga. Some of the kriyas and pains that accompany Kundalini awakening are also the result of energy pressing against contracted areas, pushing for release.

Some patterns of physical symptoms, such as those of Krishnamurti when he felt his head was being opened every night, or Irina Tweedie, when overwhelmed by sexual energy, seem to be purposeful invasions of energy to perform a certain task on the body. Gopi Krishna emphasized that this task was to transform the body to meet the demand of evolution for another kind of human who would be a "genius", having direct access to the wisdom of cosmic consciousness. Aurobindo and others have discussed this as a cellular transformation of the body, creating a new kind of human being. Many people with Kundalini symptoms report a feeling of "being worked over" by an energy or a source they cannot describe.

As indicated in chapter four, it is possible that many patterns of energy release may be attributed to the stimulation of certain areas of the brain that are receiving higher charges of energy than normal and sending messages along various neuronal pathways which are received by the nervous system and translated into energy charges, jerks, vibrations, etc. In addition, eastern theory would suggest that the subtle body system is being activated and cleared during this process, and the invisible nadis that transport energy throughout the subtle body system are being opened and purified by Kundalini energy. Breathing exercises, acupressure, acupuncture, and yoga asana are useful ways to open the flows within this complex system.

If the body is in pain, feels stiff, or is frequently subjected to strong vibrational patterns body therapy may help because it opens the body, releases traumas and memories, and enables breath to flow more freely and fully. Practices such as movement therapy, dance, massage, yoga, Tai Chi, acupressure or breathwork can be supportive and enable people to utilize higher levels of energy. It is advisable to learn them from teachers and therapists who understand and relate well to spiritual processes. An attitude of exploration is useful, because not everyone will respond well to the same kinds of bodywork. Some people will feel very nourished, relaxed or energized through treatments. Paradoxically, others may find their bodies too sensitized to handle any kind of touch, and discover it is best to forego such practices in order to tone down energetic phenomena. As energy intensifies in the body it is essential to find ways to express it rather than contract against it. Dance, song, running, movement, exercise, and creative activities are helpful.

Staying on the Ground

Following the deep transpersonal processes accessed through body therapies, altered-state imagery, hypnogogic states and similar processes it is helpful to do grounding practices, which bring one back fully into body-awareness and reality-orientation. People who pursue mystical states are frequently accused of having their "heads in the clouds", a clear indication one needs to learn to ground more completely on the earth plane. This can be done by holding their feet while they concentrate on breathing in all the way down to the soles. Or it is useful to walk, stomp, dance, or pretend to have the feet of a lion hugging the ground. Grounding can be as simple as taking time to have a cup of tea and discussing how to integrate an experience into everyday life in practical terms, rather than leaving someone in a "spaced-out" condition after a therapy session. It can be done with visualizations, such as pretending to be an oak tree, stretching your arms into the sun and your roots into the ground. It can be done by hugging a tree, tending a garden, working with clay, kneading dough, baking, engaging in athletic activities, hiking and building sand castles (in the sand).

In order to live our lives in ways that bring forth our spiritual insights and are aligned with our depths we must build a strong physical and psychological container that is comfortable being alive on this planet. Without this we may be subjected to disorientation, inflation, and terrible angst. It is clear from the lives of some of the Christian saints, as well as in the stories of psychotherapists who treat anorexia and other body-denying conditions that those who spend years separating their spirit from their body are often subjected to extreme ill-health and even premature death. When we honor the tasks of day-to-day living, and care for the health of our bodies we begin to build a container in this world that can carry the impact of spiritual awareness into the human dimension. Impulses toward starvation and extreme asceticism undoubtedly emerge from the demonic or dark side of this experience, related not so much to transcendence as to hatred of the human condition. True enlightenment brings appreciation for human existence and compassion for its limitations.

The order, discipline and regularity of life in a spiritual community, such as an ashram or monastery, has a practical purpose of helping people with a tendency toward mystical or etherial states of awareness to have tasks that reengage the body and mind in the simple realities of life. In addition, responsible spiritual communities promote a moderate and moral code of living and a life of service to others, which support the psyche in the Kundalini process. On the whole, people I have known who followed consistent structure such as work or family life, seemed better able to integrate these higher energies than those who had little else to occupy their minds. Too much structure would be oppressive during the intensity of spiritual awakening, but moderate discipline and consistent work are immensely supportive.

If their lifestyle is not satisfying, those who are in the Kundalini process are likely to feel internally pushed to make changes that better support their physical and emotional needs. Sometimes major changes occur, as people leave jobs, relationships and homes and move to the ocean or the woods, to India, or to other environs to which they feel drawn. I have noticed such a totality in these kinds of decisions; it as if an unseen force is sweeping one into one's destiny. In such cases it is helpful to have a strong spiritual teacher or guide, a commitment to using rationality in caring for one's physical being, and friends or a support system of people who understand what is happening. It is really terrifying to be completely disoriented or seriously ill while isolated or surrounded only by people who do not recognize the spiritual dimensions of the psyche. The healthier the personality structure and the body before the awakening the better one can deal with radical upheavals, and follow such callings successfully. Being grounded in one's own being (the capacity to feel centered and whole), and being grounded in a practical appreciation of reality are thus very important allies to this process.

Living With Kriyas

It is clear that numerous varieties of kriyas often accompany this process, and that some of them appear to be related to growth and others to pleasure. These may include intense heat and energy streaming up the spine or radiating from the body, tremors, spasms or spastic movements, violent shaking, twisting movements, anal or uterine contractions, jaw clenching and emitting of vocal noises and animal sounds. The entire body can become either rigid or limp, and there may be intense pain, sensations of expansion or contraction, out-of-body experiences, twitches and a seemingly endless and imaginative range of other movements and responses, most of which were previously explored in chapter two.

Regarding kriyas occurring as jerks and spasms, Swami Sivananda wrote: "You may get jerks of hands, legs, trunks and whole body. Sometimes the jerk is very terrible. . .It is nothing. It can do nothing. . . It is due to sudden muscular contraction from the new pranic influence, new nerve-stimuli. Remember that new nerve currents are formed now owning to the purification of nadis from sadhana. The jerks will pass off after some time." He commented that a tremor that may occur during meditation is due to prana being taken up to the brain, and is simply a stage in the process. He said "the sudden jerks in meditation come especially when the prana becomes slow and the outward vibrations make the mind come down from its union with the Lord to the level of physical consciousness".[2]

Kriyas probably occur as well when intensified levels of energy are impacting various areas of the brain, which respond automatically to the stimulus in their characteristic ways. The emitting of sounds and tones may also be correlated with brain stimulation, or with the release of certain blockages in the chakras. To reduce kriyas one might reduce the energy stimulus temporarily by avoiding meditation and other practices that increase energy flow, and utilizing more active methods of expending energy such as exercise and creative self-expression. One needs to live in an expanded energy field, integrating the energy, accepting and responding to the unknown and unpredictable. As physical and emotional contraction decrease, so will the range and intensity of kriyas.

Although kriyas are commonly thought to be responses to blocks in the body, or involuntary relaxation responses, I have observed them flowing intensely during altered states of consciousness and believe they may occur at times when one's awareness is in the subtle body rather than the gross body. It may be that an energy exchange is going on between the two and no awareness is there to hold the gross body in it's accustomed rigid pattern. It is as if one has surrendered to the flow of an energy field and is being carried like a piece of bark on a river. These kinds of kriyas are often smooth and rhythmical and may leave a sensation of blissful tingling in the body, along with an aroused and energized physical system when they are completed.

Illness & Pseudo-Illness

Latent illness erupts, or a pseudo-illness sometimes arises during the Kundalini process that cannot be adequately diagnosed by medical doctors. People complain of headaches and bands of energy tightening around the skull or burning the top of the head. A few men and women have what appears to be a false pregnancy, with the belly swollen (called "Buddha belly") periodically for a number of months. Some people have chest pains and numbness, symptoms very similar to those of a heart attack. This is likely due to the Kundalini energy moving through the anahata, or heart chakra. It may be that the nervous system, the digestive tract or the hormonal system is seriously disrupted.

B.S. Goel also noted among his problems such symptoms as automatic twitching and concentration between the eyebrows, a burning and pulling sensation in his eyes as if they were being tugged at by magnets, an increased pulse-rate, his tongue coated white with thick saliva, difficulties in passing urine, and seeing a red aura spread throughout the brain when he closed his eyes and tried to concentrate. But he said that to him the most important indication of Kundalini was that after each state of severe suffering, he automatically shifted to a state of peace, bliss and stability. These states alternated automatically throughout his process.[3]

The lives of many mystics include periods when they were subject to peculiar illness. Evelyn Underhill pointed out in Mysticism that even though they had robust intelligence and intellectual ability such saints as Plotinus, St. Bernard, St. Catherine of Genoa, St. John of the Cross, and the Sufi poets Jame and Jalalu'ddin suffered poor physical health. She added that "More, their mystical activities have generally reacted upon their bodies in a definite and special way producing in several cases a peculiar kind of illness and of physical disability, accompanied by pains and functional disturbances for which no organic cause could be discovered, unless that cause were the immense strain which exalted spirit puts on the body adopted to a very different form of life."[4]

Swami Narayanananda related specific physical illness to what he termed partially awakened Kundalini moving by improper paths. He said the awakened shakti often absorbs excess heat and cold in the body, along with poisons and pains from various body parts, and that when the Kundalini-shakti absorbs cold, its activities become very dull, and its movements very painful and unpleasant. He attributes this slow movement of energy through various chakra areas as the cause of problems such as "looseness" and "lack of control" of the genitals, liver malfunctions, stomach pain and disorders, heart troubles and heaviness of the chest, breathing troubles and asthma, heaviness of the head with a "dull brain", and colds.[5]

On the other hand, he believed when Kundalini absorbs heat and carries hot currents to different body parts one may have "lascivious desires", genital irritation, "continuous secretion of semen, until he is exhausted and weak", and experience conditions such as nervous debility, wet dreams, piles, jaundice, cough, dyspepsia, loss of memory, loss of vigor, fear, hatred, and premature aging. He reported that such hot currents can injure nerves and veins of the anus and cause improper blood circulation, or influence the bladder, causing constipation and intense burning. In addition they may cause heart palpitations and burning sensations in the heart, lungs, spleen and stomach. He said that during exposure to wind and cold weather the currents have difficulty penetrating above the heart-center and may travel instead toward the left hand, which will become numb for awhile.[6]

If over-heated currents reach the mind, he said, one suffers sleeplessness, headaches, loss of vitality, peevishness and possible "brain derangements or insanity." His recommendation for these mental diseases was to use a wet loin cloth, or to keep the region of the anus and genitals under a cold water bandage for 24 hours, changing it every 15 or 20 minutes. (Perhaps this is the equivalent of the western "cold shower"!) In his opinion, in the loins this shakti can cause lumbago, and in the abdomen, colic. If it remains in the stomach one can get chronic dysentery. When treatment is given to one body part the problem will move to another, and medicines provide only a temporary cure. He said stomach complaints are usually the first problems of spiritual aspirants, and medicines tend to make the cure more complicated.[7]

If Narayanananda's evaluation of these problems is correct, it is reasonable for individuals with Kundalini difficulties to be especially careful about the balance of heat and cold in their bodies, and avoid extremes of temperature in food and environment. He stated that these diseases could be easily cured by purifying the Kundalini-shakti, keeping it always in a normal state of working through regular pranayama practice in the morning and evening, and by adjusting food, drink, bath, weather, etc. to proper temperatures.

The pranayama he recommended is a form of alternate-nostril breathing, where the throat is locked and the inhaled breath held between the heart and the throat until it is released. One breathes through the right nostril for five minutes, and then through the left nostril, until gradually confidence and endurance enables one to breath up to 30 minutes through each nostril. (He warns never to do this pranayama during pregnancy.)

It is useful to know a variety of pranayama exercises and yogic asanas, which are taught at most yoga centers, because some of them specifically modulate body temperature, or affect particular body organs. These practices should not be followed compulsively or obsessively once Kundalini is awakened but individuals should experiment to discover the practices that have beneficial effect on their own well-being and use them to strengthen and moderate the pranic energies. In similar ways acupressure and acupuncture treatments can balance the system and alleviate many symptoms.

According to Swami Sivananda there are other remedies for some of the Kundalini symptoms. He wrote of both positive and negative sensations, commenting that in meditation "You will feel that power is radiating from you. Your consciousness will be deeper. Thoughts of God will start the spiritual currents in the body. If heat is produced in the head, apply butter, a malak or Brahmi oil. Take cold baths. Take butter and sugar-candy."[8]

It is not uncommon for some ashrams to provide chocolate as a counter-effect following intense meditation programs, and some meditators report that the purpose is to replace lecithin in the body, which tends to diminish during prolonged states of altered consciousness. The use of oil massage has also been recommended for the relaxation of involuntary spasms by Baba Hari Dass.[9] When Irina Tweedie complained to her guru about the ice-cold feeling on the top of her head when she did a head stand, her guru recommended hot tea with a bit of butter in it "to prevent dryness of the brain." [10] One subject commented that frequent baths, tranquility tanks, ginger soaks or mud baths were very soothing and helpful.

Sivananda explained discomforts that may come during meditation such as numbness, jerks, and ticklishness, as the body's effort to hold on to new vibrations. When the hands are numb he advised that one massage each arm with the palm, neither stirring nor opening the eyes.

He stated that in order to become a perfect yogi and experience the "wonderful samadhi" one must control mind and breath, and continuously practice yoga. To achieve realization quickly he advised advanced aspirants to stop all work, to remain in a solitary place on the river, and to live on milk and fruit.They should plunge wholeheartedly into their practice of meditation, sleep only two or three hours a day, and begin this practice at the beginning of winter in Nov-ember.He wrote that it is the act of complete surrender that will bring grace to the yogi, which removes all obstacles, snares and pitfalls in the spiritual path.[11]

Most Westerners are not going to become "perfect yogis", live by a river and exist on only milk and fruit, and even if they did it is not likely to resolve all their difficulties. But it is interesting that people sometimes feel pulled by their inner psyches to do these types of yogic practices as Kundalini awakens. Many report much less need for sleep. Most of my subjects spontaneously became vegetarian. Sivananda's advice may seem contradictory to the comments of other teachers regarding balance, and the need for order and discipline. The difference here is perhaps one related to the goal, and to the fact that his words are aimed at "advanced" yogis, who have already traversed much of the path, and probably follow rigid rules of order and self-control. There are times when a spiritual aspirant wants only to go deeper, to put all of heart and soul into this inward process, pushing beyond all previous limits. This seems to be the direction of Sivananda's advice in this passage. It is most helpful to have a protected environment and a guide if one is to pursue this path, and most disturbing to do it alone, with no spiritual guidance.

Sleepiness & Trance

In contrast to reports that yogis often need very little sleep, Swami Muktananda ascribed symptoms of sleepiness, heaviness and lassitude to Kundalini, saying that some will fall into a deep sleep, but that this is a positive sign which passes and should not be alarming.[12] This symptom was also commonly reported by the Western subjects, along with lethargy and falling into trance.

Jung described some of the physical symptoms of Kundalini, including sleepiness, as conditions observed in many who moved into transformative stages of development. He said that when these disturbances arose, it was as if either the structure of the brain were changing or certain cells in it were destroyed. (The restructuring of the cells is commonly defined in yoga as a correlate of the Kundalini process; however stimulation of certain areas of the brain can also cause lethargy and trance.) Jung said that he knew from experience that regressive libido resembled a drug, working like a poison or toxin. He wrote "People whose libido is regressive feel terribly sleepy, they can hardly open their eyes and they feel generally unwell; the whole functioning of the body is upset. . .Very little is known about these things, but we know positively that in regressive moods, the viscosity of the blood is measurably decreased, and of course, the alteration in the blood affects the whole body."[13] He reported that latent diseases may be released by this condition, such as lingering infections, since the resistance of the body is reduced, and suggested this may account for the frequency of angina under certain psychological conditions.

These remarks may explain some of the characteristic sleep disturbances and sudden illness of people going through Kundalini awakening, which is invariably accompanied by the regression of libido. The yogis might attribute these conditions to increased shakti but there is no doubt that the deeply altered states of consciousness plunge one into a profoundly regressive state, in the sense that one is regressed from or deeply removed from ordinary consciousness.

More Dynamic States

Muktananda also described a more dynamic view of the physical sensations of Kundalini, saying that in a seeker who is steadfast and full of devotion to his guru, Kundalini may pulsate with its grand, joyous and ecstatic vibrations in extraordinary ways. At these time the seeker may spontaneously dance, sing and weep. One may even shout, groan, roar like a lion, make animal sounds, chant Om loudly or say mantras spontaneously. Parts of the body may begin to move, and he/she may hop like a frog, spin, twist, run in circles, roll on the ground, slap the face, roll the head round and round, adopt different yogic postures and mudras, shake, sweat, do yogic locks, pull the tongue in or up against the palate in the kechari mudra, or roll the eyeballs upward. Different kinds of pranayama may happen automatically. There is involuntary kumbhaka, or retention of the breath.

Like most gurus, Muktananda's prescription for treatment of Kundalini symptoms was primarily discipline, meditation, the avoidance of fear, and surrender to the guru, a classical yogic viewpoint. The guru is to be the container, in a way similar to that of a therapist when someone is in a deep psychic process---he/she is the hope, trust, and strength throughout the crisis. He advised students to avoid anger, resentment, and comparisons with others, and to control bad habits. He also suggested living in the company of Siddhas (Masters), avoiding aimless talk and false gossip, refusing to indulge in self-willed behavior, avoiding others leftover food and not touching people unnecessarily. He warned that too much talking and the company of useless people destroys the storehouse of shakti.

The challenge for people enmeshed in Western civilization is obvious here. [14]
The interrelationship between mind and body underlies much of the advise in yogic literature regarding Kundalini processes. This makes yogic literature appear somewhat vague from the perspective of Western medical treatment, which tends to isolate and treat symptoms of disease rather than exploring the hologram of a lifestyle as it relates to illness and health. One's behavior, self-control, attitudes, emotions, and relationships are the significant factors emphasized when Kundalini presents difficulties. This is a common understanding of Eastern medicine, which treats patients in a holistic style, questioning what it is in their lives that contributes to physical illness, disease and good health. From this perspective one who has physical difficulties with this energy has not been adequately prepared psychologically or emotionally, and may also lack the strength and clarity that comes from following yogic cleansing practices, breathing exercises, correct living and asanas.

Themes of preparedness, moderate living, self-control, trust in the process, avoiding unnecessary stress, avoiding unhealthy company and developing a relationship with a guru, whether it be external or internal, echo throughout the literature. There is little about dealing with symptoms in such a way as to make them disappear. Ultimately, the intention is that through the inner work and attitude and the grace of a guru or higher source one will experience bliss and profound wisdom, so there is little rationale for making the energy stop.

In the West, some yoga teachers advise those made uncomfortable by this process to shorten meditation and eliminate pranayama exercises temporarily; to eliminate meat (or begin eating it again); to give up alcohol, cigarettes, caffeine and other addictive substances; to eat natural and alive foods (vegetables, greens, fresh fruit); to practice hatha postures; and to simplify their lifestyle. These are all ways of experimenting with slowing down or inhibiting the intensity of the energy, or enhancing the body's ability to sustain higher energies. The Ayurvedic medicine of India is concerned about balancing and harmonizing pranas in the body, so herbal remedies as prescribed by an Ayurvedic physician may also be helpful.

When all else fails try talking to the energy. One subject I interviewed asked it to leave her alone when she was driving or out in public, and thereafter had no more "spacing-out" symptoms in either situation. This suggests the value of a "relationship" with this otherness. Dialogue is known by many therapists to be a way of aligning ourselves with deeper psychic structures, winning the cooperation between our many aspects of self.

Sarah, who practices voice-dialogue with clients experiencing Kundalini, frequently has the energy speak through the client as if the goddess was a sub-personality. This enables the client to own and integrate some of the aspects of the deeper Self, and reflect more deeply on the reasons for any difficulties the energy has generated in the system. (Another option is to dialogue with a troublesome symptom or body part and ask it why it is creating pain or difficulties.) Creative processes such as art, clay modeling, dance, and movement can also help clients to get in touch with physical or emotional blocks and move into them and through them. Richard Moss wrote in The Black Butterfly (1986), about singing out his emotional states, and making up songs and movements to express them, as a method of transcending them.

It is clear that the physical aspects of this process cannot be addressed separately from the psychological aspects, which may in fact be true at the deepest level for any disease or ailment. On the other hand if latent problems do emerge, appropriate medical diagnosis should be sought. Mystics are as prone to life-threatening illness as any other segment of the population and it would be foolhardy to attribute every symptom to the Kundalini. There are specific kinds of illness that carry Kundalini-like symptoms, as well as vulnerable body systems that become ill as a consequence of the heightened energy in the body, and appropriate tests are often needed. But if medical examination is inconclusive, and symptoms appear to be floating or short-lived rather than consistent, those who are engaged in this process need to release fear and anxiety and may wish to address the emotional blocks that might be constricting the free flow of spiritual energy.

To Eat or Not to Eat

Yogic texts emphasize the importance of proper diet, generally recommending moderate eating, and vegetarian fare. Fasting is not generally advocated. However Gopi Krishna described erratic swings in appetite during periods of his Kundalini difficulties, ranging from eating four to six times the amount of food he would have eaten at a sitting before the Kundalini awakening, to desiring no food at all for days. He said lack of appetite was a common occurrence. If he disregarded his scheduled time to eat he at times lost all appetite and taste, sometimes becoming nauseous.

In one instance, after weeks of not eating because of a strong aversion to food, Krishna tried to swallow a few morsels and wash them down with water. He felt a sudden unbearable stab of pain in the abdomen and around the sacral plexus, so intense that he fell prostrate, writhing and twisting on the floor. The pain left after a few hours. A few days later, while his son was eating rice in front of him, his appetite returned.

He decided that the intervals between attempting to eat were too long, and he would try to eat small amounts every three hours. He found he could hold this amount of food down, but he continued to have convulsions, pain sensations along nerve paths and delirium. He believed he was going to die. At the height of this crisis he fell asleep for the first time in weeks and dreamed a vivid dream in which he saw himself seated with a meal in front of him consisting of a half-filled plate of boiled rice and meat, which he ate with enjoyment. When he awoke he asked his wife to prepare this dish and serve it to him every two hours and by nightfall he felt a slight relief and was able to sleep through the next night. The next day he ate every hour, then moved to an hour a half, but added fruit and curd to the diet. Gradually the delirium vanished and insomnia gave way to an excessive desire to sleep. He began eating four to six times the quantity of food he had eaten earlier in his life, and to select the constituents of every meal, choosing a combination of acids and alkalis, sugars and salts, fruits and vegetables, in a manner that helped him to digest enormous quantities.

Not long after this dietary shift Krishna's condition stabilized and he was able to return to work and other responsibilities of life. He attributes his many dietary problems to "a poisoned state of nerves, an inevitable result of the awakening in the first stages, for which there is no known antidote except proper feeding in spite of the aversions, done in a manner as may be indicated by the habits and the condition of the system." [15]

He advised that high quality, easily digestible, completely natural foods should be taken in small amounts at regular intervals, normally at least every three hours. He believed a nutritious diet was essential in order to enable the nervous system to rid itself of impurities.

Krishna wrote that aversion to food is a common feature in sudden awakening, and that the abrupt release of this force and its movement through the nerves causes acute disturbances in the digestive and excretory systems. Some hatha yoga exercises teach aspirants to empty the stomach and colon at will to prepare for emergencies that may accompany this experience.

Narayanananda strongly advised one to avoid foods and drinks that are too hot or too cold, as they will impact the movement of Kundalini with the problems he attributed to the shakti's tendency to absorb heat or cold and cause various physical illness. An exception is if hot or cold drinks are needed to balance extreme weather temperatures, although he suggested one live in a moderate climate. He recommended a similar approach to bathing, using hot water in cold weather, and cold water in hot weather, and moderate temperature otherwise. He also believed a body needed to be "in between leanness and fattiness" if Kundalini is to function normally and rise to higher centers, and he recommended a moderate diet with avoidance of alcohol. Fruits and vegetables should be selected according to their availability by season.[16]

In my experience a strictly vegetarian diet tends to make the body feel more light and less earth-bound and is therefore advantageous for people who tend to be too mental and pragmatic, and have difficulties going into meditative states. For this reason, and also because of values which oppose the killing of animals or concern about the effect of chemicals injected in animals before they are slaughtered, many spiritual aspirants never eat meat. I have heard from followers that their teachers recommend meat occasionally for people with distracting Kundalini symptoms in order to ground them, or help them become more body-conscious. Several subjects I interviewed reported that returning meat to the diet reduced uncomfortable symptoms. In other cases the sensitivity to the killing of animals is so acute that one feels ill or depressed after eating meat. Some noticed that eating regular meals made them feel better, sometimes eating as frequently as every three hours. Several subjects went through periods of extreme loss of appetite.

Most subjects who were not already vegetarian felt an inner compulsion to follow a vegetarian or semi-vegetarian diet after the awakening of Kundalini, especially finding no appetite for red meat. It is as if the body wants to maintain lightness and openness, and feels more comfortable without meat in the system. Elimination of drugs and alcohol also often occurred spontaneously, in some cases with people compulsively taking these items and throwing them out of the house.

Physician Gabriel Cousens, who describes his own Kundalini awakening, and outlines a nutritional program for the maintenance of spiritual energy in <u>Spiritual Nutrition and the Rainbow Diet</u> (1986) makes a case for the harmony of a vegetarian diet to support subtle body energetics. He describes a natural harmony between plants and human, since plants take in carbon dioxides, a product of human respiration, and convert it to oxygen and carbohydrates. He writes that "Each colored plant, as food, is a condensed spectrum band of sunlight color for us to take in for the balancing of our chakras and the physical organ, gland and nervous systems. When we take in a full spectrum throughout the day, we benefit by having our total chakra system balanced energetically by our plant friends. This is the principle of the Rainbow diet".[17]

He states that the correct alkaline/acid balance is 80% alkaline-forming foods (vegetables and fruits which are high in calcium, magnesium, potassium, sodium, and iron) and 20% acid-forming foods (proteins). He recommends fasting, food-combining (a method of eating foods together which digest well together), and under-eating. (He cites studies which suggest this may prolong the life-span.) Cousens states that the awakening of Kundalini energy seems to increase the need for glucose, which can be met by including complex natural carbohydrates in the diet. If the energy is too active, he reports the glucose from honey can calm it down, acting as a "pranic shock absorber".

Cousens' book includes many ideas for balancing and harmonizing the physical, emotional and spiritual dimensions of the being through correct diet, drawing from Ayurvedic medicine, Chinese concepts of yin and yang, macrobiotics and his background as a physician.

Visual Problems

The reports of several subjects and biographical accounts record difficulties with vision apparently related to Kundalini. They have experiences such as the eyes closing spontaneously and refusing to open, or temporary blindness. Great sensitivity to light is common, and sometimes there is pain in the eyes. Usually these symptoms pass quickly.

Muktananda described a time when he felt that the pupils of both his eyes became centered together, and he began to see one thing with two eyes. In the scriptures this is called bindu bheda. After this happened, a blue light opened in his eyes. He wrote that when this process starts, some aspirants feel they are losing their sight. In his case his eyes rolled around and up and down violently. Others could see it happening and were frightened. As the eyes revolved, the optical chakras were pierced, and he felt pain in both eyes and ears. He says that ultimately this condition leads one to clairvoyance. [18]

I have not seen anything in the literature to indicate treatment to alleviate these specific difficulties, but in various yoga asana classes I have experienced a number of yogic exercises for the eyes, including rolling the eyes in a circle; rapid eye-movement in four directions and up and down, rubbing the hands together to generate heat and energy and then cupping them over the eyes, and staring at the moon or at distance objects until the eyes tear (which is said to develop psychic abilities). There are also acupressure points around the eyes, and a proper acupressure treatment of the facial muscles is very relaxing.

General Guidelines

With so much advice on the proper nurturing and control to facilitate positive Kundalini experience, it is not surprising that modern Westerners, with their varieties of biases, sensate pleasures, material attachments, and undisciplined life styles would have difficulty managing this energy effectively. It is clear that the very firm structure of the ashram or spiritual community is designed to facilitate smooth passage through spiritual processes, and is the antithesis of secular society, although even in ashrams many difficulties may be experienced. Most of us would resent the curtailment of our freedom to eat and drink what we wish, enjoy sexuality, follow our moods spontaneously, and cling to our mind-set about the meaning of life, even when such promises as spiritual enlightenment beckon. It is painful when the physical aspects of Kundalini force us to confront the reordering of our lives. Some wish only to find a way to cut off the entire process, which may be possible by plunging wholeheartedly into secular living, but this is likely to make us feel cut off from our deeper roots.

Probably most who are not practicing yogis or part of another spiritual tradition, try to create a compromise between honoring the spiritual impulse and living the worldly temptations, seeking slowly a transition that will satisfy the inclinations of the deeper Self. It appears from the literature and reports of subjects that the physical symptoms eventually pass, as long as one is willing to endure, to trust, and to bring balance and new energy into his/her life. Generally the advice is to practice yoga, live with self-discipline, eat moderately and avoid stimulants and meat,avoid indulgence in negative habits and relationships, avoid excessive stimulation and keep the mind tranquil. In addition one might explore bodywork and self-expression to open blocks in the system or relax tensions. Allowing ample time for the energy to flow has been useful for some subjects, rather than trying to control or block it. This can be done by resting or meditating for a given period each day. Creating a relationship with it, that is talking to it as an ally or companion, and relaxing into it, can bring one into bliss. Many of us are not accustomed to high energy charge in our bodies and tighten against it or react as if it were painful. When we can align to it and expand our consciousness to include it we can find it is a source of pleasure. We might compare it to being contracted against an orgasmic experience, versus flowing with it. The same experience can be felt as painful or pleasurable. Once trust is built the energetic phenomena are rarely painful. The pain is often caused by contraction, or occurs when energy is trying to move through injuries or severe blockage in the body.

It appears from the case histories that during difficult phases of the Kundalini process people should not be alone. Krishnamurti insisted two friends sit with him during these times, even though they did not interact or interfere, nor even understand the process. They did prevent him from hurting himself occasionally when he felt compelled to run, or would stand up and fall over due to the intensity of his pain. Krishna, Kennett and Goel all stressed the value of having persons who stayed with them through the process. Muktananda, Tweedie, and Radha depended on the support of their gurus. I believe one of the most important things a therapist or friend can do is to provide a supportive environment, and act as a silent non-judgmental observer or a good listener. During any crisis those who have such friends or partners in their lives are immensely reassured by them.

When one has illness which seem to be related to Kundalini it is of course important not to ignore them, so medical evaluation may be necessary. But when a diagnosis cannot be determined, it may be best to delay treatment for a reasonable period of time. Medications and exploratory surgery can only aggravate the difficulties for a Kundalini client. Sometimes a latent illness is generated by Kundalini and must be treated medically. Sometimes symptoms for which causes cannot be determined pass spontaneously through the system. This is why it is so important for physicians to have a rudimentary knowledge of this process.

Energy discharges and other conditions such as heat and cold rushes, or eating disorders, tend to come periodically, and to pass spontaneously. Some spiritual teachers such as Ramakrishna, Krishna, Krishnamurti, Muktananda, and Tweedie experienced extreme difficulty for a period of time, and many Westerners report the same. Others have only minimal discomfort. We can only speculate about the factors underlying these diversities. They may be related to the speed or depth at which the awakening is unfolding, the length of a yogic or other spiritual practice, the ability of the brain to respond to energetic changes, intensity of commitment to the process, maturity or stability in one's lifestyle, personality type, previous psychological and physical conditions, previous therapy or bodywork, the intervention of a guru who is facilitating the process, the kinds of karma to be relieved, the number of past lives in which one has had Kundalini experiences, and other factors beyond our comprehension. It would be interesting to compare the experiences of people who had practiced yoga asanas and pranayama for 20 years with an equal number of cases who had not practiced yoga.

I believe it is not accidental when an opening occurs, but that awakening is orchestrated by the deepest core of the inner Self. However, it seems likely that those in initial stages of this process may not have the same experiences as people in later stages, and that those who have   serious psychological problems may be overwhelmed by this eruption. This energy pushes one toward completions through physical and emotional transformation, and no one claims the ability to predict its timing or its outcome for any individual. It is an encounter with the numinous, and the personality's ability to recognize and integrate such an encounter has a great impact on further development of the psyche.

Breath: The Great Generator

Understanding the relationship between breath and Kundalini is important for several reasons. First, many people who seem to have difficulties with Kundalini have practiced pranayama techniques, and most books which discuss pranayama say it can be a dangerous practice if done overzealously, or without proper preparation and guidance. Because these practices are so readily available in books and classes today it is possible to do them without this preparation and to experience problems as a result. Over-zealous breathing practices have been blamed for many difficulties including perspiration, trembling, black-outs, hallucinations, blood-shot eyes. excessive heat in the body and bleeding gums.

Secondly, there are significant similarities between these yogic practices and modern breathwork practices, where breathing patterns are altered and used to bring one to altered states of consciousness. This may be experienced in hypnotic states as well as with bodywork therapies and breathwork. Again, knowing that a client follows such practices can enable a physician or therapist to more accurately diagnose a Kundalini experience.

Finally, I have wondered whether breath practices may be useful to someone who has already awakened Kundalini as a method of gaining some control. Lee Sannella advises against this, seeing pranayama as a risky practice. In an interview with Baba Hari Dass I was advised that people require differing breathing practices according to their temperament and where they are in their development. This is one reason the direction of a yogic master is so often recommended. Swami Narayanananda cites pranayama as essential to controlling physical problems related to improper movement of Kundalini in the body.

In the yogic tradition pranayama is learned in sequential steps, appropriate to various stages of practice, and when one masters the easier techniques, one is taught more advanced practices. There are six purification exercises done with the breath, which are usually practices learned before pranayama techniques, in order to cleanse the nadis or arteries of impurities. A series of contractions of the throat, abdomen and anal sphincter muscle, called bandhas or yogic locks, are often performed prior to or concurrent with pranayama, to hold the breath in the body. The ultimate purpose of pranayama is the harmonization and control of the various energies of the body, leading to the awakening of Kundalini energy with proper management of the energy as it releases upward through the spine. The practices of kriya yoga specifically aim at releasing this energy by contracting the anal sphincter and following the movement of the breath upward from the base to the crown chakra. It seems that yogis who practice these techniques may experience Kundalini during meditation and experience great self-awareness, peacefulness, bliss and samadhi without having the uncontrolled disruptive experiences of the uninitiated.

According to Pancham Sinh, translator of the Hatha Yoga Pradipika "Pranayama is nothing but a properly regulated form of the otherwise irregular and hurried flow of air, without using much force or undue restraint; and if this is accomplished by patiently keeping the flow slow and steady, there can be no danger." He indicates that it is impatience for yogic power that causes "undue pressure on the organs and thereby causes pains in the ears, the eyes, the chest. etc. If the three bandhas (the yogic locks) be carefully performed while practising the pranayama, there is no possibility of any danger." [19]

According to Swami Vishnudevananda, pranayama is one of the most important practices in all forms of yoga. Through pranayama one is able to control the nervous system and obtain gradual control over prana or the vital energy of the mind. "We constantly drain our life force or pranic energy by our thinking, willing, acting, etc....Yogis count life not by the number of years but by the number of breaths." [20]

Prana is carried to all parts of the nervous system through pranayama, taken in through inhalation and stored in nerve centers, especially in the solar plexus. This increases the yogi's vitality. Yogis declare that the correct habit of breathing, and following a natural diet, would regenerate the race and eliminate modern diseases of civilized man, such as high and low blood pressure, heart disease, asthma, and tuberculosis. These practices also increase will power, self-control, concentration, moral character and spiritual evolution, assisting the yogi to manage both physical and emotional conditions.

According to the ancient Gheranda Samhita, factors that influence the effectiveness of pranayama practice include performing it in a proper place, establishing a consistent and correct time, eating moderately and purifying the nadis. It warns that if yoga is commenced in the hot, cold or rainy seasons one will contact diseases, and recommends beginning in spring or autumn. [21]

A yogi who does pranayama is advised in the Gheranda Samhita to eat rice, barley or wheaten bread, and beans that are white, clean and free from chaff. Also allowable are patola (a kind of cucumber), and a number of other vegetables. "Pure, sweet and cooling food should be eaten to fill half the stomach: eating thus sweet juices with pleasure, and leaving the other half of the stomach empty is called moderation in diet." One should avoid bitter, acid, salt, pungent and roasted things, curd, whey, heavy vegetables, wine, palmnuts, and over-ripe jack-fruit, certain beans, stems, gourds, berries, onions, lotus and other items common to the Indian culture. Food that is hard (not easily digestible), putrid, very hot, or very stale, very cooling or very exciting should not be taken. [22]

It also recommends that the yogi avoid much traveling, the company of women, warming by the fire, early morning baths (before sunrise), fasting, and anything giving pain to the body.

There are a number of advanced pranayama techniques, which are generally not described in books but are passed down by teachers. These involve various kinds of breathing such as panting, rapid exhalations, breath retention, holding of the locks while focusing on the sixth chakra, turning the head slowly in each direction, holding the breath and rotating the stomach, and following the breath upward along the spine as in kriya practices. Deep meditation sometimes releases the spontaneous practices of pranayama, even in one who has not learned the techniques, and I have also seen them occur in breathwork, once a person moves beyond conscious control of the breathing.

Breathing practices are also significant in the Zen Buddhist tradition. In a description of how to practice Zen breathing by Kennett Roshi, Shakyamuni Buddha is described as having been successful in achieving enlightenment within hours of practicing the correct method of breathing, which is naturally known to children. This method involves following the natural flow of the breath, and consciously, at the beginning of meditation or if awareness is lost during meditation return to the following elliptic pattern:

> Inhalation starts at the base of the spine and continues up the spine to the crown of the head; exhalation starts at the crown of the head and continues down the front of the body to the pubic area where inhalation takes over at the base of the pine. Thus the breath goes in a circle, inhalation up the back of the body and exhalation down the front, and this irregular breathing is the turning of the Wheel of the Law.[23]

One is advised to follow the breath consciously two or three times and then to leave it behind and let the breath settle naturally into the rhythm that is right for the individual. This is a gentle breathing process, much less invasive than pranayama or breathwork, perfectly safe and useful for centering and concentrating energy. In my opinion more intense breathing exercises are also useful for centering and managing the inner energy, but they should be used with caution by one who has inadvertently opened the Kundalini. In my own experience I can do gentle pranayama and kriya exercises for a short while, but if I practice more than 15 minutes my energy becomes very intense, there may be pain in the spine, and I feel "strung out", or I become very cold. Other factors, such as physical injuries, or emotional trauma seem to make these energy flows uncomfortable for some people.

It is possible to trigger emotional difficulties and Kundalini crisis through overzealous practice of pranayama when one is not "purified" in mind, body or emotional discipline to handle the high intensity of energy it can generate. It seems inadvisable to recommend this technique for those who tend toward compulsive and overzealous practice, unless they live in an ashram setting with a qualified spiritual teacher.

It is helpful for individuals dealing with Kundalini to understand pranayama techniques and the dietary advice that supports them because they are designed to create a physical system that can best support Kundalini. These techniques develop mastery and control of inner processes. Breathing through the left nostril is said to cool the body system, and breathing through the right nostril is said to heat it. The right nostril is also said to raise emotions, and the left to calm them down. The breath, properly directed, has the power to clean and open the physical system, free it from physical and emotional disturbances, relieve radical internal or external temperature change, and stimulate equanimity and inner peace. It is a doorway into mystical experience. There are many specific advanced pranayamas developed to modulate temperature, moods, organic difficulties, and mental distractions.

There is evidence that breathwork produces many of the psychic contents and changes credited to pranayama. One may experience a wide range of physical releases, images, emotional catharsis and spiritual openings. Pranayama seems to prepare the yogi in much the same way, but without the drama, for one is taught to sit and simply observe whatever comes up, where in breathwork the tendency is toward expression and cathartic release. In both processes it is staying with something -- going completely through an awareness or experience without getting attached to it, neither trying to enhance it nor to avoid it, which seems to produce release and transformation of the personality. Often, in a spontaneous Kundalini experience it seems the person is going through similar inner attempts toward transformation, and what makes it most difficult is the lack of boundaries, or direction; one needs safety in order to contain and experience the process without getting entangled in it. In a yoga practice, a Zen practice, or a breathwork session one knows the timeframe and the intention of the practice, and this holds them in a container which allows them to deal effectively with any fear or difficulty, especially if a teacher is working with them. One who is isolated in this experience, or surrounded by people who think it is abnormal, suffers greatly from the lack of context and boundary. Therapists can help such individuals to create both.

Body Therapies & Kundalini

In the West the practice of using bodywork along with concentration on the breath is becoming more common, and responses to various kinds of bodywork may range from discomfort to emotional catharsis to experiencing transpersonal energies, lights and visions.

Anma Massage and Acupressure

Kennett Roshi wrote that one who meditates often has more difficulty tolerating invasive forms of body therapy, and she recommended a specific gentle bodywork called Anma massage, which can be self-administered, or the use of acupressure, to assist with the subtle tensions released through meditation. She stated that Jin Shin Do (a form of acupressure), regardless of the attitude of mind of the one who is doing it, may have a slightly coarse and manipulative feeling about it to the meditator, as if the "energy flows" are sometimes temporarily channeled backward through the meridians or are run back and forth to scour out the blocks. "Of course," she adds " there are times when this is precisely what is needed: I have personally seen great good accomplished through the use of these releases. Some of them seem particularly suited to assisting a person in recalling memories of early traumatic experiences and even karmic memory traces of unresolved problems from previous lives. As such, I believe they could be of considerable use in psychotherapy." [24] My research and personal experience suggests that Jin Shin Do assists greatly to open nadis or energy channels in the body, balance energy, strengthen body organs, and encourage transcendent experiences.

Kennett described a subtle and gentle mudra system used at Shasta Abbey, but warned that unless it is practiced with the mind of meditation, and faith in something greater than oneself it is useless. She saw the practice as a sacramental act tapping into energy much greater than that contained in the meridians, and called this energy the "Love of the Lord", beyond any limits of physical anatomy. Thus the points used in Anma massage are not restricted to the areas of the traditional meridian systems, and do not require the practitioners to have their hands directly on the body. However she saw direct touching necessary at times because "it is sometimes important to know that one is loved by man as well as by the Cosmic Buddha, and there is no more effective way of knowing this than to feel the warm touch of a loving hand on your body." She also stated that in this system: " Finally, it is not even necessary to use mudras at all; the energy can be directed and tensions in the meridians can be cleansed solely through the power of meditation or contemplative prayer."[25]

Side effects of Anma treatments can include the arousal of sexual energy, or a greatly increased sensitivity and vulnerability, so that one becomes so aware of the condition of all things and so emphatically linked to them that pain is felt when a flower is picked or strain is placed on a spring. If one is being treated for a serious illness it may appear that all the vital energy has retreated within, so that he/she appears to be weaker or deteriorated. During these times she advises forgoing the responsibilities to work or family, reducing the social life to one or two trusted friends, and living in "an atmosphere of quiet simplicity." Unlike a mental illness, this condition should not include a disturbance of the thought processes. Such heightened sensitivity is relatively rare and Kennett wrote that it is usually part of a major breakthrough in religious understanding. She indicates that "It is not a cause for worry and should be allowed to take place unhindered... In time the ability to deal with everyday matters will return in full, and with it a greater strength, efficiency and wisdom than one had previously known."[26]

In addition to using a meditative mind and absolute love and respect while doing the mudras, Kennett warned that the person receiving the treatment must be willing to face whatever may arise in the body and mind, accept it, and embrace it with love and with the faith that at the origin of every desire and act, no matter how bizarre and destructive, there is something pure and undefiled. Otherwise the treater will needlessly expend tremendous energy and become drained, exhausted and possibly more susceptible to illness.

Reichian and Neo-Reichian Therapies

Styles of bodywork at the opposite end of the scale from the gentle Anma massage mudras are Reichian and neo-Reichian therapies, which combine breathing processes and vigorous body movements along with the manipulations of the therapist to free the physical system from blocks or "armoring" which restrain energy and prevent people from feeling completely energetic and alive. Wilhelm Reich, a controversial physician who studied with Freud and practiced as a Freudian analyst in the early years of his career, was the founder of this style of Western body-oriented psychotherapy. He developed an interest in the physical aspects of an individual's character, and believed that successful therapy meant the client was completely orgasmic, able to expand and contract the body fully. He believed that the structure and demands of society inhibited this capacity, and caused neurosis.

Reich studied and experimented with the body and determined that "armoring" kept physical sensations from coming to awareness, and that this armoring occurred because the organism made energetic decisions at the time of a trauma that caused it to carry or hold on habitually to muscular tension and contraction. He concluded that psychological learning was not enough but that the body also needed help in order to experience complete health. He developed a theory of various character types correlated with typical patterns of armoring.

Eventually Reich identified an energy he called "orgone" energy, in its cosmic, primordial state, and labeled "ether" when it was expressed in the human body. "Cosmic orgone energy functions in the living organism as specific biological energy. As such, it governs the entire organism; it is expressed in the emotions as well as in the purely biophysical movement of the organs." [27] Orgone was a primal cosmic energy of the universe, according to Reich, and it was possible that the physical reality underlying concepts of "God" and "ether" might be this same orgone energy. He defined cosmic orgone energy as being primordial, universally existent, all-permeating, the origin of all energy and matter, being biological energy in the living being and the origin of the galactic system in the universe.[28]

Orgone energy flows up and down the body, parallel to the spine, according to Reich. Rings of armor are formed at right angles to this flow and operate to sever it. In Reichian therapy deep breathing is used to build an energy charge in the body that can dissolve the armor, and physical pressure is placed on the chronically tense muscles by the therapist. Cathartic expression is encouraged, along with working through whatever resistances or emotional restrictions arise.[29] According to psychologists James Fadiman and Robert Frager:

> Reich felt that the process of armoring created
> two distorted intellectual traditions which form
> the basis of civilization: mystical religion and
> mechanistic · science. Mechanists are so well
> armored that they have no real sense of their
> own life processes or inner nature. They have a
> basic fear of deep emotion, aliveness and spon-
> taneity. They tend to develop a rigid, me-

chanical conception of nature and are interested
primarily in external objects and the natural
sciences. . . Mystics have not developed their
armoring so completely; they remain partly in
touch with their own life energy and are capable
of great insight because of this partial contact
with their innermost nature. However, Reich
saw this insight as distorted, because mystics
tend to become ascetic and antisexual, to reject
their own physical nature, and to lose contact
with their own bodies. [30]

Reich saw religion as counter-productive to human health,
and was also frequently at odds with society because of his radical
views of sexuality, and his insistence on the existence of orgone
energy, going so far as to build a machine to capture it. But his
comments and descriptions of orgone clearly match the descriptions
of prana in Eastern scriptures. And he developed ways of working
with the breath and body that break through armoring and release vibrations, pleasurable energy charges, feelings of hot and cold,
prickling, itching and emotional arousal, in much the same way that
meditation and pranayama practices release physical blocks. Some of
his comments are remarkably in tune with Eastern scriptures:

In penetration to the deepest depth and the
fullest extent of emotional integration of the
Self, we not only experience and feel, we also
learn to understand, if only dimly, the meaning
and working of the cosmic orgone ocean of
which we are a tiny part.[31]

The conceptual worlds of 'God' and 'ether' show
so many similarities that they must have a
common origin, regardless the fact that God as
an esthetic quality and ether as a physical
quantity so far have never met, and could not
meet within the framework of human thought.
. . It seems all the more peculiar and
significant because God and ether have so
many similarities in the world of human
imagination.[32]

It is probable that the energy Reich identified is both pranic energy and Kundalini energy, depending on the intensity and level of consciousness that is experienced, and that people engaging in bodywork with a Reichian base, including Bioenergetics, and many neo-Reichian bodywork spin-offs, are potentially able to release enough armoring to open the system to Kundalini. However the limitation of doing this work with a body therapist who is chiefly focused on releasing sexual expression would be that the intensified pranic energy would end up primarily expressed through the lower chakras, bringing more sex and power and stability into one's life (or possibly more difficulties in dealing with these energies), but not fully energizing and expressing the upper chakra energies.

Although his goals were usually expressed in terms of sexual energy Reich did value the releasing of the heart energies. According to Baker, holding in the chest is equated with heartbreak, bitter sobbing, rage, reaching, and longing. These are deep emotions which need to be expressed and relieved in order for a genuine expression of love to become possible. Baker commented, "It must be remembered that most of what passes for love is really not love at all but is based on the anxiety or hate present in armored man where all natural impulses, particularly love, are inhibited." [33]

Another interesting correlate of Reichian therapy and yoga is the stages that occur in sequence as layers of armoring are removed. According to Baker: "First, anxiety occurs. Then emotion is released -- rage, contempt, spite, crying, etc. After the emotion is expressed, there is a sense of relief. Third, contactlessness appears. There is no desire to move and the patient is temporarily stuck. A stage where the repressed and repressing forces are equal has been reached."[34]

He points out that inner loneliness or deadness may emerge in this process, including an inability to make human contact, and orgasm anxiety. He believes, in contrast to the yogic theories promoting sexual continence in order to retain energy for higher experiences, that these conditions indicate "the last form of neurotic contactlessness to show itself and the final hurdle that must be surmounted before health is established..." In addition, he points to an emptiness of life or experience that accompanies orgasm anxiety, along with " superficial communications and a disinclination to speak of genital desires, a sudden deepening of reserve, fears that the body will come apart, falling dreams and fantasies, flight from meaningful relations with the world (including sexual relations), and a return to infantile reactions and to earlier symptoms. . ." [35]

Baker's approach to resolving contactlessness is to disturb it by increasing the push outward, or reducing holding, or both, making the patient aware of it, and describing to the patient "the difference between the patient's behavior and the ideal he sets for himself and the emptiness in which he lives."[36]

These symptoms are remarkably similar to some of those reported by mystics and people in Kundalini processes and it is possible Baker's approach to breaking these impasses could be used effectively with them; however, this might be counter-productive for the spiritual goals of those who practice yoga, which generally advocates renouncing worldly attachments and pleasures, particularly sexuality. Reichian therapy encourages people to become more expressive and more alive in every aspect of their life, rather than to channel energy specifically to spiritual purposes. I believe these contrasts highlight a major struggle for individuating Western spiritual seekers -- whether it is best to freely live and express their entire beings or to withdraw and withhold themselves in order to heighten spiritual awakening. It is possible that such splits are resolved through higher levels of integration when people have passed through the Kundalini stage of awakening, and are capable of using heartfelt connection with others as a spiritual practice.

Psychologists and neo-Reichian therapists Gay and Kathlyn Hendricks encourage the releasing of energy through all the chakras, and do neo-Reichian work with a focus on energy and space, rather than limiting the focus to body musculature. They believe this creates an environment that enhances the potential for spiritual experience. Clients appear able to expand and focus their consciousness into subtle and causal realms of experience, becoming more "alive" in dimensions beyond the physical body. I have observed several people move into spiritual experiences when doing the Radiance Breathwork developed by the Hendricks', and experience the subsequent transformation of living with higher levels of energy.

Reich, like Freud, created a system to expand human concepts of consciousness and facilitate Self-awareness, but both were limited in their vision due to personal traumas of their own childhoods and the sexually repressive society of their time. They laid a groundwork in lower-chakra psychology that was expanded to include issues of the upper chakras by Jung and the many humanistic and transpersonal therapies that followed.

Fire Meets Fire:
Sexuality & Spiritual Awakening

In sharp contrast to Reich's views, yogic literature makes it abundantly clear that celibacy is the highest choice if one follows a spiritual path, not because of any great issues of morality but because of the need to marshall and redirect pranic energies, and because of the distractibility and attachment generated by desires for the opposite sex. References to this ideal often arouse tension in Western spiritual seekers, who may react with feelings of anxiety,self-denigration, guilt, denial and hostility. Instead of acknowledging celibacy as a tool that is useful for some at some stages of the process they overlay cultural dogma on the concept and consider it avoidance of evil.

Control of the senses is the ultimate skill for yogis who wish to contain and direct their energies beyond material concerns, and some Sanscrit scriptures maintain that no one who is sexually active has any hope of attaining the highest levels of spiritual awakening. In the male-dominated society of Vedic India many monks tended to view a female as evil simply because of the distracting temptations which were associated with sexual attractiveness, and some monks refused ever to look at a woman. Women in India still suffer from discrimination and separatist attitudes to a great extent because of the anxieties of spiritually-striving males who see them as obstacles on the path to liberation.

The recognition of the value of sexual energy in the tantric tradition introduced a new option for a brief period of history, in which the female might be embraced as a goddess, and the path to freedom be engaged through ritualistic use of the senses, including highly evolved sexual practices in which energy could be raised mutually and merged simultaneously between male and female partners. There is evidence that this was also the understanding of earlier matriarchal cultures which included goddess cults. This secret and advanced ritual was intended only for those who had already achieved significant stages of spiritual consciousness, and were accomplished in the arts of concentration, meditation and mastery of the senses. It's purpose was not to encourage sexual practices but to enable the seeker to transcend sexual attraction or desire, and to channel the secretions of sexual intercourse upward through the sushumna so they could be used to transform consciousness and revitalize the body. Such teachings are not generally condoned today and are considered an embarrassment by many spiritual, political and intellectual leaders in India.

Sexual and materialistic excesses such as those of Bhagvan Rajneesh who taught tantric practices in both India and the U.S. have further damaged the reputation of this ancient art, which is greatly misunderstood in the West. In fact most Westerners who have heard the term "tantra" mistakenly believe it is only concerned with sexual practices, as if it were a rather glorified elaboration of the Karma Sutra. But in fact sexual rituals were never a major part of the right-handed tantric tradition and in many cases were considered only in symbolic visualizations or used by only a small number of advanced yogis who had mastered many other levels of sensate detachment, and could easily achieve samadhi. The Buddhist tantric tradition is also rich in visualization, discipline. structure, and ritual, and is focused on enlightenment and living for the good of all sentient beings.

Where it is still practiced, sexual tantra is as secretive as ever in India, but occasionally it is available in the West in ab-breviated version, brought by a handful of people who practice yoga or teach ways to enhance sexuality. There is often moderate to no concern about the spiritual aspects, the preparedness of the aspirant or the ritualistic elements of the practice, which must make it a far different experience than it would be if practiced in the purist tradition. True tantric practice was never meant to be for indulgence of the senses or improving one's sexual life. It was used to awaken and move energy in a way that transcended all further need for sexuality or other earthly pleasures and attachments (although it has probably rarely been practiced this way with much success!) What it teaches is control and surrender, along with methods of using breath and concentration to channel sexual energy upward through the spine into the crown chakra. Semen and female secretions are changed into a form of energy called ojas, which is the essence of the life force and is capable of restructuring human biology.

I am not qualified to discuss in depth the essence of tantric practices, but I believe it is important to acknowledge their existence as a viable path for spiritual experiences, and to point as well to the lack of a requirement for celibacy in many mystical traditions. Tibetan lamas and Muslim or Indian Sufi teachers often have wives and families. In fact, a Sufi "Pir" or teaching lineage is traditionally passed from father or mother to son or daughter. Jewish Kabbalah, Buddhist, Shamanic and Native American traditions do not view celibacy as a prerequisite for enlightenment. A number of Christian saints were married and had families. These facts may offer some perspective to those meditators who believe they must suppress all sexual urges.

Sexual energy frequently intensifies during spiritual awakening because it is a central part of the very life force one is encouraging. It is clear that powerful sexual experiences can occur as part of this opening, and Kundalini subjects reported a wide range of reactions and responses to the process. Many continued active sexual lives. One deeply intensified her spiritual experiences through sexual engagement. The following attitudes and practices have been reported by people who have awakened Kundalini.

1. Some practice celibacy consistently.

2. Some feel intensified sexual energy and release it with great joy with a partner.

3. Some people feel swamped with waves of sexual energy and are frightened or embarrassed by it, but wait for it to pass and do not act on it.

4. Some have sexual experiences with partners which move them well beyond the confines of ordinary consciousness and generate radical new openings and altered-state experiences.

5. Some use sexuality as an outlet for intensified energies so they can relax and release tension.

6. Some have little or no interest in sex, or feel great fluctuations in their desires. Or they may feel physically uncomfortable, with their energy "out of control" if they become sexually aroused. Most will experience a desire for celibacy during certain stages of Kundalini awakening.

7. Some break their celibacy occasionally, finding that it relieves depression or stress to do so.

8. Some practice containing the energy, limiting sexual activity to once a month or less, simply to manage energy and desire more consciously.

9. Some feel Kundalini has little or no impact on their sexual lives.

10. Some report awakening Kundalini or feeling intense and uncomfortable pranic energy following sexual involvement with an awakened partner.

11. Some report occasional or frequent spontaneous orgasms occurring with no external stimulus.

12. Some generate sexual energy and channel it upward through the chakra system in order to experience whole-body orgasmic sensations, or what seems like "brain-orgasms" to several people.

13. Some believe in sublimating all sexual desire into creative activity and work.

Clearly the variations are great and there is no tendency to follow one single pattern. Although many "saints" advocate and practice celibacy, and may themselves have found the thought of sexual involvement a hindrance in their spiritual work, there is no real evidence that sexuality prevents spiritual awakening. However it is possible there may be levels of realization that one cannot penetrate while still involved in such activities. Certainly preoccupation or obsession with sexual concerns will generate less energy in the direction of enlightenment and may keep one attached to the gross body, and sex undoubtedly is a more addictive attachment than most other sensate pleasures. It also seems unlikely that one who can penetrate reality to the level of Nirvikalpa Samadhi would care to have the distraction of a sexual partner at the moment. This is unnecessary and irrelevant to an experience which lies far beyond the senses. I expect that sexual tantric practices lead people more commonly into subtle-body energies and bliss, and not into the higher stages of samadhi.

From a therapeutic perspective there is no clear direction, other than to encourage self-acceptance, and respect for the individual desires and needs of the aspirant. It is clear that some people who practice yoga and adopt rigid sexual attitudes are suffering from deep sexual conflicts and fears and have found a convenient way to justify them. Such patterns of self-denial and self-rejection interfere not only with the ability to be psychologically healthy but with the capacity to attain spiritual fulfillment as well: the energy cannot properly awaken and move, the heart can-not open, and no surrender is possible. Individuals are best advised to seek inner intuition as to which path or practices to follow at any given time, letting go any tendency to be guided by rigid belief systems and fear.

Most who have awakened and learned to live with higher levels of spiritual energy will probably find sexuality to be uncomfortable and heavy if it is done out of obligation, or with partners who cannot match them energetically. Sex as an act of release loses its flavor in the face of the ecstatic vibrations that accompany the energy of the Self. On the other hand, when sexual energy is exchanged between two people who know how to engage and blend this energy at all levels it can take them to new and rare heights, as if they are merging separate selves, and allow them to reenter life with extraordinary vitality and well-being.

Ultimately, spirituality should not become life-negating but life-empowering, and those who engage it need channels for expression that encourage it to expand and be lived on the planet. Some ways this may occur are through service, creative expression or relationship. There is a time to sublimate all of oneself to the influence of the divine, and a time to bring one's awakened consciousness of the divine into the living patterns of human existence.

References: Chapter 7

1 Krishna, G. (1970 rev.) Kundalini: The evolutionary energy in man, Boulder: Shambhala, p. 51.

2 Sivananda, S. (1969) Spiritual experiences (Amrita anubhava), Himalyas: Divine Life Society, p. 70.

3 Goel, B.S. (1985) Third eye and Kundalini, India: Third Eye Foundation.

4 Underhill, E. (1961) Mysticism, New York: E. P. Dutton, p. 59.

5 Narayanananda, S. (1950) The primal power in man or The Kundalini shakti, Gylling, Denmark: N. U. Yoga Trust & Ashrama, p. 124.

6 Op. cit., p. 125-127.

7 Op. cit., p. 127-128.

8 Sivananda, Op. cit., p. 60.

9 Hari Dass, B. (Personal communication, Dec. 30, 1986).

10 Tweedie, I. (1979). Chasm of Fire. Great Britain: Element.

11 Sivananda, Op. cit., p. 60.

12 Muktananda, S. (1978) Play of consciousness. Ganeshpuri: Gurudev Siddha Peeth, p. 31.

13 Jung, C. G. (1968) Psychological commentary on Kundalini yoga. Spring. New York: Spring Pub., p. 96.

14 Muktananda,S. Op. cit., p. 40.

15 Krishna, G. Op. cit., p. 195.

16 Narayanananda, S. Op. cit., pp. 132-137.

17 Cousens, G. (1986) Spiritual nutrition and the rainbow diet. Boulder: Cassandra Press. p. 113.

18 Muktananda, S. Op. cit., p. 125.

19 Sinh, P. (trans.) (1981) The hatha yoga pradipika, Delhi: Sri Satguru, p. i.

20 Vishnudevanada, S. (1960) The complete illustrated book of yoga,New York: Julian, p. 246.

21 Vasu, R. (trans.) (1914) The gheranda samhita, Delhi: Sri
        Satguru, pp. 37-38.
22 Op. cit., pp. 40-41.
23 Kennett, R. (1979) How to grow a lotus blossom. Mt. Shasta,
        CA.:Shasta Abbey, p. 187.
24 Op. cit., pp. 57.
25 Op. cit., pp. 80-81.
26 Op. cit., p. 84.
27 Reich, S. (1946/1979) Character Analysis, New York: Pocket.
        p. 393.
28 Op. cit., p. 50.
29 Baker, E. (1969) Man in the trap.New York: Macmillan.
30 Fadiman, J. and Frager, R. (1976). Personality and personal
        growth, New York: Harper and Row, p. 127.
31 Reich, W. (1961) Ether, God and the devil & Cosmic super-
        imposition, New York: Farrar, Straus & Giroux, pp. 51-52.
32 Op. cit., p. 49.
33 Baker, E. Op. cit., p. 68.
34 Op. cit., p. 70.
35 Op. cit., pp. 69-70.
36 Op. cit., p. 71.

CHAPTER EIGHT

THOSE SURGING WAVES OF EGO IDENTITY: THE EMOTIONAL CRUCIBLE

A dream --I am in a boat full of people, docked
in shallow water. I get off. I put my hand
along the bow and it begins to turn over. I try
to catch it and can't. In a minute it is upside
down and sinking. People and things keep
floating up from the depths. I and others
watch as hands and legs reach up and we seem
much larger than the boat and pull people out.
It's like fishing toys out of a bathtub. I am
anxious that someone may have drowned but
the water is only about 8 feet deep so people
can be pulled upright. Finally it seems
everyone is out of the water and the boat
floats up empty. I pick it up like it is a toy,
tip it to drain out excess water, and set it back
on the sea. It appears no one drowned. . . .
Subject, Chris.

Immense waves of emotional turmoil may swamp the
individual who is struggling to integrate the spiritual Self. There are
many possible sources for this upheaval. Some of it may simply be
biochemical reactions to intensified energy. But never doubt that a
great inner struggle is at hand. All the old values and beliefs are up
for grabs, as the world perspective shifts. Those egoic attachments,

even for the comforts of home and family, the security of work one
enjoys, the desires for travel or relationship or whatever else has
shaped the motivations of the personality, begin slipping away,
falling back into the unconscious. They may seem irrelevant or
empty. One feels naked, isolated, separated.

Paradoxically, great waves of bliss, a sense of belonging,
and unitive awareness may flood the psyche, alternated by blackness
and a confrontation with the existential void. It becomes possible to
recognize the dynamics of the personal ego and the unreality of
attachments with a starkness far beyond the ability of rationalization.
When surrendered into nihilistic bliss this does not seem such a loss,
but when the ego returns to shape a way to live in Western society, a
massive struggle for integration is called for. Emotions rise and fall
like a surly ocean and one is doomed to navigate them.

Fear

One of my favorite pieces of advice regarding effective
treatments for spiritual crisis is this statement by Da Free John:

> Heartfelt release of fear is the secret of passing
> through the spiritual process without going
> mad. To the degree that you are full of fear,
> you limit your experience -- and if experience
> is forced upon you, then you have no ability
> while fearful to view it sanely, to relax and
> surrender within it. You cannot surrender by
> relaxing and trying to feel better. You can
> surrender only by giving yourself up, relaxing
> your self-hold, surrendering your mind
> altogether to the Transcendental Consciousness
> in which it arises, and yielding your body to
> the All-Pervading Current of Life, of which it
> is but a temporary modification.[1]

Da Free John wrote that the emotional problem of self-di-
vision is the root of all suffering and delusion. People are not relaxed
in the heart, and are afraid and contracted against the experience of
being in contact with divine being which is manifest everywhere. His
writings suggest that the way toward integration lies in embracing all
of life as the Divine, staying open to the moment and whatever it
brings. He said that allowing oneself the freedom to love and be

ecstatic is the only way to happiness, yet most people are so contracted against this that no amount of Kundalini energy can touch it. The only solution for this "emotional recoil" is to "enter into a presumed association with god as the intimate, heartfelt Associate or companion of your life." He called this the only cure for the loveless heart and the life of suffering. [2]

Many people suffer from a tendency to be self-negating, and a difficulty in freely experiencing and expressing love. The persona is adapted as a protection against recognizing this contraction or block -- it carries the image and often the belief system regarding who we are, and how we fit into life, providing a role and an illusion of belonging. If Kundalini awakens and one is contracted against the consciousness it brings, it appears that nothing of value can happen, although much struggle may still occur. Westerners who have resolved issues related to identity, relationship and self-actualization in their personal lives are probably better equipped to integrate the Kundalini experience, because they have learned to face uncomfortable truths about themselves and to respond to the inward impetus for growth and change. Those who are trapped by more rigid patterns or come from a negative spiritual tradition, where God is associated with punishment and judgement, are more likely to fear this activity is some evil force punishing them or possessing them.

In addition to fears about oneself, some people feel a terror regarding the energy itself, as if they are being invaded or possessed, especially if they have never considered a potential association between physical energy and spirituality. For people in traditional or fundamentalist religious systems it is shocking and guilt-inducing to have spontaneous sexual fantasies or orgasmic convulsions when praying. I have found clients to be greatly surprised and relieved to learn that it is not uncommon for sexual energy to arise when one is intensely engaged in prayer and meditation. It is not the work of the devil but the activity of the subtle body energy field interacting with human physiology. The first stirrings of Kundalini are sometimes felt as increased vibration, itching, or tingling in the genital area, and the deeply altered and relaxed consciousness of sincere prayer or meditation encourages this energy to awake.

Although Free John's "heartfelt release of fear" and the "creation of a relationship with God" is advisable, it may be difficult for the average person to attain. In the interim the most effective ways to address fear are to understand the process, find confidants who support and understand what is happening, and accept the experience. It can help to explore creative and active methods of confronting the fear -- personifying it as the "child" within or as a sub-personality, drawing it, dancing it, having a dialogue with it. There is a fearful self and a wise self in each of us and we need to clarify who we wish to be in charge, without negating the voice of either.

Anger

In an article written in "The Dawn Horse" newspaper, an interviewer asked Irina Tweedie, author of Chasm of Fire, about a passage in her book where she related beating a mouse to a pulp in an outburst of anger. "How did your guru explain this?" he asked. She replied "This sudden anger is one of the symptoms of Kundalini. At that moment, I realized with horror that I could have killed a human being. But when I talked to Bhai Sahib about it, he very calmly said 'Oh yes, those things do occur'. When the Kundalini awakens, one can have the most terrible moments of irrational anger. One goes beyond it, of course. Later on, the symptoms are different."[3]

Da Free John and Aurobindo have offered advice on moving beyond constricted feelings through witnessing. Aurobindo said that in the face of negative emotions "Somewhere deep down we shall feel the Witness in us who is not touched -- who is never touched-- who does not suffer. There are falls and there are rising and each time one rises up stronger. The only sin is to be discouraged."[4]

Da Free John said we must notice that it is we who are making us unhappy, emotionally disturbed or limited -- we discover this by observing ourselves no matter what we are doing. He encourages people to be present as "unobstructed" feeling instead of contracting against feelings, saying that when there is no contraction what is felt is absolute bliss, and this will create a new interpretation of the universe: "You will not interpret manifest existence to be evil or suffering or sinful, or others to be unloving, or life to be terrible. Instead of that, you will regard all of manifest existence to be pervaded by Bliss -- not merely Bliss coming at you from every direction, but Bliss radiating from every direction in the place where you stand. This Bliss has no center, no bounds, no limits. It is free energy."[5]

The contraction one experiences when locked in anger and fear may be released through opening of the heart chakra, which is a significant phase of the spiritual process in many esoteric traditions, signifying the movement from lower to higher chakra energies. When this occurs the personality can more easily cope with the emotional issues of the lower chakras that may activate during Kundalini movement, and attention turns more naturally toward spiritual interests. It becomes possible for love to direct the process.

Meditation on the heart chakra is a yogic method of addressing this transformation, and acupressure treatments focused on the heart meridian may also be useful for this kind of release.

Depression & Mood Swings

Many meditators have been surprised to discover that following experiences of bliss and peace in meditation, and believing they have made gains toward a spiritual life, they suddenly encounter moodiness, doubts, anxiety, guilt and depression. In addition, as spiritual commitment deepens it seems as if a splitting away of ordinary consciousness may occur as connection is made with the inner Self, and then life as it was previously lived is no longer satisfying, and activities of the old persona have no congruence with the inner being. Alienation from friends may occur if they cannot understand the process.

While the former identity feels unnatural, identification with the new Self may bring ambivalence or inflation. Spiritual ideals such as liberation and non-attachment are usually unappealing to the ego and may be discounted as fantasy or impossibility. As people become more conscious of the process the sacrifices and difficulties become more clear. They may feel torn between wanting to release worldly desires, and feeling panic as non-spiritual interests fall away. They may feel bliss and joy in meditation, flatness and deadness in living.

B.S. Goel wrote of his despair over the psychic fluctuations and bouts of uncontrollable weeping he endured. He was haunted by fears of death and insanity until he had to give up his work. His self-confidence plummeted. He wrote: "A genuine case of Kundalini arousal is in the grip of veritable hell during the initial five or six months. The states of confusion and bewilderment are so intense that they are beyond the reach and understanding of any intellect. The fears of death and insanity are very acute. The reason for such a situation is that the mind organized on the old ideas and formations is shaken completely and gets disorganized. . ."[6]

Goel eventually noticed that such periods of suffering were characteristically followed by a sudden inexplicable state of relaxation for a few hours. He believed the tendency to ups and downs was a process of becoming caught in worldly delusions, which are being burned away by the rising Kundalini. When the pain becomes unbearable the inner guru makes a contact to release this obsession and produce sudden peace, stability and bliss. In his experience the pain was so intense during the downward pull that he could not remember or hope for peace again, but wept uncontrollably, or ran for help.

It is reassuring to know from the autobiographies and case histories that many spiritual aspirants who suffer from such traumas do move beyond feelings of doubt and despair, because in the West when individuals are caught up in these feelings there is no place to go culturally for reassurance. Traditional Western culture would simply agree that spiritual aspirants should forget their introverted processes and get on with living. Standard approaches to dealing with depression in therapy may include medication, helping clients to express anger, or promoting behavioral changes. In my experience these are not particularly healing approaches for Kundalini clients, unless they are triggered by obvious life circumstances.

An intervention more in tune with the process would be to observe and witness the moods, and to teach clients to carry the tension of opposing forces patiently until the unconscious allows them to shift. They need to know their feelings are commonly experienced by mystics, and to be encouraged to go on with their life the best they are able and trust the moods will pass. They need to be reminded of the joys or bliss, the highest of their experiences, and reassured these will return. The lives of mystics suggest that one cannot exist permanently in a stage of bliss until all karma and personality issues have been released, and this is a life-long process.

Some of the subjects found it helpful to adopt an attitude of acceptance and of surrendering their feelings to God, or they cited meditation, acupressure, breathwork, massage, hot baths, understanding friends, vigorous expression of feelings and making love as having the potential for relieving depressions. In the yogic literature the ability to wait out these moods, to practice right living, to continue with disciplined practices, to read scriptures, and to depend on the guru are more traditional methods. Aurobindo (1971) said "All limitations can be surmounted. . . by calling in a higher power and consciousness than that of the personal mind and will. The higher consciousness can by what it brings correct or rebuild what is defective in the personal nature."[7] He believed one of the first tasks necessary for spiritual seekers was to achieve a settled peace and silence in the mind, and equanimity in the being, trusting that happiness comes from the satisfaction of the soul rather than of the emotions or the body, which can never be satisfied.

Theosophist Alice Bailey advised that one may pass through great difficulties by learning to stand with steadfastness in spite of all that one may do and feel, realizing that the cyclic condition is related to the pairs of opposites and is part of the life manifestation of existence itself. She believed that during cycles of reincarnation the soul experiences periods of being outgoing and extraverted, followed immediately with lives of introversion and introspection, with apparent lack of interest in relationships and environment. Between these two extremes we may flounder, for many lives, until the opposites are blended. Then the dual roles of a spiritual aspirant become clear and both aspects come together so that one may concurrently live a life of both service and reflection.

While this process takes place, Bailey wrote, a definite work moves forward in the etheric body, energies of the lower centers becoming refocused above the diaphragm. She identified the solar plexus as the most potent center, the clearing house for the personality forces, and said it is the movement through this center that causes the most upheaval.[8]

Aurobindo also wrote of a depression and moodiness that may follow the first connections with higher consciousness, after one falls back into an ordinary state. This can cause the psyche to be overwhelmed by depression, disappointment and despair, or to feel stagnant, as if no further progress can be made on the spiritual journey. Other depressing factors may be the awareness of personal imperfections or a sudden eruption of doubt. In such states "One feels as if the very ground were cut away from under one's feet and that one had nowhere to turn to for solace or encouragement. One comes sometimes even to think of giving up the yogic life and returning to the ordinary ways of worldly dreams. All this is a state of bleak forlornness and corroding gloom."[9]

He suggested that the remedy comes when one refuses to brood over the fall and recovers through making "contact with the psychic being and infusing it's fire and light into the physical mind. Once the rays of the soul penetrate and permeate the physical mind it will tend to lose its habitual tendency to doubt and depression and develop the capacity for sustained aspiration, devotion and self-offering. Step back from the physical mind, which is the home of doubt and dependency and try to take one's stand in the inner consciousness."[10]

Since this experience can shatter the entire base on which the ego stands -- all the previous beliefs, relationships, and psychic structures of life -- people should not be surprised or self-critical if they find they are caught in panic or despair . Aurobindo said "There can be no doubt that you can go through -- everyone has these struggles; what is needed to pass through is sincerity and perseverance."   He advised remaining in the higher part of consciousness, putting a pressure on the lower impulses to change. Once this becomes a habit "the progress is easier, smoother and less painful."[11]

Love --Variations on the Theme

In addition to radical mood swings, and the many negative emotions, love is another emotion which therapists might note that causes havoc for some people during Kundalini awakening. Goel cites an irrational love projection on the daughter of a friend, and one subject interviewed experienced a similar infatuation with her therapist. Heart openings produce intense loving energy, often projected on a teacher or guru, sometimes felt as an overwhelming wave of compassion for the entire world. Mystics will channel this passion toward a love of God or of nature. In addition, the newly-awakened energy may affect others, causing romantic projections.

Bailey wrote that of the problems of disciples, those arising from the awakened heart center are perhaps the most common and most difficult to handle.

In the early stages, this inflowing love-force establishes personality contacts which veer between the stages of wild devotion and utmost hate on the part of the person affected by the disciple's energy. This produces constant turmoil in the disciple's life, until he has become adjusted to the effects of his energy distribution, and also frequent disruption of relationships and frequent reconciliations.[12]

The problem is overcome when one learns to stand firm at the center, loving impersonally. The problems that spiritual leaders frequently have with individuals and groups Bailey attributes to this problem of the heart energy and its impact on others.

Several subjects were given teachings about love from inner guides in their process, and others experienced feeling unconditional love. This is a primary and fundamental aspect of God, according to most spiritual teachings, and learning to be with it in its purest state is part of the integration of the spiritual life. Unconditional love is not a familiar experience for most of us, and loving without a particular object is difficult to maintain, thus projections are engaged.

The personality just naturally wants someone special to give it to. Learning to love God as expressed in every aspect of the universe is one of the highest intentions of the spiritual practice, and one of the most difficult to attain. Richard Moss emphasizes the act of realizing unconditional love as the second step in transmuting and refining negative energies (the first step is the realization "that all experience is relative and the direct consequence of its underlaying energy dynamic.") He wrote:

> Love is the great transmuting force that can take any fixed energetic/existential pattern and allow it to resolve into harmony on a much greater scale. *Without unconditional love as the center from which to concentrate our Beingness, the ability to shift and transmute energies can become just another manipulation of our ego power.* It is critical to understand this.[13]

He acknowledges, however, that one cannot make unconditional love happen by thinking about it. In his personal process he engaged in what he called a "knock-down-drag-out fight" by sitting with his negative energy until it transmuted even if it took a week. He said "At first the state I was working to transmute would intensify and my being would seethe like a volcano, and then as I stayed with this I would become blank. Still I kept returning my awareness to the heart and waiting."[14]

He became convinced that if he drifted off to other thoughts or had a wonderful creative insight it was simply a displacement of awareness into acceptable territory and was not transmutation. So he would continue in this intense introspective state until he experienced a deep feeling state of well-being that emanated from his chest." Then I would reexamine the issue from this higher state to see the assumptions about reality that had allowed it to configurate in the first place. I found that in this expanded state I could marry divisive issues to each other and could appreciate the energy process inherent in their activation."

As he followed this practice it became more comfortable, even automatic, and seemed to go beyond emotional issues into what he calls issues "of the soul itself". He discovered that "the existential fear that at times would sweep through me early in the awakening process was in fact a miraculous sensation of embodiment to a higher level of my being. The even deeper patterns and reality frames began to transmute into a more and more unconditional and eternal sense of Self." [15]

What Moss developed in this process is much like a tantric practice of being completely with an emotion until it transforms into its elemental energy beyond form, and moving energy from lower chakras into the deepest level of the heart chakra, where unconditional love can transform it. Unconditional love is without judgement, values or design. It is more an intense presence, encompassing and blessing all that is, without boundary or parameter. It is the emotion or feeling component of the consciousness/energy of Kundalini. One cannot "do" it -- one can only become immersed within it.

The Struggle to Be

As we assess the emotional difficulties experienced by one dealing with Kundalini energy remember that most people react with stress and anxiety to change, and the changes engendered by this opening can profoundly and permanently alter the inner structure of a man or woman. One can easily become stuck in the middle, unable to go back to the old perspective and afraid to plunge forward into the new.

In addition, one may be confronted with what Aurobindo (sounding like C.G. Jung) termed the "shadow" or the "negative persona", a being attached to one, sometimes appearing like a part of oneself and sometimes a force in the environment, "which is just the contradiction of the thing he centrally represents in the work to be done."[16]   This energy "seems to oppose, create stumblings and wrong conditions, in a word, to set before him the whole problem of the work he has started to do." The Mother has stressed the same phenomenon, stating that with the possibility of a victory, one always carries inside the opposing elements:

> When you see a very black shadow somewhere, something that is truly painful, you may be sure that you have the possibility of the corresponding light. . . .Always you will find that within you the shadow and the light go together: you have a capacity, you have also the negation of that capacity.. . . It is up to you to know how to utilize the one to realize the other.[17]

Although the work to integrate these forces is essential, the potential for stepping aside from the emotions and turmoil engendered by this confrontation and mastering them as yogic teachers encourage, is supported conceptually by Jung. He said :

> People lose themselves entirely in their emotions and deplete themselves, and finally they are burnt to bits and nothing remains -- just a heap of ashes, that is all. The same thing occurs in lunacy: people get into a certain state and cannot get out of it; they burn up in their emotions and explode. There is a possibility of detaching oneself from an emotion, however, and when a man discovers this, he becomes man. In manipura he is in the womb of nature, extraordinarily automatic; it is merely a process. But in anahata a new thing comes up, the possibility of lifting himself above the emotional happenings and looking at them. He discovers the purusha in his heart. . . In the centre of anahata Siva again appears in the form of the linga, and the small flame means the first germ-like apparition of the Self. . . It is the withdrawal from the emotions; you are no longer identical with them. If you succeed in making a difference between yourself and that outburst of passion, you begin to discover the Self. In anahata individuation begins.[18]

Many of the emotional turmoils described in literature about Kundalini are echoed in Jung's comments about working with the deep unconscious. He saw regression becoming increasingly dangerous as advanced stages of psychological development are reached. "We are generally inclined to think that it is ideal and desirable to develop toward a higher condition, but we forget that it is dangerous, because the development usually means sacrifice, it costs blood. . . There are cases where the psychological development of an individual leads to his destruction, where he cannot stand the tension. That is why all the mystery cults, or Yoga teaching,warn their adepts to be careful; these things have to be surrounded by extraordinary precautions, one has to protect oneself. One has to follow the rules and fulfill all sorts of conditions to avoid falling into terrible danger."[19]

Yogic literature offers many rules for managing this process, although primarily it advises reliance on a guru. One of the oldest documents offering some advice on Kundalini management is the Jnaneshvari version of the <u>Bhagavadgita</u>, which recommends casting off egoism, practicing self-examination, and trusting the strength of the Self. In describing how one crosses over the "river of illusion" and enters into union, this scripture describes difficulties in doing this by one's own efforts. In order to acquire the self-control necessary one is advised to fix the mind in the innermost place of the heart, curing the tendency to run after external objects (which is only possible when the senses are restrained). With the mind silent in the heart and attention fixed, the life breath should be transmitted into the sacred syllable (Om) and brought up by the central path to the brow center, then held with firm resolution until the three elements of the sacred syllable are merged together in the crown center. The focus is on practices which create mastery and self-restraint, developing devotion to God, and attaining enlightenment. Devotion involves seeing all as the manifestation of God; respecting all as one; being humble and free of conceit.[20]

Yogi Alain Danielou has provided another list of practices designed to develop equanimity and mental purity. He recommends creating a pure place within, and establishing a pure direction. In his writings purity means control of the senses, absence of fear, contentment of mind, charity, ritual sacrifices, penance, simplicity, non-violence, truth, endurance, and forgiveness. He recommends abstaining from self-assertion, possessiveness, attachment, enmity, envy, greed, sensuality, anger, and agitation. One should also follow food restrictions, seek contentment, austerity, and self-development, and think constantly of divinity. [21]

The main obstacles that disturb the mind of a spiritual aspirant, according to Danielou, who quotes from the <u>Yoga Darshana</u>, are ill-health, irregular life, lack of success, lack of stability, laziness, material difficulties, lack of convictions, wrong ideas or wrong knowledge. The five secondary obstacles are physical pain, melancholy, unsteady limbs, and irregular in and out breathing. Other problems include unregulated eating and sleeping, breaking the rules of chastity, having an imposter as a guide, disregarding the true guide, atheism, desire for physical attainments, belief that attainments mean realization, having rituals performed by others, and pretension to being oneself a guide. In contrast to yogic methods of controlling emotional states, it is interesting to note that in recent years alternative therapies dealing with deep emotional traumas encourage complete catharsis and emotional expression. Gestalt practices, bodywork, and breathwork are among these approaches. Stan and Christina Grof, who have pursued an in-depth study of spiritual crisis and Kundalini, utilize in Holotropic Therapy hyperventilation and the use of evocative music to change consciousness through intense and dramatic release of emotion. They define the main principle of their work as "to encourage the experiencer to surrender fully to the emerging emotions, sensations, and physical energy, and find appropriate ways of expressing them through sounds, grimaces, postures, and movements, without judging or analyzing the experience...This work continues until the experiencer reaches a state of resolution and relaxation." [22]

It is difficult to reconcile these opposite approaches of emotional mastery and cathartic release in dealing with emotions, both offered as activities to assist spiritual awakening, unless one looks at the psyche as having the possibility of releasing completely and moving beyond the trauma of previously lived emotional pain and blocks. There is a critical difference between being lost in an emotional trauma for weeks or months, and being focused on it in a therapeutic setting for a few hours. In Holotropic Therapy, breathing practices are in some ways akin to tantric practices that use the senses to take one beyond ordinary limitations.

In a meditation practice, when confronted with a painful memory, one is generally advised to observe it and hold back emotional surrender to it, although in practice uncontrollable weeping or anger may erupt, despite the best intentions of the subject. Letting it move on is the primary objective, avoiding the tendency to get caught in the drama.

In Holotropic Breathwork one releases fully to the expression, but with the intention of allowing it to move on, releasing oneself from the conditioned patterns that have previously limited or influenced the personality. The therapist is advised not to interfere in any way. As these experiences are transcended, new potentials for higher states of consciousness emerge. It is possible to leap beyond the personality during these altered-state processes, and see the entire experience from an expanded perspective. The Grof's emphasize the importance of distinguishing between the two entities of body-ego and Self, when engaging in transpersonal processes; otherwise the result can be ego-inflation or psychopathology. They also recommend using cathartic practices in a group setting, and if people are in a state of crisis, providing an environment free of stress.

Whether choosing to use Holotropic therapy or mastery of detachment as an approach for emotional healing the factors to consider are personality style, disposition, health, ego structure, emotional stability, and available support systems.

Chanting as Emotional Release

Chanting (swadhyaya) and repeating the names of God (japa, or mantra) are also emphasized in some yogic scriptures. According to Ron Jones, psychologist and Siddha yoga teacher, chanting was the main practice recommended to followers by Muktananda because "It brings up joy, it focuses the mind and it organizes the psyche by tuning up all the chakras. It is a more active way of participating with the opening, and automatically introduces a form of pranayama."[23]

Muktananda said chanting focuses the mind on God, and makes one intoxicated all day, raising a seeker to a state beyond the mind. It makes the mind one-pointed and can also induce samadhi. Chanting draws one toward understanding of the inner self, increases inner radiance, mental vigor and agility, nourishes the inner being, imparts spiritual strength and purifies the mind and heart. He states "If you meditate and neglect chanting, then your heart will remain as dry as wood." [24]

None of the case subjects emphasized chanting or mantra recitation specifically as factors in their process, but TM meditation, which was an introduction to meditation for many of them, is based on mantra repetition and others practiced yoga which sometimes included chanting experiences. Several subjects remarked on the importance of sound and inner tones in their process. Experimental studies on the outcome of chanting with people having difficulties with Kundalini might provide some interesting material for research.

Therapy with the self & the Self

C. G. Jung recognized the need in many Westerners for a personal spirituality, a genuine experience of the numinous, writing that the Western tendency to project all religious experience outside of oneself may rob the soul of it's values, making it incapable of further development and causing a person to get stuck in an unconscious state. He believed that as long as religion is only faith and outward form, and religious function is not experienced in the soul, nothing of importance can happen, and he said "the mysterium magnum is first and foremost rooted in the human psyche...It is high time we realized that it is pointless to praise the light and preach it if nobody can see it."[25]

Since much of Jung's work with the deep unconscious offers insight into the natural tendency of the psyche toward a spiritual perspective, it suggests potential applications for working with the Kundalini process. Jung mentions yoga and Kundalini energy frequently in The Collected Works, referring to images associated with Kundalini appearing in the dreams and art of patients.

Speaking of how Kundalini is awakened during a lecture in 1932, Jung said it is an instigation from above which arouses her, and one must have a purified spirit in order to do so. He stated that in psychological terms, that would mean that you can approach the unconscious only in one way, namely, by a purified mind, by the right attitude, and by the grace of heaven. An inner urge must lead one to it, a guiding spark that forces one on.

> And that spark is the Kundalini, something absolutely unrecognizable, which may show perhaps as fear, as a neurosis, or apparently also a vivid interest, but it must be something which is superior to your will. Otherwise you don't go through with it; you turn back at the first obstacle, as soon as you see the leviathan you run away. But if that living spark, that urge, that need, gets you by the neck, you cannot turn back, you have to face the music.[26]

Neurosis, fear and interest are definitively NOT Kundalini, although as pointed out earlier it is not uncommon to experience them as part of the awakening process. But in many ways Jung captures the crux of the experience -- the power and inevitability of being seized by an urge greater than oneself.

Jung also felt at the time that Westerners take a route to the unconscious that is the opposite to that taken by Easterners, the Western process bringing us down into the unconscious, while the chakra system posits the movement as rising upward. His efforts to describe and define this difference, his view that the superconsciousness of yoga and the unconscious of analysis were the same, and his tendency to put aside the Hindu world view in his efforts at interpretation make his theoretical work of limited value.

Nonetheless Jungian approaches to the psyche can help a client to respect and integrate this process. Images, symbols, themes and dreams of the individuation process are strikingly similar to those of the Kundalini process. Jung spoke of the relationship between analysis and religion in terms which could well define the confrontation with Kundalini, calling it "an extended conflict in which the man as analyst and the religious man confront one another and search each other's depths. This confrontation becomes an enterprise which shuttles back and forth adjusting, recommencing; a proceeding which digs even deeper only to undo at each stage the composure we should love to achieve by saying, yes, this time, the delusion is it."[27]

Jung also expressed a grave concern over the possibility of the psyche becoming lost in the unconscious, and said it is a "psychic catastrophe when the ego is assimilated by the Self." He said "The image of wholeness then remains in the unconscious, so that on the one hand it shares the archaic nature of the unconscious and on the other finds itself in the psychically relative space-time continuum that is characteristic of the unconscious as such." It is vital that the ego exist in absolute space and time or else its adaptation can become disturbed and "the way (is opened) for all sorts of possible accidents."[28]

If the Self assimilates the ego, one has merged into infinite chaos with no place to come home to. Conversely, if the ego assimilates the Self, inflation runs rampant, for the human has usurped the gods. The challenge is to create bridges between the two planes, so that the values of the deeper Self can be integrated into the patterns lived out by the ego self. Jung believed that "the more numerous and the more significant the unconscious contents which are assimilated to the ego, the closer the approximation of the ego to the Self, even though this approximation must be a never-ending process."[29] It is clear he perceived this as a profoundly spiritual undertaking.

According to analyst Jolande Jacobi the term individuation process defines the possibility of development of a psychically whole individual, incorporating both conscious and unconscious components of the psyche in balanced and creative interaction. She defined the foremost task of this process as "to raise the God-images, that is their radiations and effects, to consciousness and thus establish a constant dynamic contact between the ego and the Self. This alliance bridges over the tendencies to personality dissociation which arise from the instincts pulling in opposite directions."[30]

Her view of the individuation process offers insight into spiritual transformation as well:

> . . .the discovery of a new life-form which goes hand in hand with the successful conduct of life as a whole depends on the degree to which a person is gripped by this transformation, adopts a positive attitude towards it, and is able to accomplish it. Very often the capacity for such a transformation does not depend on the objective bigness or smallness of the personality, but on the extension or "reconstruction" of its psychic "dimension". It is a situation of moving from an "ego-centered" attitude to an "ego-transcending" one, in which the guiding principles of life are directed to something objective. . . .The individuation process in the Jungian sense means the conscious realization and integration of all the possibilities congenitally present in the individual. It is opposed to any kind of conformity and, as a therapeutic factor in analytical work, also demands the rejection of those prefabricated psychic matrices in which most people would like to live.[31]

Like individuation, Kundalini follows a unique and individual pattern, and refuses the acceptance of conformity. The Kundalini process is unlike individuation for the yogi however, in the sense that the yogi attempts to surrender his or her entire being into the infinite, merging with the supraconscious. This is a task Jung did not recognize as healthy for the psyche. His work aims at keeping the ever-present dialogue going between Self and ego, integrating and working effectively with each side of consciousness.

The risks of identification with the numinous are great for the average person. One of the most difficult aspects for the Westerner in this process is that of going as deeply as the heart wills into the numinous, and still maintaining the balance to live among the demands and stresses of modern society. Ultimately, when the transformation is completed, it may be possible to live more fully from a deeper state of consciousness. But to reach that state of purity can take decades, and lifetimes, and in the meanwhile whoever is engaged in this experiment can benefit from the insights of analytical psychology in learning to balance the demands of two opposing psychic elements.

Jacobi further distinguishes the individuation process from ideas characteristic of spiritual systems, by saying individuation has in no sense a "moral" goal in the accepted meaning of the word. "It does not aim at perfectionism, but only at helping a man to become in the truest sense what he in fact is, and not to hide behind the ideal mask which is so easily mistaken for his true essence, although by so doing, he makes it all the more likely that the evil repressed behind it will break out." [32]

Jung's psychology focused primarily on the tasks of the second half of life, the time when the ego comes to terms with death, finds completion for the meaning of the individual life, and brings from the deep unconscious the material to complete wholeness. It may be especially appropriate therefore to use the techniques and processes of Jungian work with people in a Kundalini crisis, because they are also dealing with the struggle to face the death of parts of the ego and paradoxically expand their sense of wholeness. The capacity to witness, to work on symbolic content and to find a way to live that is in harmony with deep spiritual processes are all analogous to Jungian analysis.

A significant experience to one caught in a crisis of either individuation or Kundalini awakening is the battle of opposites -- forces arising from the unconscious that seem in direct conflict with the position of the ego. Yoga has attempted to address these "temptations" through strict discipline and order prescribed as preliminary practices before awakening Kundalini. Jungian psychology addresses these conflicts more directly as they appear in the process; when consciousness and the messages of the unconscious are in opposition, and no reconciliation seems possible the analysand is encouraged to persevere until a tolerable solution occurs, and a third possibility emerges that does justice to both sides.[33] Jung commented in a lecture series on the interpretation of visions that one can only withstand the onslaught of the opposites "by not being volatile in any way; you have to be heavy, like stone, to stand the movement that begins when you are their victim." [34]

Jung also demonstrated that right-brain processes such as art, sculpture, dreamwork, and writing poetry or journals were keys to holding one's center when assaulted by the emerging unconscious material. These practices encourage the emergence of a symbol that contains the possibility of transformation, amplify the capacity to witness one's own process and objectify some of the elements of it, allow a more free flow of material that might otherwise stay blocked, and may even develop new neural pathways in the brain. The flood of creative activity sometimes associated with Kundalini may be as much a spontaneous and unconscious survival and growth mechanism as a grand flowering of genius.

The Knots & the Selves

Jung's model of individuation presents a concept of self that is broad enough to include the entire spectrum of collective experiences. It promotes encounter with spirit and acknowledgement of the numinous aspects of human existence. But if we move on to the nature of the Kundalini experience, we must consider the Eastern idea that self is established in the mind-body complex only until Self-realization occurs,which then establishes it as consciousness, bliss and union with cosmic consciousness. One who is thus aware knows that Self abides in all beings and all beings in oneself.

Clearly we are now moving from identification with personal self to identification with collective Self, a situation Jung warns against. Perhaps this is the crux of the psychological dynamics of Kundalini awakening. The pain and upheavals of Kundalini awakening are similar to those of individuation, where the former persona and false selves are abdicating their role in favor of the unification of personality around the deeper self. A similar process occurs during the Kundalini experience, accompanied by an intense disruption of energy and a movement of the psyche to reject identification with the very body, mind and emotions we have previously claimed as our own. The wholeness of our self is disintegrating in order to allow us to experience Wholeness -- the primal and eternal wholeness of the universal Self. Now we are grappling with an awareness that claims our very existence is only a play of energies contracted within an illusionary space and time.

As indicated earlier, yogic literature refers to three granthis or knots in the subtle body system, which link physical, subtle and causal bodies and carry especially intense charges of energy. These are identified as the knot of Brahma, the knot of Vishnu, and the knot of Rudra or Shiva. usually associated with muladhara, anahata and ajna chakras, respectively. Tantric gurus warn that if psychic energy is forced through these knots before a practitioner is adequately prepared, physical and nervous system disorders will erupt. Psychic blockages called lingas are associated with each knot. Ajit Mookerjee wrote: "To clear the Brahma knot is to get established in totality; to clear the Vishnu knot, to perceive the existence of a universal life-principle; to clear the Rudra knot, to attain the non-dual state, realization of oneness, the universal joy."[35]   The breaking of these three knots are major steps achieved in detaching the mind from illusionary existence and making Self-realization possible.

These three stages appear to correspond to stages of change in consciousness. It is possible that the psychic center of an individual who has not opened the Brahma knot corresponds to what psychologists identify as the "false self" or the unreal self. It is locked into survival, sexual and power drives -- preoccupied with appearances, superficial accomplishments, immediate pleasures or pains, defensive positions and other lower chakra energies. People with narcissistic or borderline personality disorders often model this level of psychological functioning, which is transformed when they unveil and activate the real self. It then becomes possible for them to live authentically and creatively, using latent potentials, and engaging in genuine relationship. (In fact, most people can slip back and forth between these two kinds of self-identifications at any moment, depending on the pressures they are dealing with.)

The psychic center after the Brahma knot is pierced might then correspond to what psychotherapists identify as the" real" self, the authentic or the actualized self. Those who are centered and directed from a sense of their "real" self live with congruence and well-being. They have self-awareness, flexibility, and creativity in solving problems.   They are fully engaging energies of the subtle body, which carry the mental, emotional and sensate activities of the individual. As these energies come into balance throughout the chakras people become "individuated", which would imply that in addition to functioning well in the world, there are glimpses of the higher Self. Symbolic material may emerge through which they become aware of a greater reality or universal truths. Psychologies of the self link inevitably to the integration of subtle-body material for this is the substance of our psychic life which must be activated for our personal wholeness to occur. The gross body is only the container for the life; the subtle body animates and energizes it with memories, emotions, thoughts, patterns, and possibilities. Piercing the knot of Brahma brings us into our full potential as human beings, establishing us in our totality.

If the Vishnu knot is pierced, the psyche becomes attuned to the principles of existence and begins to deal with the Self as it is known in yoga. This Self has access to the psychic, visual and archetypal worlds and yet transcends them. The Kundalini experience, fully lived through, includes the process of integrating causal body awareness, of recognizing existence beyond the personalized patterns of subtle body. This is comparable to living in the Tao in the Chinese tradition, not the ego living there but clear presence being there. This transition is almost too much for the personality to bear, implying as it does a giving up of all justification for the existence of the real self, the right to be "me", an individual or unique being, in control of my environment. To identify with this deeper or primary "Self" is to release the delusion of control and surrender to a higher stream of energy and consciousness which guides and motivates ones life.

When this kind of awareness emerges pressures are forced on consciousness to complete the task of individuating or transcending the subtle body samskaras still incompleted. Those who are prepared to move on into higher levels of causal experience will live no longer from an individual sense but from a sense of universal consciousness, an acting out for the good of others whatever collective needs are felt in the unique connection an individual has through the deeper Self. Thus people like Aurobindo, Ramakrishna, Yogananda, Krishnamurti, Anandamayi Ma and others who are enlightened are moved to act, as if by a force outside of themselves, to create a movement in universal consciousness, such as all great spiritual masters have done. This is a non-dual state called Rudra.

Clearly Jesus was not acting out of his experience of individuation, but from a much more profound place of awareness. The problem for the ego in following such a model is that such an action can never be chosen, or led by the ego. If it is attempted it will always be distorted. Therefore just because someone tries to model their lives after a spiritual leader or saint does not mean they have achieved non-dualism, and in fact such modeling often leads to delusion and inflation. It is only a lengthy process of awakening and transformation of one's personal self that allows such developments, all in its own timing. The majority of those who awaken Kundalini are not going to engage this process and transcend the ego at the level required to make a complete transition to this kind of consciousness. That would undoubtedly be the piercing of the third granthi or knot. But I suspect it is sometimes the energies pulling them in this direction that cause such psychic havoc.

Therapists can deal with incompletions in individuation and help clients to find bridges between aspects of the causal world with its powerful psychic, visionary and numinous contents and the ordinary reality in which we all must live. People who have broken this third granthi or knot and live with a deeper knowledge as the center of their psyche would have no interest in or need of therapy.

If we look at the development of consciousness through this three-tiered pattern of the granthis or knots, we can hypothesize that people with psychotic or personality disorders who have religious delusions have come in contact somehow (possibly because of very weak ego boundaries or natural psychic potentials) with this third level, the causal body, and may be charged with its considerable energy and vision. This becomes distorted and dangerous because there is no real self to moderate self-discipline, goal-setting, relatedness, creative activity -- all the tasks which the real self must do to establish a successful integration of subtle body energies in the world. This stage of development simply must occur in some way. Otherwise it is akin to a primitive consciousness being charged with power it cannot distribute or modulate, and becoming identified with universal forces beyond any capacity to digest them.

Perhaps to a degree some of those who reported intense spiritual openings on LSD experienced a similar process. Those who had neither context not spiritual practice to hold the ego in check, and little individuation to sustain such processes, could only become infatuated with the drug itself, follow it as if it were a Messiah, and plunge into experiences over and over again which had no hope of assimilation. Often their lives and their goals changed because their perspective was altered, but they had no hope of becoming enlightened on the drug.

I do not believe Kundalini awakening causes psychosis, but it presents material from the collective and the numinous world so intensely that a stable psychic structure is needed to hold it (a fact which is also true of the LSD experience). Almost all of the work of psychotherapists with Kundalini clients is to help them achieve such a structure, while accepting and supporting the new awareness that has emerged. A larger psychic container is needed. Tools that are useful to this end are found in psychologies that recognize the unifying capacities of the personal self and the transcendent energies of the deeper Self, such as Jungian analysis and Psychosynthesis. Yogic or tantric perspectives are supportive because they provide a cosmological perspective wide enough to encompass the multi-dimensional realities of the Self.

Visions & Voices

Numerous visions and images may accompany the Kundalini process, many of which were described in an earlier chapter of this book. None of them are indicative of psychosis. Yogis and tantric Buddhists utilize these images extensively, and a considerable yogic and tantric iconography has developed around the various chakras, including the symbols of the elements, the gods and goddesses, and the frightening images of demons and destruction that appear during meditative states. In tantra these are real forces and powers which the psyche must encounter and integrate as part of the spiritual path.

Some of the images common in yoga and in the art and dreams of subjects in the Kundalini process have been interpreted by Jung in relationship to the individuation process. They are links with the collective unconscious, often reflecting archetypes. These correlations do not mean that individuation and Kundalini awakening are identical experiences, only that the psychic reaction to intensive change is accompanied by similar images of dying and rebirth.

In early stages of spiritual awakening visions or symbolic images might be considered figments of imagination, or representations of the changes one is undergoing psychically. In later stages, however, much of the biographical material suggests that one may actually be encountering guidance or learning lessons from masters on another plane of consciousness.

Giving medication to control such visions may be either useless or dangerous. Providing a loving, supportive atmosphere where the images can be safely shared allows more integration, and eventually this stage of the process will end, for the ultimate religious experience is not about visions, but is beyond form. Visions are frequently produced, however, as a link between ordinary reality and supraordinary consciousness. Whether the mind is projecting them, or entities from other dimensions providing them, one is best advised to pay attention but avoid attachment; simply observe and release the experience.

Visions may also show clearly the energies emerging as a particular chakra awakens and provide insight into the physical, emotional or psychic events that accompany this movement. It is possible that physical symptoms, imagery and emotional difficulties coalesce around particular chakras as each encounters the powers of the Kundalini energy, and that looking at the material provided by the unconscious through vision could help one to integrate and understand more clearly what is happening. This is a very unexamined concept, since the intellect is not generally used in the yogic tradition to analyze the numinous content of spiritual experiences. But when one is trying to integrate Western conditioning and mentality with Eastern experience, these bridges may be reassuring and lead ultimately to some understanding of the interrelationship between psyche and spiritual experience.

On the other hand the evidence of my subjects suggests that if visions do occur this stage passes quickly, and one may be best advised to simply observe and let it pass, rather than psychoanalyze it. Aurobindo advised against talking about experiences, saying that sharing weakened them and brought down the consciousness; but it seems from the case histories in the literature that having at least one understanding confidant is nurturing to this process. Muktananda was not in favor of concealing spiritual experiences, and encouraged setting up sharing sessions for Westerners in his ashram. He believed this guided and encouraged students and heightened their experiences.

The psychotherapist who is seeking a way to integrate the visual experiences of a Kundalini client can draw on Jungian and yogic resources for interpretation, including the Tibetan Book of the Dead, a classical description of the imagery that accompanies death and rebirth. There seems to be a dramatic variation among individuals in the production of such phenomena and the usefulness of it in the spiritual process. Visions are much less significant in earlier stages of spiritual development, and are reported by some yogis to be a hindrance and distraction on the path, yet they had profound impact in later stages for Caitanya who became lost in his visions of Krishna, for Kennett Roshi who assimilated her third kensho through visionary experiences, for Muktananda, Da Free John, Krishnamurti, and most of the other subjects of this book. The proper relationship to such profound visions is to bear a humble witnessing to them rather than to psychoanalyze them. The mind can do nothing to improve on the experience of the numinous, and unfortunately tends to reduce it.

However, analytical psychology repeatedly demonstrates the value to the psyche of the transforming symbol. Jung wrote that this symbol helps to heal the neurosis which is at the root of the dissociation of the personality. He said "the consciousness goes to the right and the unconscious to the left. As opposites never unite at their own level. . . a subordinate "third" is always required in which the two parts can come together, and since the symbol derives as much from the conscious as the unconscious, it is able to unite them

both, reconciling their conceptional polarity through its numinosity"[36]
This comment echoes the yogic image of ida, pingala and sushumna nadis, experienced as a vivid visual image in B. S. Goel's case. The blue pearl described by Muktananda may initiate a similar resolution of opposites, as did the vision of purusha and prakriti in Chris's case. There was not a significant use of symbolic imagery in the majority of cases I studied; however, reactivating a spontaneous numinous image and bringing it into consciousness deliberately could be useful in this process, helping people to achieve integration, in ways similar to the individuation process.

Hearing voices, or being aware of a guiding presence and receiving information from it, are also experiences commonly reported in the stories. Usually the voice contains a simple message such as "call to commitment", or "peace be with you," or offers specific instructions. Sometimes it directs people to write autobiographies or explore certain aspects of their lives. The voices of the Kundalini process are soothing, directive, and healing and these distinguish them significantly from the haunting voices of disassociative psychic elements that disturb psychotic people. The sounds and music heard in this process are also indicative of deep, profound connections with supraconscious vibrations, as discussed in some detail in an earlier chapter. The most useful approach to such opportunities is to witness them and receive them used as guidance for personal life, without inflation or assumptions regarding their truth for everyone else.

By respecting the inner voice one can learn to tune in to a deep inner awareness, a sense of the Self with its wise perspective regarding ones life and actions, which is reassuring and psychologically strengthening throughout this process. This voice becomes the center of trust and foundation for one's life. It will never impose the shoulds and sanctions of society, nor encourage any destructive impulses, and should these occur they indicate the emerging of a sub-personality, a yet unredeemed psychic fragment that must be dealt with. Psychotherapists can help the Kundalini client acknowledge the true voice of the Self, and turn to it like a beacon in the night.

Remembering & Reliving Past Lives

Several of the stories of Kundalini awakening included a unique kind of visionary process, the spontaneous remembering of a past life. This also happens to people who are not engaged in spiritual processes, as evidenced by many volumes written on the subject, and memories can easily be induced through hypnosis and other relaxation techniques. Sometimes the remembering of a past life provides a fresh perspective on ingrained personality patterns, explains difficulties and allows completions that need to occur in the psyche or personal life, or sets the tone for a new movement.

Although some people believe in past lives as a literal, sequential occurrence, we might hypothesize also that they come to us allegorically, or genetically, or from the collective unconscious so that we have access to a past experience or archetypal pattern lived through by someone else that is activated to assist us at a particular time, as in the case of a dream. Past lives feel more real subjectively however, than dreams or mere images, for it is possible to experience the emotions and body sensations as if one were reliving certain events, even if one has never had such experiences in the present life.

Kennett Roshi recommends a highly structured process for assisting people in cleansing the karmic residue from past lives, under the guidance of a priest and with the assistance of loving friends who use mudras. The first hours in the enlightenment of Buddha reportedly involved the remembering of past lives, showing him the cause of suffering in attachments, enabling him to see the truth of impermanence and suffering and the reasons for his own birth, old age, disease and death. Although understanding past lives is not a prerequisite for enlightenment, it is "the natural way in which the Buddhas teach the trainee the cause of suffering and how to avoid the clouding of his realization which would result from repeating the same mistakes that started the chain of suffering long ago."[37] Karmic memories also tend to deepen compassion and empathy.

In addition to hearing of these stories from those in Kundalini processes, I have seen them emerge frequently during breathwork sessions and acupressure treatments. They are easily elicited through deep altered-state experiences. Kennett believes the most remote of past-life memories often show the cause of suffering in its most powerful and subtle forms, and indicate an attachment one is likely to repeat in this life unless one pursues meditation and other spiritual training. Memories of past lives can come forth to help one convert tendencies of the present life, especially if more than one past life is remembered within several months.

Bhai Sahib, Irina Tweedie's guru, also referred to past-life memories in his advice to her, saying that fearful images she experienced were relieving past-life karma, and that horrible dreams sometimes act out the karma of past lives so that a subject will not have to do so consciously.

I have personally found past-life regression to be a way of deepening my understanding of my own spiritual process and experiences, especially recalling of spiritually-oriented past lives and one in which Kundalini energy was active. These regressions provided insight into my personal process and gave me an inner sense of where my psyche is going in its spiritual work in this life. I found that I could access a state of consciousness I had not yet known in this life, which provided an imprint or a "felt sense" of myself to be drawn on when needed. This can be a useful support as one begins to integrate the awakening process, let go of old identifications, and look toward a new future with a changed world perspective.

References: Chapter 8

1   Da Free John (1979) Compulsory dancing, Clearlake, CA.: The Dawn Horse Press. p. 91.

2   Op. cit., pp. 20-21.

3   Anonymous, "The Dawn Horse" (1986 Nov/Dec), p. 6.

4   Satprem (1970) Sri Aurobindo or The Adventure of Consciousness. Pondicherry: Sri Aurobindo Ashram Trust.

5   Da Free John, Op. cit. p. 5.

6   Goel, B.S. (1985) Third Eye and Kundalini, India: Third Eye Fd. p. 145.

7   Aurobindo, S. (1971) Letters on Yoga, 4 parts, Pondicherry: Sri Aurobindo Ashram, p. 1670.

8   Bailey, A. (1953) Esoteric Healing, New York: Lucis, p. 127.

9   Aurobindo, S. (1950) Letters of Aurobindo, first series, Bombay: Sri Aurobindo Ashram, p. 79.

10 Op. cit.

11 Aurobindo (1971) Op. cit., p. 1679.

12 Bailey, A., Op. cit., p. 123.

13 Moss, R. (1981) The I that is we. Berkeley: Celestial Arts, p. 25.

14 Op. cit.

15 Op. cit., p. 26.

16 Satprem, Op. cit., p. 250.

17 Op. cit., p. 251.

18 Jung, C. G. (1975) Psychological Commentary on Kundalini Yoga -
   lectures one and two --1932. Spring. New York: Spring Pub.
   p. 30.

19 Op. cit. p. 30.

20 Pradhan, V. G.(1969) Jnaneshwari: A song-sermon on the Bhag-
   avadgita,Vols. 1-2. London: Blackie & Son,pp. 183--201.

21 Danielou, A. (1955) Yoga: The Method of Re-Integration, p. 22.

22 Grof, S. and Grof, C. (1986). "Spiritual Emergency: the Undertand-
   ing and Treatment of Transpersonal Crisis", ReVision 8, 7-31,
   p. 17.

23 Jones, R. (personal communication, Dec. 6, 1987).

24 Muktananda, S. (1978) Understanding siddha yoga, pp. 101 -- 104.

25 Jung, C. G. (1968) Op. cit., p. 12.

26 Jung, C. G. (1975) Psychological Commentary on Kundalini Yoga -
   lectures one and two --1932. Spring. New York: Spring Pub.
   p. 13.

27 Jung, C. G. (1976) The Symbolic Life: Miscellaneous Writings
   (R.F.C. Hull, Trans.) Collected Works. Vol.18, New York:
   Princeton University, p. 126.

28 Jung. C. G. (1959) Aion (R.F.C. Hull, Trans.) Collected Works.
   Vol. 9 New York: Princeton, University, p. 24.

29 Op. cit., p. 23.

30 Jacobi, J. (1967) The Way of Individuation. London: Hodder &
   Stoughton, p. 53.

31 Op. cit., p. 83.

32 Op. cit., p. 118.

33 Jacobi, J. Op. cit., p. 20.

34 Jung, C. G. (1968) The Interpretation of Visions: Excerpts from the
   Notes of Mary Foote, Spring. New York: Spring Pub., p.100.

35 Mookerjee, A. (1983) Kundalini: The arousal of the inner energy.
   New York: Destiny, p. 53.

36 Jung. C. G. (1959) Op. cit., p. 180.

37 Kennett, J. (1979) The Book of Life. Mt. Shasta, CA.: Shasta
   Abbey, p. 96.

AFTER AWAKENING: OXHERDING IN THE WEST 293

CHAPTER NINE

AFTER AWAKENING: OX-HERDING IN THE WEST

This book is a tapestry woven from the threads of many teachings, reflecting the dramas and the deepest insights of lives spent in meditation and surrendering to the possibility of numinous experience. I have attempted to include the flavor of the whole of it, as nearly as I could discover during six years of research. Yet this is only a foundation, and a sparse one at that, for the mystery of Kundalini bridges science and mysticism, ancient history and modern experiences, bringing up questions about what is human and what is divine. We are using the limited constructs of the left-brain to place interpretations on realms it is incapable of knowing. I recognize that this left-brain dimension of my mind would like to be reductionistic and provide simple answers to clarify the mystery and uncertainty in this process. The right-brained part of me would paradoxically design a grand monument and have everyone grasp intuitively what cannot be said in language alone.

One question I have pondered often in this process is "What is the difference, if any, between great saints such as Ramakrishna or Yogananda and those who have more modest spiritual paths such as the subjects of this book?" Is it presumptuous to lump the experiences of therapists and nurses, housewives and businessmen, students and physicians, with those of people who achieved significant status as models of enlightenment and peace?

And some sages have suggested that inexplicable dark and disturbing conditions of the psyche such as mental illness or the charismatic and evil power of people like Hitler can be attributed to the eruption of Kundalini in distorted and disproportionate ways. I disagree with this perspective. Although the chaos of an awakening in a disturbed mind would certainly put the psyche under extreme pressure I find it impossible to believe that anyone who lives in the process for a considerable length of time will not ultimately experience some ecstasy, and a deeper compassion for humanity. Hitler was clearly insane, and carried as well the archetypal energy that was repressed in the shadow of the time and place in which he came to power. Powerful forces can be constellated in the psyche that have nothing to do with Kundalini awakening.

Gopi Krishna attributed the capacity of thought to the psychic energy supplied by nerves which flow to the brain. He believed that once Kundalini is awakened metabolic body processes are accelerated and the entire nervous system produces a radiation that pours into the brain causing it to evolve like "an embryo in the womb". Ultimately this transforms consciousness and a "superior type of mind is born". Such development can only occur through Kundalini awakening, according to Krishna. In fact, he called Kundalini the energy responsible for all remarkable and inexplicable phenomena that has ever been noted in human experience ranging from insanity to psychic and artistic gifts to genius.

The equation of Kundalini and genius raises pressing questions for those who study this phenomena. Can genius be "created" by encouraging spiritual practices? Have all who demonstrated genius experienced Kundalini? Do such questions promote elitism and cause unhealthy ego tendencies?   Krishna felt the future of the planet depended on the ability of science to understand this fundamental energy and to apply it in ways that would stimulate expanded consciousness, creativity and genius which could be applied to solving social and ecological problems. This indeed may be the evolutionary direction of this process, but in terms of the ego a certain risk is imposed when great accomplishments are seen as the consequence of spiritual awareness. Such striving can perpetuate the dualistic intellectual divisions so frequently encouraged by the rationalistic mind. It makes of spiritual awakening an achievement, an ambition and a grave responsibility. There are advantages to this viewpoint as it may attract persons with strong will and intentionality to the spiritual quest, but I have observed that when striving for perfection, accomplishment and superiority the egoic mind can be greatly inhibited in achieving spiritual progress: traditionally seekers are expected to develop modesty, humility and egoic surrender. Many enlightened saints reached their goal through devotion and intense love of the divine and withdrew their minds from worldly achievements.

I prefer to view Kundalini awakening not as an accomplishment but as an opening, a development of spirit, mind and body, which deepens one's understanding and appreciation of the wonders of existence, and leads the psyche toward peaceful coexistence with the natural cycles of living and dying. I expect it creates an expansion of right-brained development, initiating new pathways and patterns through which emerge enhanced creativity, vision, spontaneity and intuitive awareness. It also allows consciousness to tap more fully into subtle and causal body realms and beyond. Its' ultimate climax pushes consciousness into cosmic awareness and stabilized bliss. Such openings have evidently always existed and have always been possible in humans, at least through recorded history. All that is needed essentially is to be more respectful of them, to encourage this growth concurrently with left-brained accomplishments, so that a greater wholeness can be achieved by individuals.

We have become so spiritually bereft as a culture that we rely on soap-opera ministers with billion-dollar empires to lecture us on morality, we no longer expect to find genuine spirituality in the pulpit nor in religious institutions, and we are quick to discredit and discourage any overt evidence of a spiritual calling among our friends and associates. Culturally there is a need to reframe our concept of what it means to be a spiritual person, accepting it as a natural response, a calling in our deeper selves, which pulls us into a harmonious relationship with our deepest potential and with the larger community of the planet. At the same time, spiritual experiences bring us into direct contact with dimensions of consciousness beyond linear thinking and limited belief systems, expanding understanding beyond those parameters of dogma, ritual and fear-inducing theories that have crippled the capacity of modern religion to touch the soul.

A genuine spiritual encounter has the potential to shatter the foundations of ego boundaries from within, and plunge us into a vast perspective -- for some, a magnificent and joyous event. It helps us recognize our contraction and separation. It causes us to know one another's pain, and that it is for us that others hurt. Jesus is not the only one who carried pain in the world. Every victim, every criminal, every being who suffers is carrying a piece of a joint enterprise. What they are willing to carry is something others do not have to carry. Whatever we carry is for them as well as ourselves. We sense our collective process guided by the flow of a limitless universe when we slip out of the ego perspective and experience universal creative energy. We release "I" and discover the "not-I" that contains us.

Such glimpses, while they change our perspective profoundly, do not generally make us knowledgeable of everything and able to read everyone's mind, nor do they cure personality problems nor obliterate the necessity for thoughtfulness and will. These are delusions and projections the ego makes on those who are spiritually awake. Awakening nurtures the capacity for love in some, but seems to contain others in a cocoon of detached peaccfulness. It seems to pass over many lives, leaving a mark in the way a spring rain nourishes the crops and clears the air. In others it is a maelstrom bringing major life changes, and dangerous physical and emotional confrontations. Not everyone who experiences Her energy and power will become a Krishnamurti, or a crazy wisdom teacher the likes of Da Free John or a God-intoxicated saint like Ramakrishna.

As in every other aspect of life, each of us brings a different character, personality, and potential into every moment of experience and each responds in unique ways. Most of those who awaken this connection with the ecstatic inner Self will return to being who they were, perhaps doing their lives with more contentment or a gentler perspective, perhaps more involved and committed in service to others, perhaps more energized and expressive, perhaps writing poetry, teaching, loving unconditionally. Hopefully, some will eventually eradicate ego tendencies, live more consistently in higher states of awareness and expand their minds to the extent they can make significant contributions to society.

Archetypes of the Spiritual Life

Hindu models of enlightenment have traditionally reflected two archetypal responses, both of them masculine in their single-pointedness. One is the guru, the other the hermit. Both are beyond all the attachments of life, the first being essential to other souls as a teacher, the other enjoying the play of forces without needing to use personality in daily life. A few have demonstrated a life of bhakti, devotion to the divine which inspires others to faith and practice. Christian saints have traditionally been social activists, although there are many hermits and bhakti's in the tradition. The Buddhist path, acknowledging that one simply returns to chop wood and cut water, suggests that people generally do return to their lives and simply try to live them a little bit better, working for the good of others. The Bodhisattva vow is to reincarnate over and over only to serve others, until every soul is liberated. The idea of service to humanity has always permeated spiritual literature of every persuasion.

As Westerners pursue spiritual processes and develop the capacity to express new dimensions of their humanity a wider range of archetypes may become available to us. We may find new ways to live -- more creative, more interactive, more respectful of the environment. We may find ways to contain our humanness and our godliness without being arrogant about either, and therefore respecting the same equally in everyone else. We may learn to experience living more as a game and a passion and as multiple interconnections and patterns of light and dark. We may find ways to relieve the heavy, oppressive and intense seriousness of day-to day living, the fierce competition, and the economic struggles that so permeate all strata of society. Taking responsibility may be less burdensome. We may lose our fear of dying and thereby intensify our response to living.

We can observe historically that change is always and in every moment the nature and pattern of existence. Every civilization, every epoch, every belief system, every day eventually passes to another while the ego desperately struggles to keep things the same, to hold back the natural processes of living and dying . The changes occurring now in terms of spiritual expansion in the West are not as radically new as they seem at first glance. They are newly stimulated but deeply encoded possibilities, which can now be integrated by a more scientifically developed culture. Every mind that is open to them helps to create the foundation for whatever changes are meant to emerge in the next hundreds of years of this planet. It is encouraging to see public polls which indicate that 4.5 million Americans have tried meditation. In time they may bring more light to the planet.

However we should not be so naive as to believe spiritual awakening brings only light. It is clear from the conditions described during Kundalini awakening that as light increases an invariable counterbalance arises. It does not appear to be in the nature of this species to live in a world that is only light, only peace; darkness and disturbance coexist as soon as dualism is acknowledged. The shadow is well known in philosophy and psychology, and appears consistently in our dreams. Conflict emerges as soon as human will is put into motion, for as each of us attempts to have our own way, expand our territory, or enforce our particular spiritual or political beliefs we are forced up against the will of others, caught up again in the play of opposites that is part of a dynamic existence. Therefore what individuals can seek, and the planet may hope for in time, is not perfection, but sanity, wholeness and balance, as each individual plays a role in harmony with the deepest Self, and is capable of connecting at least momentarily with inner peace, compassion, unitive consciousness and bliss.

Great spiritual teachers are not all "purely" good and "perfect" beings, but perhaps are perfectly disciplined, not in a harsh and punitive style, but simply capable of choosing a communal good over and above a personal desire, having annihilated to a great extent the personal desires that drive the average soul to distraction. It is not likely that human beings will rapidly develop this capacity to release personal desire -- it is unrealistic to anticipate and expect it. If one considers the teaching of yoga scriptures, without desires there would be no one choosing to be birthed on the planet at all. From a psychological perspective it is dangerous to experience dispassion prematurely, and can lead to emotional sterility, existential angst and despair unless there is a corresponding depth of connection with the deeper Self.

The majority of those who awaken Kundalini will not choose to annihilate their egos, but will follow a path more akin to individuation, creating a way in their lives to integrate insight, harmony and productivity into their various lifestyles. They may interject greater depth, ecological awareness and compassion into their environments. They may teach, serve or play in more light-hearted and nurturing patterns than were available to them before. Their intelligence and creativity may expand. They may make it possible to develop a genuine understanding of the spiritual potential of humanity, and encourage this recognition in a culture that has been sadly blinded to it. Hopefully they will discover ways of acknowledging the shadow without allowing it to unconsciously damage or destroy others. I see this as the most likely model in the West for the integration of Kundalini experiences.

Kundalini is the pure energy of life force, part of the infinite consciousness that creates all form and extends beyond the limits of our mental concept of time and space. Whether it awakens by accident or design it has a potential to connect us directly with rich experiences and wisdom, if we are ready to open ourselves to it. An initial satori or samadhi experience appears to be just the opening, a powerful flash of seeing or merging into bliss or awareness that can certainly change entirely our view of human life, our behavior, our capacity to love. But this is only the slightest crack into what is available to us. There appears to be endless potential for extension and expression in the spiritual life, just as there are seemingly endless life styles, patterns and personalities to be expressed on the planet by human beings over the millions of years allotted the human species.

Kundalini is fundamentally associated with the spiritualizing of body and mind, expanding the capacity of the human to experience and hold the infinite. It is a slow development, as all evolutionary changes are slow. It is often painful both physically and psychologically as it involves both dissolution of blocks to expansion and the giving up of identity, beliefs, and attachments. This is what the de-structive aspect of the Hindu goddess Kali represents, the letting go and surrendering of ego identity as we know it. The pain of this is further exacerbated when one's experience is misunderstood, rejected or advised against by peers. It is a transformation difficult to navi-gate successfully without understanding, and the willingness to sur-render one's heart and mind to a higher source, and traditionally the guru has acted as navigator.

Facing Spiritual Confrontation

This process confronts our view of reality at it's deepest core. The life force erupts with the intensity of an earthquake, and the psyche is left to shift through the rubble. Those who have opened accidentally into an experience they are not ready to fully embrace may seek help to cool it down, to distance themselves from the trauma. To some extent this may be possible through working with emotional issues and blocks, eating balanced meals, becoming intel-lectually or emotionally involved in secular goals and interests, and forgoing meditation and all other forms of altered-state practices. I have spoken with people who seemed to have temporary openings that abated after some time because of their preoccupation with other matters, and lack of sustained interest in spiritual practices. I suspect that for those people who have genuine Kundalini openings rather than pranic releases or stress reactions that resemble Kundalini, there would be great difficulty in inhibiting the symptoms, or they might disappear temporarily but reopen easily at a later time.

If you are reading this from the perspective of a healer or a transpersonal therapist, your task is to facilitate and support the direc-tion of the soul. If a client is genuinely seeking to cooperate with the Kundalini opening, many processes can be used to facilitate the breaking down of blocks, and to reach the capacity to open and sur-render to the natural direction of this force itself. One can learn to manage and direct the energy. Clients must learn to differentiate clearly between inner-world experience and the outer consciousness. This separation is essential if one is to avoid mental problems or in-flation. But there is a transformation of outer consciousness occur-ring nonetheless, as perceptions, attitudes, the capacity to witness, and the range of compassion and clarity grow.

In addition, the Kundalini experience works on all the impu-rities in the personality, forcing one to confront and release negative patterns and personality traits. It draws one more toward introversion and introspection, stimulates the attraction to spiritual practices, and causes one to see the unity more than the divisiveness of life. If one learns to flow with this energy, respect it, and cooperate with the process we may suppose it will slowly lead one toward an integrated and lasting transformation of consciousness and personality. The outward symptoms and difficulties may ultimately fall away and the energy be active at a more subtle level, leading one into deeper states of light, bliss and wisdom while meditating, or practicing awareness in day to day life.

It would seem, if this is possible, that everyone would seek it. But the problem is that the spiritual life is painful, slow and difficult in the earlier stages, the ego is asked to abandon itself, and it feels as if survival is at stake. Discipline and structure is demanded. One clearly sees that all the ordinary joys of life are diminished, and it is hard to believe something better could arise from all the ashes. At any point on the journey we can abandon hope, or become sidetracked by the attraction of some new external diversion, or unfinished instinct or karmic business.

I propose that there are levels of evolution in this process, and the majority of them are correlated with an intensified prana in the body or the opening of various chakras, and of the three knots or granthis. These openings generally occur as one progresses on a spiritual path, addresses resistance and psychological issues, or practices yogic or tantric techniques and other meditations, but they may occur spontaneously because of some kind of psychological and physical readiness that is not apparent to outside observers. An awakened teacher can stimulate and/or monitor the process. But it is clear from the cases presented that one does not have to be on a classical spiritual path in order to engage this experience.

Even in psychoanalysis one experiences major energetic and emotional changes as complexes are addressed and resolved, symbols are integrated, and repressed emotions are released. Numinous experiences such as visions, lucid dreams, synchronistic events, waves of peace and love, and encounters with the Self may emerge. Spiritual practices, particularly meditation, bring similar psychic evolution and tear down repressive egoic structures. The dangers of inflation are present in both circumstances, and this is one of the dangers of labeling an experience "Kundalini" prematurely, when heightened prana is more likely the cause of the phenomenon. Such labeling invites a delusion that one is complete in one's spiritual work and ready to "save the world", which will dramatically inhibit progress.

Neither is it wise to equate all Kundalini experiences with enlightenment, even if the energy itself is the life force of universal consciousness, as described by the yogis. The literature and my experience with subjects suggest to me that the phenomena associated with Kundalini is a preliminary stage or transition through which the body and psyche prepare over years for a deeper and deeper experience of energy and awareness.

I expect "enlightenment" is rarely a single, final and complete encounter with the numinous, but that we experience glimpses and intimations and consciousness in varying degrees of intensity as we are able to contain and integrate them. Even the smallest encounter can completely redirect our life, and bring some satisfaction to the thirsty soul. We enter through a door and grasp an entirely new reality. But we live in an ever-expanding and eternal universe and it is Self-limiting to make assumptions that we have understood it all.

One of the significant facts of this research is that it was relatively easy to locate ten subjects who have had intense and life-transforming experiences with Kundalini energy, although none of them were practicing yogis or monks in the traditional sense. I have spoken with at least forty others who also fit the criteria but for various reasons were not included in this research. Several hundred people a year contact the Spiritual Emergence Network, an international referral source which specializes in helping people through spiritual crisis, and many of them describe what could be Kundalini experiences.[1]

The implication is that a number of people in western cultures are finding paths to spiritual awakening not commonly known or supported by western spiritual traditions. It suggests that the rigors of monastic life, celibacy and disciplined spiritual practices are not essential to awakening, although they may be helpful, and that people living more ordinary lives can have mystical experiences previously ascribed only to saints. It is important to bring this experience into the realm of ordinary life, so that people who aspire to mystic experience will be encouraged to follow this natural impulse of the psyche, instead of believing that only extraordinary and saintly people (so defined by the tenets of some specific church hierarchy) are capable of it. Inevitably this will bring more genuine spirituality into the culture.

---

[1] The Spiritual Emergence Network was founded by Stanislav and Christina Grof at Esalen Institute in 1980. In 1984 it was moved to the Institute of Transpersonal Psychology, 250 Oak Grove Ave., Menlo Park, California . Telephone:(415) 327-2776. In 1990 it will become an independent non-profit organization.

Collective Awakening

Many mystics and teachers suggest that the increased reports of Kundalini awakening at this time in history suggest a larger purpose at work, a universal planetary movement.. The earth appears to be trembling in the foreboding presence of major upheavals as we approach the 21st century. There are dire predictions of cataclysmic environmental changes, along with the ever-present annihilating threat of nuclear war and the continual pressures of war, oppression, starvation, crime and economic collapse in every sector of the hemisphere.

Today, in the 90's, we are watching with astonishment the collapse of Communism and the emergence of freedom in Eastern Europe. This is a radical upheaval, to a remarkable extent non-violent, coming from the core of millions of people who have long felt trapped in an unresponsive political system. Only a few months earlier the possibility of such enormous shifts in ideology was inconceivable. That this kind of ideological shift can occur so rapidly offers hope for all of the stuck places on the planet -- ideologies that hold many in the throes of poverty, starvation, guerrilla wars, and criminal activities. Perhaps such spontaneous movements, impacting the entire world, are part of the universal aspect of Kundalini. Certainly great confusion and chaos will reign for some years as the countries of Eastern Europe struggle to create a new economic and political system, and the entire continent moves to form the United States of Europe. The possibilities in Europe have far surpassed any kinds of previous predictions, and no on can say what will eventually emerge.

Not only politically but environmentally, monumental and inconceivable adaptations may lie in our immediate future. At every level we are poisoning the environment, from the ocean to the ozone layer to storage within the earth of deadly gases. Major earthquakes, shifting of the earth plates, and weather changes that promote drought are only a few of the predicted disasters psychics say may herald the "New Age". If these predictions should ever come to pass human life will only continue because of human beings with strong characters, flexibility, creativity, cooperative attitudes, inner resources, values which promote communal survival above individual acquisition, and the inner strength that is nourished by engaging that which is divine in us. Spiritual communities are emerging around the globe at this time, and individuals in many unlikely places are having shamanic visions, Kundalini awakenings, psychic intuitions and a passion for teaching what they know to others. Slowly the vision of what it means to be human and divine is changing, merging, awakening, and teaching us more about our capacities and potentialities.

Perhaps the individuals engaging in the tumultuous event of spiritual awakening are prototypes for what the planetary consciousness must ultimately face:

-- purification of the unconscious patterns that allow us to destroy, abuse and violate one another;

-- awareness there is one humanity and one planet with one set of resources we all share that could only be connected to one spiritual source;

-- reawakening of our capacity to connect psychically and experientially with that source and experience bliss and joy and wisdom directly;

-- and willingness to live in moderation and nurture our planet in healthy ways which sustain all life.

There are numerous patterns with which to identify the human microcosm with the planetary macrocosm, for universally our thought forms as a species create the quality of life on this fragile sphere hurtling through space, sustained by the same pranic sources on which we all depend.

Kundalini awakening is awakening into awareness of this energy which can be used to heal, transform, energize and evolve higher levels of consciousness. Once we are fully alive as a spiritual species we will know how to sustain change and develop from within us a quality of life that can cooperate with the forces of nature to nurture our planet for future generations. We do not yet know what is possible and can only play with imagination to visualize a healthier and saner planet, peopled by a wise and loving species in touch with the natural ecstasy of the inner being. Such changes are unlikely to be the consequence of following one great teacher, many of whom we have known already. They will result when many individuals are willing to turn their egos inside-out and plunge deeply into the more firmly rooted core of the Self, in order to activate the fundamental values of human existence. This is the long-term potential of such awakenings, whether they occur after great disciplined effort, or spontaneously. They teach of the possibilities inherent in transformational change which we need to understand in order to move to the next stage of planetary development.

This does not mean that all who have awakened Kundalini energies are already so wise. Universal energy has always been neutral, has the capacity to be used for better or worse purposes by an individual who does not have the strength to go completely through the purifying process it offers. There are always forces in human consciousness that tempt us with power, greed, envy, sloth and all the seven deadly sins. These "sins" are human failings, our shadows, which keep us in ignorance because we cannot go all the way through this process as long as we actively focus our attention on them. And everyone falls, over and over. At this stage of development it is prudent to acknowledge with compassion and love who we are, where we are weak, where we can become stronger.

As we push toward awakening, and try to engage in activities that sustain and deepen it, we may possibly become more than we were. When we break into the ecstasy of pure awareness, at those moments we cannot be anything else but light, but how impossible it seems to live there all the time, and how natural to fall back into our ordinary imperfections. Never underestimate the difficulties of such a process -- for individuals, for the planet. The lessons are all around us. It is in the Christianity that became the Inquisition, in the Islam that kills infidels, in the failed guru who betrays his followers, in governments ruled by special interests, in corruptions that follow in the footsteps of good intentions. No matter how noble our ideals and purposes, we slide over and over into destruction and inhumane choices, in order to protect our position, our desires, our points of view. Spiritual awakening cannot prevent this, at least not in the early stages with which we are primarily involved: it simply gives us an added incentive to transform those renegade elements of ourselves that keep us from being in the peace and ecstasy hidden inside our deepest core.

The more I open myself to observe the true condition of the planet, the depth of the pain that is the norm for much of the human species, and the portents for the future, the less surprised I am at the growing number of individuals who are "awakening" and going through ordeals much like ancient initiations which shift their consciousness. Perhaps all of us need this experience, and need it quickly. Or perhaps the earth is being seeded for something to come in the distant future, and we are only being asked to experiment and to study spiritual processes at this moment in time. Whatever it's purpose we cannot afford to allow psychology, philosophy, science or religion to ignore or reject these processes. We need to develop tolerance, respect, understanding and support for individuals who are pioneering these uncharted territories. We are all learning together, we share a common destiny, and we are winding hand-in-hand through the labyrinthine energy fields that will ultimately lead is into the sacred light and purpose of the human soul.

GLOSSARY

ajna chakra 6th chakra, located between the eyebrows, also called the third eye; considered the "command post" for all the chakras.

anahata chakra the 4th or heart chakra; the emotional center.

ananda transcendent bliss, spiritual ecstasy.

apana breath as it is inspired, prana with a downward tendency.

asana yoga postures or poses that strengthen the body

Atman the Self

bandhas muscular contractions of throat, solar plexus and anus sometimes included in the yogic mudras, asanas or pranayamas.

bhajan singing devotional songs.

bhakti love, devotion.

bij or **bija** seed, the significant sound associated with a particular energy force, often associated with the chakras.

Brahman the supreme God; when spelled brahman, may refer to a member of the Hindu priest caste.

chitrini a subtle channel within the sushumna nadi which runs from the root chakra to the crown of the head.Chitrini carries downward flowing energy and is called the source of universal sound.

cit or **chit** consciousness as pure intelligence.

citsakti same as jiva, the soul or the Self

citta or **chitta** mind-stuff, the substance that mediates memory and habits.

darshan seeing or being in the presence of a scared idol, place or teacher, and experiencing the blessing therein.

deva or **devi** demi-god or angel, god or goddess.

dharma the teaching of the Buddha; the law governing world order.

hara (Japanese term) triangle formed from the base of the sternum, down the sides of the rib cage extending downward to the naval.

ida white 'lunar" channel or nadi coiling around the sushumna, beginning at the base of the spine and ending at the left nostril.

Ista chosen and loved form of God.

Isvara the creative aspect of the Divine.

japa mental repetition of a mantra, or the name of God.

jiva, or **jivatma** the individual as a human being; the individualized and embodied consciousness or soul.

jnana wisdom, understanding. Jnana yoga is the yoga of wisdom.

kanda the muladhara psychic center.

karma action similar to cause and effect; although there is no external law-giver individual souls through their own choice continually reap the consequences of previous actions in this and other lives.

kensho (Japanese term) refers to enlightenment, seeing fully one's own nature, an experience beyond the grasp of intellect.

kirtan chanting, singing and dancing in worship.

klesas afflictions, sufferings, negative tendencies

kosas five subtle body sheaths or layers of decreasing density that surround the material body.

kriya the path of action; also involuntary body movement caused by the regular or increased flow of pranic energy.

kumbhaka retention of the breath.

Layayoga absorption into higher consciousness by merging individual consciousness with a Divine object of contemplation.

makyo (Japanese term) any unusual visual or physical phenomena that disturb the single-minded focus of spiritual practice.

Manipura chakra the third chakra, at the solar plexus, related to the element fire.

mantra a sacred sound supposed to have power, used to focus the mind, induce reflection on the divine, provide protection in ordinary life or for occult purposes.

maya the process by which the true condition of the world is veiled through differentiation and limitation of phenomena.

muladhara chakra the first chakra, located at the base of the spine, identified with security issues, and the location where Kundalini energy is coiled.

mudra yogic gestures made with hands symbolizing universal principles.

Om mystical syllable representative of the Divine, the core tone of the universe from which all sound and creation emanate.

pingala the "solar "subtle channel within the sushumna winding from the base of the spine and ending at the right nostril.

prana the vital energy of the inner or subtle body, the life-force or shakti.

pranayama yogic breathing practices that play a vital part in meditation and expand or redistribute pranic energy through the breath.

pratyahara practices of withdrawing mind from the senses, turning the attention inward.

Purusha the primary Cosmic Spirit, the counterpart of the female principle, the Being beyond the universal or cosmic person; also used as the soul or pure consciousness.

sadhaka a spiritual aspirant, seeker, one who is disciplined.

sadhana spiritual disciplines and daily practices.

Sahasrara chakra   the seventh chakra, above the crown of the
   head, symbolized by the thousand-petalled lotus. The place
   here Kundalini unites with Siva and pure consciousness may be
   experienced.

Sakti or Shakti   the dynamic and creative aspect of the
   Ultimate Principle, the power that permeates all
   creation, the feminine counterpart of Siva.

shaktipat   the process of initiation by a guru through a
   transmission of energy that awakens energy in the
   initiate.

siddhis   psychic attainment or powers

Siddas   great master of yogic powers.

Siva or Shiva   pure consciousness; the transcendent divine
   principle.

sushumna   the central subtle channel through which Kundalini rises
   in the human body, located inside the spinal column.

svadhisthana chakra   the second chakra, located below the navel
   and just above the genitals, governing sexuality.

tandra   a conscious but dream-like state where one may
   experience visions.

third eye   the point in the middle of the forehead, between the
   eyebrows, where cosmic consciousness opens; the Ajna
   chakra.

Vaibhuri   a spontaneous flow of higher wisdom.

vajra nadi   an upward flowing nadi in the sushumna that
   regulates electrical energy flow.

vayu   air or wind.

visuddha or vishuddha   chakra located at the throat,
   associated with expression and creativity.

Yantra   a form or symbolic design, similar to a mandala, usually
   containing magic symbols useful in healing and for other
   metaphysical purposes, or for meditative contemplation.

Yuga   an age of history. There are four yugas in 12,000 years: the Kali,
   Dwapapra, Treta and Satya, corresponding to the Greek ideas of
   Iron, Bronze, silver and Golden. The Kali Yuga, or age of
   materialism ended about 1700 A.D. and we are now in the
   apara Yuga, a 2400 year cycle of electrical and atomic energy
   development. (Yogananda, (1945) Autobiography of a Yogi,
   p. 192.)